Smart, Connected, and Portable Biosensors and Bioelectronics for Advancing Human Healthcare, Disease Diagnosis, and Therapeutics

Smart, Connected, and Portable Biosensors and Bioelectronics for Advancing Human Healthcare, Disease Diagnosis, and Therapeutics

Editors

Jong-Hoon Kim
Woon-Hong Yeo

MDPI

Basel • Beijing • Wuhan • Barcelona • Belgrade • Novi Sad • Cluj • Manchester

Editors
Jong-Hoon Kim
Mechanical Engineering,
Washington State University
Vancouver, WA, USA

Woon-Hong Yeo
Mechanical Engineering,
Georgia Institute of
Technology
Atlanta, GA, USA

Editorial Office
MDPI
St. Alban-Anlage 66
4052 Basel, Switzerland

This is a reprint of articles from the Special Issue published online in the open access journal *Biosensors* (ISSN 2079-6374) (available at: https://www.mdpi.com/journal/biosensors/special_issues/portable_biosens).

For citation purposes, cite each article independently as indicated on the article page online and as indicated below:

Lastname, A.A.; Lastname, B.B. Article Title. *Journal Name* **Year**, *Volume Number*, Page Range.

ISBN 978-3-0365-9158-2 (Hbk)
ISBN 978-3-0365-9159-9 (PDF)
doi.org/10.3390/books978-3-0365-9159-9

Contents

Brian Senf, Woon-Hong Yeo and Jong-Hoon Kim
Recent Advances in Portable Biosensors for Biomarker Detection in Body Fluids
Reprinted from: *Biosensors* **2020**, *10*, 127, doi:10.3390/bios10090127 1

Kangkyu Kwon, Shinjae Kwon and Woon-Hong Yeo
Automatic and Accurate Sleep Stage Classification via a Convolutional Deep Neural Network and Nanomembrane Electrodes
Reprinted from: *Biosensors* **2022**, *12*, 155, doi:10.3390/bios12030155 25

Zequan Zhao, Yin Lu, Yajun Mi, Jiajing Meng, Xueqing Wang, Xia Cao and et al.
Adaptive Triboelectric Nanogenerators for Long-Term Self-Treatment: A Review
Reprinted from: *Biosensors* **2022**, *12*, 1127, doi:10.3390/bios12121127 39

Yupeng Mao, Yongsheng Zhu, Tianming Zhao, Changjun Jia, Meiyue Bian, Xinxing Li and et al.
A Portable and Flexible Self-Powered Multifunctional Sensor for Real-Time Monitoring in Swimming
Reprinted from: *Biosensors* **2021**, *11*, 147, doi:10.3390/bios11050147 67

Wei Du, Lucas Miller and Feng Zhao
Numerical Study of Graphene/Au/SiC Waveguide-Based Surface Plasmon Resonance Sensor
Reprinted from: *Biosensors* **2021**, *11*, 455, doi:10.3390/bios11110455 79

Aniello Maiese, Alice Chiara Manetti, Costantino Ciallella and Vittorio Fineschi
The Introduction of a New Diagnostic Tool in Forensic Pathology: LiDAR Sensor for 3D Autopsy Documentation
Reprinted from: *Biosensors* **2022**, *12*, 132, doi:10.3390/bios12020132 87

Xiaoxiao Kang, Jun Zhang, Zheming Shao, Guotai Wang, Xingguang Geng, Yitao Zhang and et al.
A Wearable and Real-Time Pulse Wave Monitoring System Based on a Flexible Compound Sensor
Reprinted from: *Biosensors* **2022**, *12*, 133, doi:10.3390/bios12020133 99

Tianyi Li, Scott D. Soelberg, Zachary Taylor, Vigneshwar Sakthivelpathi, Clement E. Furlong, Jong-Hoon Kim and et al.
Highly Sensitive Immunoresistive Sensor for Point-of-Care Screening for COVID-19
Reprinted from: *Biosensors* **2022**, *12*, 149, doi:10.3390/bios12030149 117

Jesse Fine, Michael J. McShane, Gerard L. Coté and Christopher G. Scully
A Computational Modeling and Simulation Workflow to Investigate the Impact of Patient-Specific and Device Factors on Hemodynamic Measurements from Non-Invasive Photoplethysmography
Reprinted from: *Biosensors* **2022**, *12*, 598, doi:10.3390/bios12080598 135

Jaskirat Singh Batra, Ting-Yen Chi, Mo-Fan Huang, Dandan Zhu, Zheyuan Chen, Dung-Fang Lee and et al.
Wearable Biosensor with Molecularly Imprinted Conductive Polymer Structure to Detect Lentivirus in Aerosol
Reprinted from: *Biosensors* **2023**, *13*, 861, doi:10.3390/bios13090861 157

biosensors

MDPI

Review

Recent Advances in Portable Biosensors for Biomarker Detection in Body Fluids

Brian Senf [1], Woon-Hong Yeo [2] and Jong-Hoon Kim [1,*]

[1] School of Engineering and Computer Science, Washington State University, Vancouver, WA 98686, USA; brian.senf@wsu.edu

[2] Human-Centric Interfaces and Engineering Program, Wallace H. Coulter Department of Biomedical Engineering, George W. Woodruff School of Mechanical Engineering, Georgia Institute of Technology, Atlanta, GA 30332, USA; whyeo@gatech.edu

* Correspondence: jh.kim@wsu.edu; Tel.: +1-360-546-9250; Fax: +1-360-546-9438

Received: 26 August 2020; Accepted: 14 September 2020; Published: 18 September 2020

Abstract: A recent development in portable biosensors allows rapid, accurate, and on-site detection of biomarkers, which helps to prevent disease spread by the control of sources. Less invasive sample collection is necessary to use portable biosensors in remote environments for accurate on-site diagnostics and testing. For non- or minimally invasive sampling, easily accessible body fluids, such as saliva, sweat, blood, or urine, have been utilized. It is also imperative to find accurate biomarkers to provide better clinical intervention and treatment at the onset of disease. At the same time, these reliable biomarkers can be utilized to monitor the progress of the disease. In this review, we summarize the most recent development of portable biosensors to detect various biomarkers accurately. In addition, we discuss ongoing issues and limitations of the existing systems and methods. Lastly, we present the key requirements of portable biosensors and discuss ideas for functional enhancements.

Keywords: portable biosensor; biomarkers in body fluids; portability; point-of-care

1. Introduction

Biosensors are a subset of chemical sensors, which transform chemical data into an analytical signal to monitor physiological and chemical analytes in the body. The chemical sensors are comprised of a chemical recognition system and a physicochemical transducer. Likewise, biosensors use a biochemical reaction as the recognition element [1] and convert a biological response into an electric signal [2]. The biosensor requires multiple components to measure these analytes and display information related to the analysis done. Figure 1 shows the schematic diagram of a biosensor composed of a biorecognition element, transducer, and signal processing unit. The biorecognition layer is the defining component that determines the specificity of the device. It's also called the bio receptor, which is a molecular species that utilizes a biochemical mechanism for the recognition of analytes. The biorecognition element binds the analytes of interest to the sensor's surface for the reaction. The reaction is then converted by the transduction mechanism. The transducer converts a biological signal to a measurable signal.

It converts one form of energy to another and can take many forms depending on design specifications. One common type of transduction mechanism used in biosensors is the electrochemical transducer. Many reactions with the biorecognition layer either produce or consume ions or electrons. This can cause changes in the electrical properties of a solution that can be measured and transduced to a signal processor. The signal processor is generally a computer or microprocessor which acquires the signal, then filters and amplifies the data. Electrical noise is inherent when processing data from the transducer. Thus, the signal processor typically subtracts the baseline noise from the transducer to amplify the signal of interest [2].

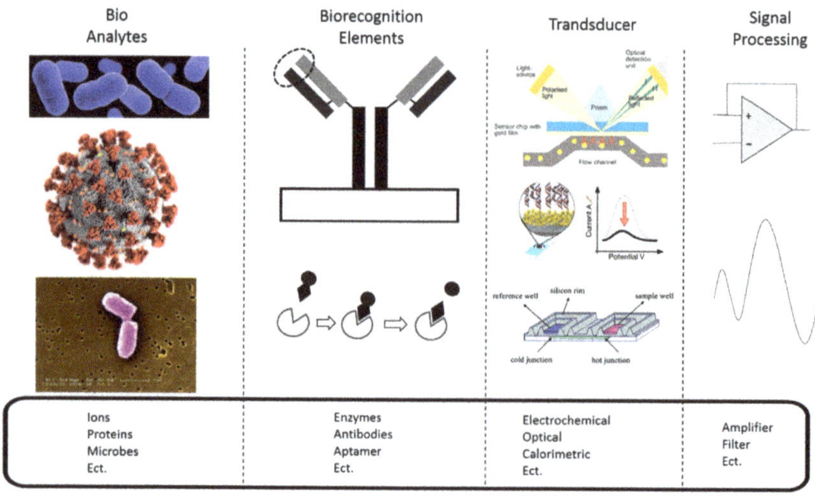

Figure 1. Overview of biomarker detection using biosensors. Bio-analytes from [3], Biorecognition elements from [4], Transducer images from [5–7].

Fabrication of biosensors is a broad topic with many different strategies and techniques, depending not only on the analyte but also on the scale of the biosensor and the longevity intended. The first true biosensor was created in 1956 by Leland C. Clark Jr. The biosensor stemmed from an earlier invention on the oxygen electrode. To calibrate the electrode, he had been deoxygenating test solutions using the enzyme glucose oxidase and glucose, which was capable of removing the oxygen from the solution. He eventually realized that this procedure could instead be used to measure glucose concentration. This was done by immobilizing the glucose oxidase on the oxygen electrode. The concentration of air could then be directly mapped to the concentration of glucose in the solution [8]. Many biosensors follow a similar path now. The oxidation or reduction reaction produces a readable signal for the electrode to read as a current. Therefore, the current can be correlated with the concentration of the analyte of interest in the solution being tested. For enzyme biosensors, the enzyme must first be immobilized in a membrane which can then be coated onto an electrode. The electrode chosen is dependent on the desired reaction [9]. A detailed explanation of the wide range of fabrication for biosensors is outside of the scope of this work, but more information can be found in the "Handbook of Biosensor and Biosensor Kinetics" with an entire chapter dedicated to covering some of the recent techniques used for biosensor fabrication [10].

Technology advances have enabled biosensors to become more accurate, reliable, and sensitive to biomarkers and analytes. As these Biosensors become more advanced, there is also a movement to make them smaller and more portable. Portable devices make them available outside of the laboratory allowing for use in the field as well as transportation to third world countries where the inability for early, rapid detection of disease has a great negative effect not only on people's lives but economies on the whole. Portable biosensors can also help prevent the spread of disease by mitigating the travel of diseased individuals. Currently, the diagnosis requires travel to a clinic as well as an extended wait period to receive the results. Subjects going in for tests can deal with white coat hypertension, which is a blood pressure difference of 20 mmHg systolic or 10 mm Hg diastolic between ambulatory and clinic blood pressures [11]. This goes to show that clinic visits can add a quantifiable amount of stress to a patient's life and can even affect test results. Therefore, the demand for portable biosensors has increased, and research is focused on the development of small portable devices that would allow rapid, accurate, and on-site detection. However, the requirements of portability are not clearly defined, especially regarding the sample preparation methods. Its perspective needs to be reviewed in detail.

The use of portable biosensors in remote environments outside of laboratory and clinical settings often correlates with an individual who may not have the same level as training those in a clinical setting. Less invasive sample collection then becomes pertinent for true on-site diagnostics and testing. For non- or minimally invasive sampling, easily accessible body fluids such as saliva, sweat, blood, or urine, have been the sample of choice as they are among the easiest types of clinical samples to obtain. Blood has been the most common sample type as a part of a routine physical examination due to many disease-associated biomarkers and its less invasive collection procedure. Thus, it becomes a good source of biomarkers for portable biosensors. Recently, other body fluids, including saliva, urine, and sweat, have attracted much attention as samples for portable biosensors due to their abundant presence, diagnostic capabilities, and noninvasive sample extraction.

In this article, we review the most recent development of biomarkers for portable biosensor systems with various sample types, i.e., saliva, sputum, blood, breath, tears, urine, and sweat. In addition, some of the recent advances in the field of portable biosensor analyzed by sample type, as well as a few issues with the field are discussed. We present metrics on portability as for the biosensors and discuss ideas for improvement in portability classifications. The difference in bio-sensing strategies and analytical performance is discussed to provide a most recent overview of the portable biosensor development, with conclusions and future perspectives at the end.

2. Analytes

2.1. Saliva

Recently, salivary diagnostics shows excellent promise as a convenient means for the early detection, prognosis, and monitoring post-therapy status, as saliva is 99% water and can be easily manipulated [12]. Screening biomarkers in the saliva is advantageous because the sample extraction is simple, noninvasive, stress-free, cost-effective, and precise. Additionally, since saliva sample collection does not require any special tools, it can even be done at home by patients themselves for continuous monitoring in necessity and easily integrated with a portable biosensor for point-of-care (POC) testing [13]. The use of saliva is broadening biosensor perspectives in disease diagnosis, clinical monitoring, and decision making for patient care. In this section, we summarize many types of salivary biomarkers for portable biosensors (Table 1). In addition, we describe the recent development of portable saliva biosensors along with their limits and ranges of detection (Figure 2).

Table 1. Summary of Portable Biosensors for Salivary Biomarker Detection.

Biomarker	Target Disease/Area	Sensor Type	Detection Limit * Sensitivity ** Specificity	Dynamic Range	Analysis Time
Lactate [14]	Respiratory insufficiency, shocks, heart failure and metabolic disorders	Modified screen printed electrode	0.01 mM	0.025–0.25 mM	<60 s
Lactate [15]	Diabetes, sports medicine, critical care	3D printed chemiluminescence biosensor	0.1 mmol/L	NA	<5 min
Lactate [16]	Clinical diagnosis, sport physiology and food analysis	Cloth-based electrochemiluminescence (ECL)	0.035 mM	0.05–2.5 mM	NA
Streptococcus [17]	Streptococcus Pyogenes	Impedimetric Immunosensor	NA	100 to 10^5 cells/10 μL cumulative incubation 100 to 10^4 cells/10 μL single-shot	NA
Avian Influenza Virus [18]	Avian influenza	Impedance biosensor	$1 \times 10^{2.2}$ ELD_{50}/mL Tracheal = 100% * Cloacal = 55% *	NA	<1 h
Cytokine biomarkers [19]	Disease detection such as cancer	Graphene-based fully integrated portable nanosensing biosensor	12 pM	NA	Real-time
H1N1 [20]	Influenza detection	Magnetic Integrated Microfluidic Electrochemical Detector	10 TCID50	NA	3.5 h
Biogenic Amines [21]	Halitosis	Diamine Oxidase Electrochemical screen printed electrode Biosensor	1×10^{-5} M	2×10^{-5}–3×10^{-4} M	NA
Cortisol [22]	Stress	Surface plasmon resonance biosensor	1.0 ng/mL	1.5 ng/mL–10 ng/mL	<10 min
PDGF [23]	Cell growth and division	Aptamer-based biosensor PGM	2.9 fM	1.0×10^{-14} M to 3.16×10^{-12} M	20 min
Saliva Conductivity [24]	Dehydration and Kidney function	Au Electrode biosensor	93.3% * 80% **	NA	Real-time
Metabolites (Glucose) [25]	Metabolite pacifier biosensor for infants	Glucose-oxidase based enzyme detection electrode biosensor	0.04 mM	0.1 to 1.4 mM	Real-time

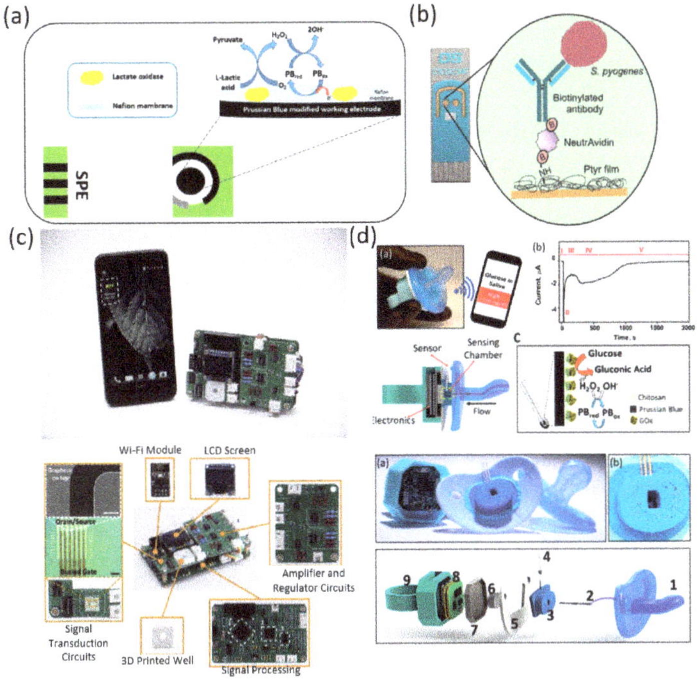

Figure 2. Portable biosensors for salivary diagnostics. (**a**) Schematic representation of SPE-PB-LOx Biosensor [14]. (**b**) Schematic of immunosensor against S. pyogenes [17]. (**c**) Images of aptameric GFET nanosensing system for cytokines detection [19]. (**d**) Glucose Pacifier sensing concept [25].

Lactate is a useful biomarker that can be tested for in saliva. It can be used to diagnose metabolic disorders, monitor diabetes, and is a useful measurement for sports physiology. Petropoulos et al. proposed a screen-printed electrode modified with Prussian Blue. The sensor detects hydrogen peroxide produced by the reaction catalyzed by the lactate oxidase enzyme immobilized onto the electrode surface. Figure 2a presents the biosensor integrated with portable instrumentation showing a working range from 0.025–0.25 mM and a limit of detection (LOD) of 0.01 mM [14]. Roda et al. reported a 3D printed mini cartridge that can be used to turn a smartphone or tablet in a luminometer. The design allows for the detection of chemiluminescence derived from enzyme reactions. To prototype the sensor, they coupled lactate oxidase with horseradish peroxidase for the measurement of lactate in saliva and sweat. The biosensor reported a LOD of 0.5 mmol/L in saliva [15]. Yao et al. developed screen-printed carbon electrodes and electrochemical chambers on a hydrophilic cloth. A smartphone is then used to read the electrochemiluminescence signals. The biosensor reports a LOD of 0.35 mM and a dynamic range of 0.05–2.5 mM [16]. Streptococcus pyogenes is a bacterium which causes an estimated 700 million of infection per year. As there are no available vaccines yet, early detection of infection is crucial to prevent serious invasive infection, which has a mortality rate of 25%. Ahmed et al. reported a screen-printed gold electrode used to create a polytyramine-based immunosensor for the detection of Streptococcus pyogenes. Biotin tagged whole antibodies against Streptococcus pyogenes were conjugated to polytramine amine groups via biotin-NeutrAvidin coupling. They showed a working range of 100 to 10^5 cells/10 µL for cumulative incubation and 100 to 10^4 cells/10 µL single-shot incubation. An image of the proposed biosensor can be seen in Figure 2b [17]. Avian influenza viruses (AIV) are naturally occurring among birds and can be spread to humans, although infection in humans is rare. However, the possibility that the virus could change and begin spreading between people is of major concern making rapid detection and identification crucial for control of outbreaks [26]. Wang et al. demonstrated an AIV biosensor and its performance on infected poultry. The design was an impedance biosensor based on a combination of magnetic nanobeads coated with AIV subtype-specific antibody. The system is also integrated with a microfluidic chip interdigitated array microelectrode for transfer, detection, and measurement of the bio-nanobeads and virus complex in a buffer. The biosensor was reported to have a LOD of $1 \times 10^{2.2}$ ELD_{50}/mL where EDL_{50} is 50% egg lethal dose [18]. Elevated levels of cytokine biomarkers in bodily fluids have been reported in patients with severe diseases such as prostate, breast, and pancreatic cancer. Hao et al. presented a graphene-based, integrated portable nanosensing device for the detection of cytokine biomarkers in saliva. The biosensor employs an aptameric graphene-based field-effect transistor with HfO_2 as a dielectric layer and an integrated processing circuit for the detection of cytokine concentrations. The biosensor reports a LOD of 12 pM (Figure 2c) [19]. H1N1, otherwise known as swine flu, is a virus that caused a worldwide outbreak starting in April 2009. The virus is easily spreading, and the World Health Organization declared a global outbreak raising the pandemic alert level to Phase 5 by 30th April 2009. Fast early detection is crucial to prevent further outbreaks in the future [27]. Ferguson et al. developed a magnetic integrated microfluidic electrochemical detector for quantification of H1N1 from throat swab samples. Integrating a multifunctional sample preparation chamber enables the testing of unprocessed samples into the biosensor without the need for external preparation or reagents. To demonstrate the device's ability, they used H1N1 detection, which had a LOD of 10 $TCID_{50}$ where $TCID_{50}$ (median tissue culture infectious dose) [20].

Halitosis is a prevalent issue for most of the adult population. It is defined as an unpleasant odor emitted from the mouth, which may be caused by oral conditions including periodontal disease, chronic sinusitis and bronchiectasis [28]. Aliphatic polyamines in the oral cavity have been associated with halitosis and can occur from the breakdown of proteins and peptides or the degradation of amino acids. Piermarini et al. proposed a Prussian Blue screen-printed electrode electrochemical biosensor for the detection of biogenic amines in saliva. The sensor uses the hydrogen peroxide produced from the reaction with the diamine oxidase enzyme. The biosensor, coupled with portable instrumentation, showed a working range of 0.02 mM to 0.3 mM and a LOD of 0.01 mM [21]. Cortisol is a hormone used for regulation of blood pressure, cardiovascular function, and other metabolic activities. Cortisol levels have become a useful measurement for overall stress levels and disease levels in patients. Stevens et al. created a cortisol detecting biosensor utilizing a surface plasmon resonance system. For detection, cortisol specific monoclonal antibodies were used to develop a competition assay with a six-channel portable device. The biosensor reports a dynamic range of 1.5–10 ng/mL and a LOD of 1.0 ng/mL [22]. Platelet-derived growth factor BB (PDGF-BB) plays a role in regulating cell growth and division. It is necessary for increased healing with fibroblast activation and granulation tissue formation in the treatment of chronic dermal wounds. Ma et al. reported a biosensor for the detection of platelet-derived growth factor-BB. It employs a personal glucose meter which has the primary aptamer of PDGF-BB bound to the surface of streptavidin magnespheres paramagnetic particles from Promega Corporation (Madison, WI, USA). The streptavidin magnespheres react with an invertase-functionalized secondary aptamer of PDGF-BB to form a stable complex which results in the attachment of invertase on the paramagnetic particles. The invertase catalyzes the hydrolysis of sucrose to produce glucose for reading with the personal glucose meter. The biosensor reports a dynamic range of 1.0×10^{-14}–3.16×10^{-12} M and a LOD of 2.9 fM [23]. Measurement of saliva conductivity can be used for the detection of dehydration. Dehydration is often associated with abnormalities in electrolyte balance allowing for a detection hydration status through the osmolality of a fluid. Hematological osmolality is a common index of hydration status. Dehydration and heat stress can lead to persistent damage to the kidneys which can lead to chronic kidney disease. Lu et al. developed a biosensor for the measurement of saliva osmolality via measurement of the conductivity of saliva samples. The sensor reports a sensitivity of 93.3% and a specificity of 80% [24]. Monitoring glucose in infants for diabetes treatment is especially challenging. García-Carmona et al. demonstrated a pacifier glucose biosensor to overcome some of the challenges of infant metabolite monitoring capable of detecting glucose in saliva. The biosensor is comprised of a Glucose-oxidase based enzyme detection electrode biosensor. It used glucose testing in adults to demonstrate the feasibility of the biosensor. They reported a LOD of 0.04 mM and a dynamic range of 0.1 to 1.4 mM. Figure 2d shows a figure of the pacifier biosensor [25].

2.2. *Sweat*

Sweat is another useful source of biomarkers for portable biosensors. Sweat sensors are often targeted towards wearable applications and allow for the noninvasive collection of samples. Human sweat is approximately 99% water with sodium chloride [12], but contains various health-related biomarkers including ascorbic acid, uric acid, metabolites like glucose and lactate, and electrolytes such as Na^+ and K^+. It is an attractive, less-painful alternative to blood samples for assessing a patient's health. In the following section, sweat biomarkers for use with portable biosensors are summarized (Table 2). In addition, we show the recent examples of portable sweat biosensor along with the limits and dynamic ranges of detection (Figure 3).

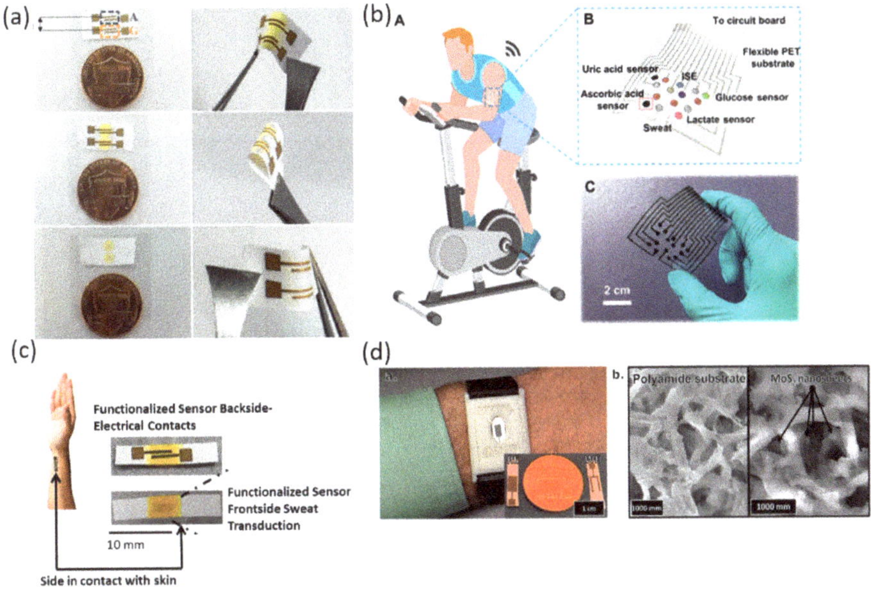

Figure 3. Portable biosensors for sweat biomarker detection. (**a**) Sweat sensor array showing fluid confinement in the active sensing region, sensor flexibility, and size comparison with one cent [29]. (**b**) Schematic illustration of a wearable sweat analysis patch mounted on human skin with a photograph of the actual patch [30]. (**c**) Wearable diagnostic sweat based biosensing and relative size of the developed sensor with RTIL and immunoassay functionalized semiconducting ZnO films on nanoporous polyamide substrates. The second part of the image shows the wicking of fluid in the active region of the sensor along with a schematic showing capture probe–target biomarker interaction in RTIL and immunoassay with ZnO thin film on a porous membrane within the wicked region of the fluid [31]. (**d**) Prototype and MoS_2 nanosheet on polyamide membrane [32].

Table 2. Summary of Portable Biosensors for Sweat Biomarker Detection.

Biomarker	Target Disease/Area	Sensor Type	Detection Limit * Sensitivity	Dynamic Range	Analysis Time
Alcohol [33]	Noninvasive measurement	Bienzyme amperometric composite biosensors	0.0005 g/L	0.0005–0.6 g/L	Real-time
Glucose [29]	Diabetes	Zinc Oxide Thin film nanoporous electrode biosensor	0.1 mg/dL	0.01–200 mg/dL	NA
Multiplexed (Metabolites/ electrolytes/temperature) [34]	Physiological monitoring	Flexible sweat sensor array with wireless FPCB	2.35 nA/μM Glucose * 220 nA/mM Lactate *		NA
glucose, lactate, ascorbic acid, uric acid, Na^+ and K^+ [30]	Multipurpose healthcare monitoring	Silk fabric–derived intrinsically nitrogen (N)–doped carbon textile (SilkNCT) flexible biosensor	Glucose: 5 μM Lactate: 0.5 mM UA: 0.1 μM AA: 1 μM Na^+: 1 mM K^+: 0.5 mM	Glucose: 25 to 300 μM Lactate: 5 to 35 mM UA: 2.5 to 115 μM AA: 20 to 300 μM Na^+: 5 to 100 mM K^+: 1.25 to 40 mM	Real-time
Interleukin [31]	Immune response	BMIM[BF4] RTIL stability enhancing capture probe immunoassay functionalized ZnO thin films deposited on nanoporous polyamide membrane biosensor	0.2 pg/mL for 0–24 h and 2 pg/mL for 24–48 h post-antibody sensor functionalization	0.2–200 pg/mL continuous detection	NA
Lactate [15]	Diabetes, sports medicine, critical care	3D printed chemiluminescence biosensor	0.1 mmol/L	NA	<5 min
Cortisol [32]	Stress	Non-faradaic label-free cortisol biosensor	1 ng/mL	1–500 ng/mL	Continuous for 3+ hours

Alcohol levels can be measured in sweat and show treatment response for conditions such as diabetes where alcohol consumption results in hypoglycemia. Additionally, alcohol is an important marker for the monitoring of drivers or individuals in safety-related work. Gamella et al. developed a biosensor based on a bienzyme amperometric composites sensitive to variation in ethanol concentration. The design enabled a dynamic range of 0.0005–0.6 g/L and a LOD of 0.0005 g/L [33]. Glucose is an important biomarker for monitoring and treating diabetes. Since alcohol and glucose are both relevant to diabetes monitoring and control, Bhide et al. presented a zinc oxide thin film integrated into a nanoporous flexible electrode biosensor to detect both glucose and alcohol. The biosensor can use low volumes of sweat for testing and both analytes have a dynamic range of 0.01–200 mg/dL with a LOD of 0.1 mg/dL. Figure 3a shows an image of the flexible biosensor [29]. Gao et al. reported a flexible, wearable biosensor capable of measuring both lactate and glucose. The sensor was used to test levels in sweat based on glucose oxidase, or lactate oxidase depending on the analyte of interest, immobilized within a permeable film. The sensor reported a LOD of 2.35 nA/μM for glucose [34]. Human sweat also contains useful ions that are often used to monitor a patient's physiological state. Sodium ions in sweat can be used to diagnose diseases such as cystic fibrosis and autonomic and peripheral neuropathy where sweat regulation is affected. He et al. developed a multiplex biosensor for the detection of ions and electrolytes (Na^+ and K^+) as well as ascorbic acid (AA), uric acid (UA), glucose and lactate (Figure 3b). The sensor reports a LOD of 5 μM, 0.5 mM, 0.1 μM, 1 μM, 1 mM, 0.5 mM for Glucose, Lactate, UA, AA, Na^+, K^+ respectively. The dynamic range is reported as 25–300 μM, 5–35 mM, 2.5–115 μM, 20–300 μM, 5–100 mM, and 1.25–40 mM for Glucose, Lactate, UA, AA, Na^+, K^+ respectively [30]. Interleukin-6 is a pluripotent cytokine secreted by lymphoid and non-lymphoid cells. It has the potential for monitoring immune response during the treatment of cancer and is known to increase glucose intake along with influencing insulin activity. Munje et al. developed a biosensor comprised of room temperature ionic liquids with antibodies functionalized sensors on nanoporous, flexible polymer membranes (Figure 3c). They used the sensor to detect interleukin with a LOD of 0.2 pg/mL and 2 pg/mL for 0–24 h and 24–48 h post antibody sensor functionalization, respectively [31]. The chemiluminescence smartphone-based biosensor seen in the saliva section can also be used to monitor lactate can be found in sweat. The LOD for Lactate analysis in sweat is reported as 0.1 mmol/L [15]. Cortisol is another biomarker found in sweat. A cortisol detecting biosensor was designed with functionalized cortisol antibodies on MoS_2 nanosheets integrated into a nanoporous flexible electrode (Figure 3d). The biosensor was targeting for a cortisol range of 8.16–141.7 ng/mL corresponding to a relevant cortisol level in human perspiration. The biosensor reports a dynamic range of 1–500 ng/mL and a LOD of 1 ng/mL [32].

2.3. Urine

Urine is 95% water with sodium, phosphate, sulfate, urea, creatinine, proteins and kidney/liver byproducts which include metabolites and drugs. It has advantages in that it can be easily obtained in large quantities and is noninvasive [12]. Additionally, the lower concentration of protein, lipids and other high molecular weight compounds allows for less complex preparation. In this section, several analytes in urine are discussed (Table 3) with the recent development of portable biosensors (Figure 4).

Table 3. Summary of Portable Biosensors for Urine Biomarker Detection.

Biomarker	Target Disease/Area	Sensor Type	Detection Limit * Sensitivity	Dynamic Range	Analysis Time
Adenosine [35]	Lung Cancer	Colorimetric aptasensor	0.17 μM	5.0 μM–60.0 μM	<20 min
Chlamydia trachomatis [36]	Chlamydia	Nanoplasmonic biosensor	300 CFU/mL	NA	Real time
Neisseria gonorrhoeae [36]	Gonorrhoeae	Nanoplasmonic biosensor	150 CFU/mL	NA	Real time
Neopterin [37]	Aging	Molecularly Imprinted Polymer integrated Potentiostat	0.025 pg/mL 0.041 pg/mL compared to reference of 35–55 ng/mL *	NA	NA
Estrogenic Endocrine Disruptor [38]	Obesity, birth defects, cancer, reproductive impairment	In-vitro Detection biosensor platform	urine 4 nM Blood 8 nM	4–100 nM, urine	2.5 h
Glucose [39]	Diabetes	Micro-Planer amperometric biosensor	NA	0–2000 mg/dL	6 s
Dopamine [40]	Doping	Stabilized lipid Membrane optical Biosensor	10^{-9} M	0 to 100 nM	<1 min
Ephedrin [40]	Doping	Stabilized lipid Membrane optical Biosensor	10^{-9} M	0 to 100 nM	<1 min

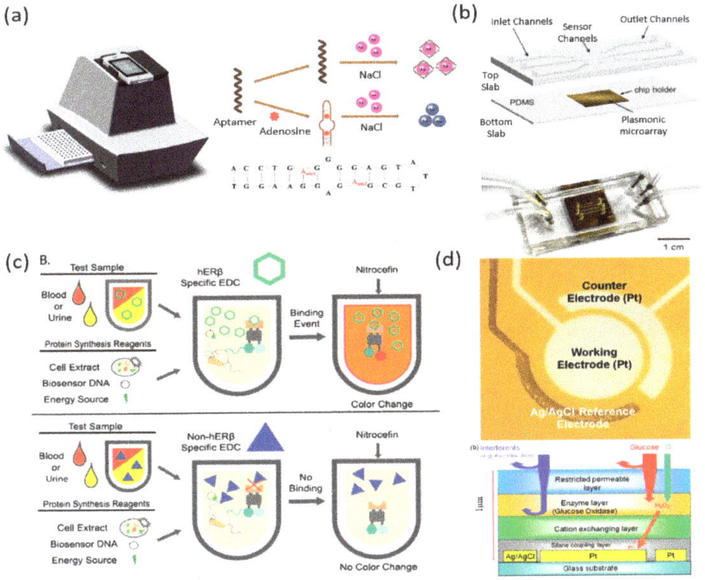

Figure 4. Portable biosensors for urine Biomarker biosensors detection. (**a**) The schematic of the bionic electronic-eye (E-eye) and the sensing mechanism of the colorimetric aptasensor for adenosine detection [35]. (**b**) Schematic and image of Soler's Chlamydia trachomatis (CT) and Neisseria gonorrhoeae (NG) biosensor integrated with a microfluidic system [36]. (**c**) The RAPID biosensor assay. The presence of estrogen hERβ-specific ligands in the sample triggers a color change in the assay, which can be observed visually or more accurately measured using a spectrometer [38]. (**d**) Glucose sensor construction showing the Electrodes layout in H_2O_2 sensor and a Cross-sectional schematic of the sensor [39].

Adenosine is a potential biomarker for detecting and monitoring lung cancer that can be found in urine. Zhou et al. developed a colorimetric aptasensor with a homemade biomimetic electronic eye for use in portable detection. The biosensor is capable of a dynamic range of 5.0 μM–60.0 μM and a LOD of 0.17 μM. A schematic of the adenosine biosensor and its operating principle can be seen in Figure 4a [35]. Chlamydia trachomatis (CT) and Neisseria gonorrhoeae (NG) are both sexually transmitted infection which is the first and second most reported bacterial infections. Soler et al. developed a portable biosensor for the detection of CT and NG in urine. It is comprised of an optically transparent gold nanohole sensor array functionalized with antibodies and a microfluidic system as shown in Figure 4b. The biosensor reports a LOD of 300 CFU/mL and 150 CFU/mL for CT and NG, respectively [36]. Neopterin is a useful biomarker as it provides information on the cellular immunity activation associated with oxidative stress. A biosensor designed by imprinting neopterin onto poly(ethylene- *co* -vinyl alcohol) as template molecules was developed by Huang et al. After imprinting, the template is removed, and the membrane can be used as a sensing element for electrochemical analysis of urine. The LOD for the biosensor was reported to be as low as 0.025 pg/mL [37]. Endocrine-disrupting chemicals such as diethylstilbestrol and bisphenol can disrupt naturally occurring endocrine control causing diseases and disorders such as cancer and epigenetic dysfunction. Salehi developed a portable biosensor (seen in Figure 4c) for the detection of chemicals that interact with estrogen receptor β (hERβ). The sensor consists of an allosterically activated fusion protein that contains the ligand-binding domain of a nuclear hormone receptor and (hERβ) is synthesized in cell-free protein synthesis. In previous work, they used β-lactamase instead of hERβ which shows the ability to change the sensor for many different endocrine disruptors. The dynamic range is reported to be 4–100 nM with a LOD of 4nM for urine [38]. Miyashita reported a urine glucose meter that uses immobilized glucose oxidase to detect glucose amperometrically. As discussed in previous sections, glucose levels are crucial to monitoring diabetes. The sensor can give results in six seconds and has a dynamic range of 0–2000 mg/dL. An image of the urine glucose meter and a diagram of its construction can be seen in Figure 4d [39]. Performance-enhancing drugs continue to be a problem in professional sports. Both dopamine and ephedrine can be detected in the urine of an individual who has used a performance-enhancing drug. Nikolelis developed a portable biosensor capable of detection of doping materials in the urine. The sensor is designed with a stabilized lipid membrane with an artificial receptor added before polymerization. The lipid film is then formed on microporous filters by polymerization of UV irradiation. The biosensor is capable of a dynamic range of 0 to 100 nM and a LOD of 10^{-9} M for both ephedrine and dopamine [40].

2.4. *Blood*

Blood has been the most widely used sample type due to a large number of disease-associated biomarkers and its less invasive collection procedure. Thus, it becomes a good source of biomarkers for portable biosensors. Blood sampling can be as simple as a finger prick with a small drop of blood used in a portable glucometer or full blood sampling which requires a trained individual to draw. Blood, plasma, and serum testing show a good correlation between pharmacologic effect and compound concentration. Blood cells are suspended in plasma and water and it contains many proteins, glucose, mineral ions, hormones, carbon dioxide and platelets [12]. In this section, we summarize many types of blood biomarkers for portable biosensors (Table 4). In addition, we describe the recent development of portable blood biosensors along with their limits and ranges of detection (Figure 5).

The effort to eradicate malaria has been able to decrease mortality by 48% from 2000 to 2015, but it still remains endemic in 97 countries. An aptamer-tethered enzyme capture assay for POC diagnosis of Plasmodium falciparum was developed by Dirkzwager et al. [41]. The sensor captures Plasmodium falciparum lactate dehydrogenase from samples and uses its enzymatic activity to generate a blue color in response. The sensor utilizes only small sample volumes of 20 μL and has a LOD in the ng/mL range. Fraser et al. present the portable biosensor (Figure 5a) by coating aptamers onto magnetic microbeads for magnet-guided capture. They employ three separate microfluidic chambers for the detection of Plasmodium falciparum lactate dehydrogenase enzyme. The LOD is reported to be 250 parasites/μL [42]. Zika is a vector-borne viral infection that can cause brain defects in fetuses. Afsahi et al. developed a biosensor for Zika detection by covalently linking graphene with monoclonal antibodies for the detection of Zika antigens. A Diagram of the sensor can be seen in Figure 5b. The biosensor responds to Zika antigens with a change in capacitance, allowing for the detection of the virus in samples. The LOD is reported to be 0.45 nM [43]. Arboviral disease, dengue hemorrhagic fever, or dengue shock syndrome can all be caused by the dengue virus. Zaytseva developed a biosensor built of generic and specific serotype-specific DNA probes. Through the use of a reflectometer, liposome immobilized in capture zones can be quantified, which directly correlates to viral RNA. The LOD is reported to be 50 RNA molecules for serotype 2, 500 RNA molecules for serotypes 3 and 4, and 50,000 molecules for serotype 1 [44]. Yersinia Pestis is the etiological agent of plague and has resulted in three pandemics. A Biosensor for detection of antibodies of Yersinia Pestis was created using a sandwich immunoassay with immobilized Escherichia coli on the optic fiber probes labeled with Cy-5 as a detection antigen. The *Yersinia Pestis* biosensor reports a LOD of 10 ng/mL with 100% sensitivity and 94.7% specificity in rabbit serum [45].

Table 4. Summary of Portable Biosensors for Blood Biomarker Detection.

Biomarker	Sample Type	Target Disease/Area	Sensor Type	Detection Limit * Sensitivity ** Specificity	Dynamic Range	Analysis Time
Malaria [41]	Whole blood	Malaria–	Aptamer Tethered Enzyme Capture assay	4.9 ng/mL	NA	<1 h
Malaria [42]	Blood	Malaria	Aptamer-Tethered Enzyme Capture (APTEC) biosensor	250 parasites/μL	NA	<20 min
Zika [43]	Simulated Serum	Zika	graphene-based biosensor	0.45 nM	NA	Real time
Dengue [44]	Blood	Dengue fever	multi-analyte biosensor based on nucleic acid hybridization and liposome signal amplification	50 RNA molecules for serotype 2, 500 RNA molecules for serotypes 3 and 4, and 50,000 molecules for serotype 1	NA	<25 min
Yersinia Pestis Antibody [45]	Rabbit serum	Etiological agent of plague	Antigen sandwich method using a portable fiber optic biosensor	10 ng/mL 100% * 94.7% **	NA	40 min
Trichloropyridino [46]	Rat Blood	Exposure to organophosphorus insecticides	Quantum Dot integrated Fluorescent biosensor	1.0 ng/mL	1–50 ng/ml	15 min
Trichloropyridino [47]	Rat plasma	Exposure to organophosphorus insecticides	Immunochromatographic electrochemical biosensor	0.1 ng/ml	0.1–100 ng/ml	15 min
Copper [48]	Serum	Copper Toxicity	Cu^{2+}-dependent DNA ligation DNAzyme PGMs	1 nM possible	10–600 mg/dL	NA
Estrogenic Endocrine Disruptor [38]	Blood	Obesity, birth defects, cancer, reproductive impairment	In-vitro Detection biosensor platform	8 nM	8–300 nM in blood 4–100 nM urine	2.5 h
Red blood [49]	Blood	Anemia	Surface Stress Biosensor	NA	NA	NA
Anti-Cancer Drugs [50]	Blood	Toxicity	Novel Tungsten Phosphide Embedded Nitrogen-Doped Carbon Nanotubes biosensor	45 nM	0.01–45 μM	NA

Exposure to organophosphorus insecticides has recently been found to inhibit the enzyme activity of acetylcholinesterase in the central and peripheral nervous systems. Trichloropyridino is the primary metabolite marker when exposure to organophosphorus insecticides occurs. Zou et al. recently developed a portable biosensor for Trichloropyridinol sensing. The biosensor contains an immunochromatographic test strip assay with a quantum dot label integrated into a portable fluorescent sensor. The biosensor exhibited a dynamic range of 1–50 ng/mL and a LOD of 1.0 ng/mL [46]. Wang et al. presented a new immunochromatographic electrochemical biosensor (IEB) for the detection of trichloropyridinal (TCP) in blood seen in Figure 5c. The sensor utilizes an immunochromatographic test strip for a competitive immunoreaction along with a disposable screen-printed carbon electrode for analysis of captured horseradish peroxidase labeling. The biosensor exhibited a dynamic range of 0.1–100 ng/mL with a LOD of 0.1 ng/m [47]. Copper ions (Cu^{2+}) are essential to human life, but at high concentrations, they can cause adverse health effects. A biosensor developed by Ming et al. using Cu^{2+}-dependent DNA ligation DNAzyme enabled Copper ion detection in a glucose meter. The biosensor reportedly has a dynamic range of 10–600 mg/dL and has a possible LOD of 1 nM [48]. The estrogenic endocrine disruptor biosensor previously described in the urine section can also be used for the detection of EED's in blood. The dynamic range is reported to be 8–300 nM with a LOD of 8 nM for blood [38].

Hemolytic anemia is a disorder in which red blood cells die faster than they can be made, causing the concentration of dead red blood cells to be much higher when compared to a healthy individual. Sang et al. developed a biosensor consisting of a multifunctional dielectrophoresis manipulation device and a surface stress biosensor to separate and detect red blood cells for the detection of hemolytic anemia. The biosensor allows for the detection of live and dead red blood cells, and the diagnosis of Hemolytic anemia can be made from capacitance reading from the biosensor. The device was successfully able to sort live/dead red blood cells. A figure of the biosensor can be seen in Figure 5d. Future tests will be needed to determine how the capacitance measurement can be used to calibrate with the severity of the disease [49]. Methotrexate is a commonly used drug in the treatment of cancers and some autoimmune diseases due to its immunosuppressive properties. Zhou et al. developed a biosensor sensor comprised of a carbon-based composite fixed to an electrode surface supporting redox cycling. The dynamic range was reported to be 0.01–45 µM with a LOD of 45 nM [50].

2.5. *Tears/Breath*

In this section, we discuss portable biosensors that use tears and breath as the specimen. Tears can provide an easily collectible convenient means for monitoring and testing biomarkers. For biosensors that passively collect tears from the surface of the eye, the collection is no more invasive than wearing a contact lens. However, if larger quantities are required, portable sampling could prove to be difficult. Human breath also contains thousands of potential disease and chemical exposure biomarkers [51]. Using breath as a specimen is very portable and noninvasive to collect. A trained individual would not be necessary for the collection. Depending on the sample volume required, collection can be as natural as breathing into a bag or through a chamber and could be repeated as often as needed. Here, we summarize many types of biomarkers in tears and breath for portable biosensors (Table 5). In addition, we describe the recent development of portable biosensors along with their limits and ranges of detection (Figure 6).

Table 5. Summary of Portable Biosensors for Tears/Breath Biomarker Detection.

Biomarker	Sample Type	Target Disease/Area	Sensor Type	Detection Limit * Sensitivity	Dynamic Range	Analysis Time
Alcohol/Glucose/Vitamins (B2,B6,C) [52]	Tear	Various disease/Health Monitoring	Alcohol-oxidase (AOx) biosensing fluidic system	NA	NA	Real-time
Glucose [53]	Tear	Diabetes	Amperometric glucose biosensor	0.01 mM 240 uA/(mM·cm^2) *	Linearity 0.1–0.6 mM	20 s
Glucose [54]	Tear	Diabetes	SCL-biosensor	NA	0.03–5.0 mmol/L	Real-time
helicobacter pylori [55]	breath	Chronic gastritis/(gastric/duodenal ulcers)/gastric cancer	Quadrupole mass Spectrometer biosensor	NA	NA	NA
Acetone [56]	Breath	Various disease/Health Monitoring	portable Si:WO3 gas sensors	20 ppb	NA	10–15 s
Volatile and non-volatile biomarkers [51]	Breath	Disease or chemical exposure	Differential Mobility Spectrometry	Toluene: 200 ppb Angiotensin: 1 pM	NA	Near real-time
CO_2 [57]	Breath	Respiratory health	Carbonic Anhydrase-Based enzyme biosensor	0.132 mV/ppm *	160–2677 ppm CO_2 linear response	12 s

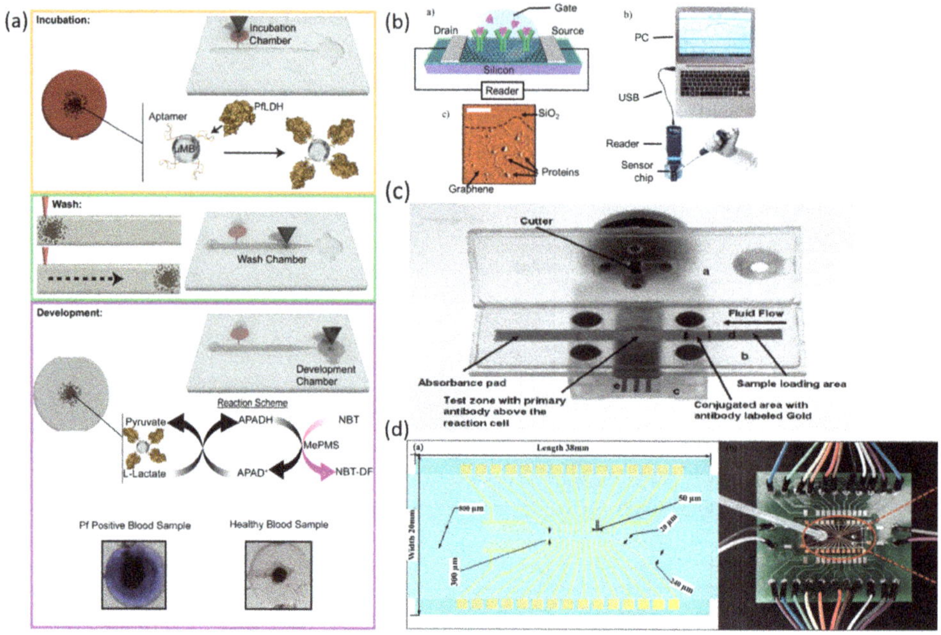

Figure 5. Portable biosensors for blood biomarker detection. (**a**) Operation and detection stages of the microfluidic APTEC biosensor [42]. (**b**) Diagram of the sensor element of the graphene biosensor chip with an AFM image of the graphene after successful protein attachment. In addition, an illustration of the entire sensor chip system [43]. (**c**) The schematic diagram of an IEB [47]. (**d**) Design sketch of the microfluidic chip; Photograph of the microfluidic chip and the peripheral control line design [49].

Sempionatto et al. developed a portable biosensor for the detection of alcohol, glucose, and vitamins B2, B6 and C in tear samples seen in Figure 6a. The biosensor consisted of an electrochemical alcohol-oxidase biosensor integrated with a microfluidic system. The sensor-enabled noninvasive, real-time testing but did not include a dynamic range or LOD in the report [52]. Yao et al. reported a contact lens integrated with an amperometric glucose sensor capable of the detection of glucose molecules from tear samples seen in Figure 6b. The sensor consisted of microstructures on a polymer substrate shaped into a contact lens. The sensor maintained a linear response to a range of 0.1–0.6 mM and has a LOD of 0.01 mM [53]. Chu et al. also demonstrated glucose monitoring with a contact lens which consists of an enzyme immobilized electrode on the surface of a PDMS lens. The system reported having a dynamic detection range of 0.03 to 5 mmol/L [54]. *Helicobacter pylori* can be detected in breath samples, which has been correlated to chronic gastritis, gastric and duodenal ulcers, and gastric cancer. Sreekumar et al. developed a noninvasive biosensor (Figure 6c) capable of detection of helicobacter pylori. The biosensor consisted of a portable quadrupole mass spectrometer (QMS) system measuring carbon-13 levels in breath samples. The results from clinical samples showed an overall agreement of 87% when compared to the laboratory isotope ratio mass spectrometry (IRMS) results [55]. Acetone in breath samples appears in a relatively high concentration of approximately 100–500 ppb. Acetone content in breath can be used as supplemental information for Diabetes treatment. Righettoni et al. fabricated a biosensor (Figure 6d) consisting of Si-doped epsilon-WO3 nanostructured films. The acetone sensor demonstrated to have a LOD of 20 ppb [56]. Exhaled breath chemicals contain both volatile and non-volatile compounds which can be indicative of different diseases. A biosensor consisting of a combination of a differential mobility spectrometer with a gas chromatograph and an electrospray ionization module is examined. The biosensor is capable of detecting aa large amount of chemical analytes but reports values of a LOD for toluene (200 ppb) and angiotensin (1 pM) [51].

Asthma, chronic obstructive pulmonary disease, pneumonia, and sleep apnea are all potentially cause respiratory acidosis. Respiratory acidosis is a condition where the lungs are unable to remove enough carbon dioxide produced by the body. Bagchi et al. reported a biosensor for the detection of CO_2 in breath by immobilizing carbonic anhydrase enzyme on an electrode assembly. The device reports a linear electrochemical response to CO_2 from 160–2677 ppm and a LOD of 0.132mV/ppm [57].

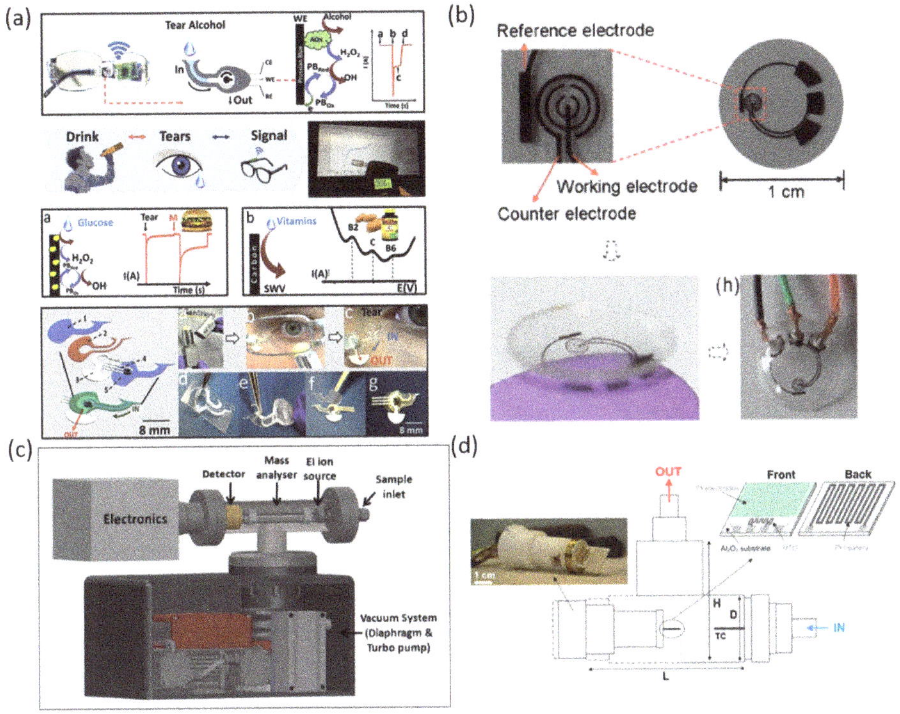

Figure 6. Portable biosensors for tears/breath biomarker detection. (**a**) Eyeglasses-based Fluidic Device [52]. (**b**) Prototype contact biosensor for glucose sensing [53]. (**c**) Schematic diagram of the portable QMS and vacuum system [55]. (**d**) Schematic and image of the portable breath acetone monitor with Si:WO3 gas sensors [56].

3. Discussion

Some of the common analytes have been repeated throughout the article (Table 6). This goes to show that not only can analytes be found in different biological samples, but that the LOD can vary widely between biosensors based on design and implementation. The commonly repeated analytes are lactate, glucose, and alcohol. Both glucose and lactate can be used for multipurpose monitoring, which can further explain why they are commonly being researched through many different biological samples. Alcohol sensing can also be used for multiple purposes, such as in the treatment of diabetes, but can be used for monitoring drivers or individuals in safety work.

As seen in the biosensors and their target biomarkers, many portable devices have been developed for pathogen detection and health monitoring. Still, the portability of the systems has not been discussed in much detail. While some portable biosensors could be moved by vehicle and set up in remote locations, others may need to be able to be worn or handheld. The portability of biosensors for on-site diagnosis can be limited due to various issues, including sample preparation techniques, fluid-handling techniques, the limited lifetime of biological reagents, device packaging, integrating electronics for data collection/analysis, and the requirement of external accessories and power. This limits the ability of researchers and physicians to identify portable biosensors, which can be applied to fields and practices. The well-defined portability for biosensors could provide users a better idea of how mobile and compact they are for field use. Here, we summarize the portability requirements for the classification categories of the biosensors in Figure 7.

Table 6. Summary of Commonly Repeated Analytes.

Biomarker	Sample Type	Target Disease/Area
Lactate	Saliva and sweat	Respiratory insufficiency, shocks, heart failure, metabolic disorders, diabetes, sports medicine, critical care, and food analysis
Glucose	Sweat, urine, and tears	Diabetes and general healthcare monitoring
Alcohol	Sweat tears, and breath	BAC for drivers and diabetes treatment for hypoglycemia prevention

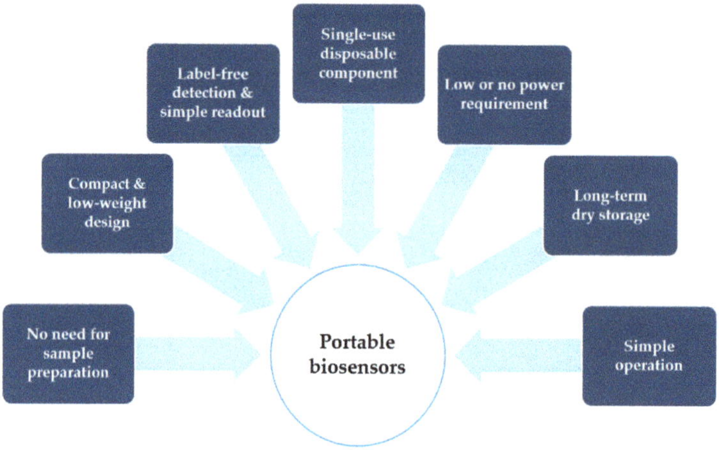

Figure 7. Key requirements for portable biosensors.

Note that all recommended requirements are not currently quantifiable and would need to be further studied and classified to create portability classification requirements. The above list also may not contain all pertinent information to the portability of a biosensor but provides recommendations for starting components to consider.

In the section of the analyte, we have seen sample preparation techniques ranging from centrifuging to chemical addition to an analyte. Biological samples contain many different proteins, lipids, and contaminants that can affect how samples need to be prepared and, ultimately, the outcome of tests. Often the analytes of interest are in a much lower concentration when compared to other substances that make up the remainder of the sample [12]. Sample preparation can be one of the limiting factors causing a biosensor system to be portable. While the biosensor itself meets the portability requirements, if the sample preparation requires non-portable laboratory equipment, the testing, diagnosis, and monitoring cannot be made remotely. Strand et al. gives an example of biosensing issues from existing sample preparation techniques. Metabolites can be found in human breath and are known to be up or down-regulated in various disease states. Measuring metabolites in exhaled breath can be used for the diagnosis or treatment of diseases, including cancer, asthma, and respiratory infections. However, analysis is currently limited due to the inability to concentrate the analytes of interest before testing. Strand developed a chip-based polymeric pre-concentration device with the ability to absorb and desorb breath volatiles for analysis [58].

One possibility to integrate portable sample preparation into a portable biosensor is to integrate microfluidics into the system. Microfluidic integrated biosensors have great potential to help make biosensors more portable. The microfluidic chip can be tiny and encompass an entire sample preparation method that may otherwise require a laboratory. Ferguson et al. demonstrate an integrated microfluidic system, which enables sequence-specific viral RNA-based pathogen detection without the need for pre-processing of throat swap samples seen in Figure 8a. [20]. Yu et al. proposed a paper-based microfluidic biosensor for uric acid determination, which gives the advantage of working with small volumes of reagent and having short reaction times Figure 8b [59]. Some microfluidic devices require external pumps or large power supply to operate, limiting the portability of the system. Chuang et al. show a microfluidic device utilizing capillary action negating the need for an external pump, further increasing the portability of sample preparation seen in Figure 8c [60].

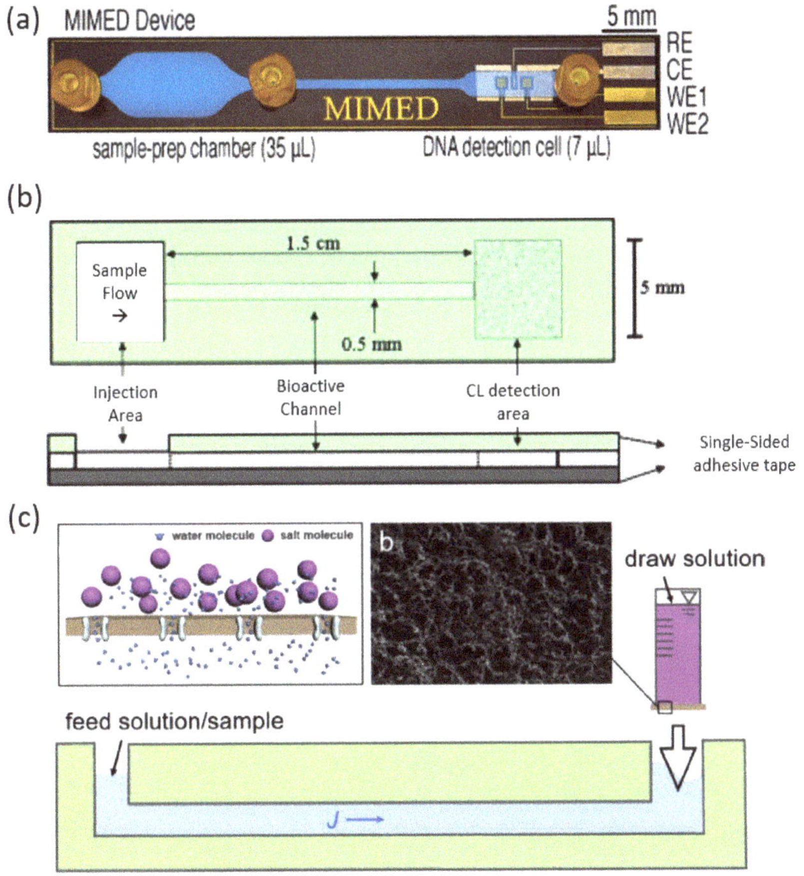

Figure 8. Microfluidic integrated biosensors. (**a**) Magnetic Integrated Microfluidic Electrochemical Detector device for detection of H1N1 [20]. (**b**) Schematic of a paper microfluidic biosensor for uric acid determination [59]. (**c**) Schematic of a microfluidic device driven by osmotic pressure [60].

4. Conclusions and Outlooks

Despite the recent progress of portable biosensors, many challenges still remain before the implementation of portable biosensors in practical applications. The following requirements need to be considered for future development. First, the sample collection and preparation method is simple, easy to use, and does not involve costly and time-consuming processes. In that sense, current lab-on-a-chip technologies, such as microfluidics, can provide a solution for this goal. Also, sample types such as saliva, sweat, urine, and breath offer an excellent opportunity for noninvasive sample collection. Second, the sensitivity and specificity improvement is an ever-lasting goal in biosensor development. This might be one of the major barriers to the application of portable biosensors. While many biosensors reported in the literature perform well in laboratory settings, they may encounter a series of problems in-field use with real samples. Thus, it is essential to develop highly sensitive and specific portable biosensors whose performance is comparable to conventional laboratory testing. Third, cost-effective packaging and manufacturing methods should be accompanied by the fabrication of portable biosensors. Microfabrication technology is widely used for manufacturing, but it needs expensive production equipment. New manufacturing technologies, such as 3D-printing, are capable of reducing fabrication costs and enabling mass production. We believe that these challenges will be gradually solved in the future, leading to successful portable biosensors, which allow us to monitor our health status at any time and place.

In conclusion, the wide variety of analytes and the associated portable biosensors provides an excellent opportunity for POC diagnostics as well as remote health care monitoring. While biosensors can be made portable, the associated sample collection and preparation play a crucial role in developing entirely portable systems that can truly expand the possibilities of diagnostics, especially in areas of limited resources and for immediate, on-demand measurement. Sample types, such as saliva, sweat, urine, and breath, offer an excellent opportunity for noninvasive sample collection. While blood provides a wide range of analytes for testing, its collection can be more invasive. The processes described in the analyte section of this paper can often be altered or expanded upon for use with different analytes to provide the ability for multiplexing biomarkers with just a single sensor. Lastly, the portability of biosensors needs to be classified. Portable is a vague statement that can cause confusion and errors in the developing field. Without classification, the practical use and viability of biosensors, sample collection, and preparation cannot be fully applied to on-site diagnostics.

Author Contributions: B.S. and J.-H.K. conducted reviews of portable biosensors and biomarkers; B.S., J.-H.K. and W.-H.Y. designed figures and reviewed all sections; all authors wrote the paper together. All authors have read and agreed to the published version of the manuscript.

Funding: J.-H.K. acknowledges the support of the National Science Foundation (CBET-1707056). Woon-Hong Yeo acknowledges the support of the Alzheimer's Association (2019-AARGD-NTF-643460) and the National Institutes of Health (NIH R21AG064309). The content is solely the responsibility of the authors and does not necessarily represent the official views of the NIH.

Conflicts of Interest: The authors declare no conflict of interest.

References

1. Thévenot, D.R.; Toth, K.; Durst, R.A.; Wilson, G.S. Electrochemical Biosensors: Recommended Definitions and Classification1International Union of Pure and Applied Chemistry: Physical Chemistry Division, Commission I.7 (Biophysical Chemistry); Analytical Chemistry Division, Commission V.5 (Electroanalytical Chemistry).1. *Biosens. Bioelectron.* **2001**, *16*, 121–131. [PubMed]
2. Reilly, R.B.; Lee, T.C. Biosensors. *Technol. Health Care* **2011**, *19*, 285–293. [CrossRef] [PubMed]
3. OADC; DNEM. Image Library|CDC Online Newsroom|CDC. 2020. Available online: https://www.cdc.gov/media/subtopic/images.htm (accessed on 13 August 2020).
4. Morales, M.A.; Mark Halpern, J. Guide to Selecting a Biorecognition Element for Biosensors. *Bioconjug. Chem.* **2018**, *29*, 3231–3239. [CrossRef] [PubMed]
5. Khansili, N.; Rattu, G.; Krishna, P.M. Label-Free Optical Biosensors for Food and Biological Sensor Applications. *Sens. Actuators B Chem.* **2018**, *265*, 35–49. [CrossRef]
6. Nordin, N.; Yusof, N.A.; Abdullah, J.; Radu, S.; Hushiarian, R. A Simple, Portable, Electrochemical Biosensor to Screen Shellfish for Vibrio Parahaemolyticus. *AMB Express* **2017**, *7*, 41. [CrossRef]
7. Vermeir, S.; Nicolaï, B.M.; Verboven, P.; Van Gerwen, P.; Baeten, B.; Hoflack, L.; Vulsteke, V.; Lammertyn, J. Microplate Differential Calorimetric Biosensor for Ascorbic Acid Analysis in Food and Pharmaceuticals. *Anal. Chem.* **2007**, *79*, 6119–6127. [CrossRef]

8. Heineman, W.R.; Jensen, W.B. Leland C. Clark Jr. (1918–2005). *Biosens. Bioelectron.* **2006**, *21*, 1403–1404. [CrossRef]
9. Nguyen, H.H.; Lee, S.H.; Lee, U.J.; Fermin, C.D.; Kim, M. Immobilized Enzymes in Biosensor Applications. *Materials* **2019**, *12*, 121. [CrossRef]
10. Sadana, A.; Sadana, N. *Handbook of Biosensors and Biosensor Kinetics*; Elsevier Science & Technology, Elsevier Science: Oxford, UK, 2010.
11. Tabeta, I.; Ueshiba, H.; Ichijo, T.; Hiroi, N.; Yakushiji, F.; Simojo, M.; Tsuboi, K.; Miyachi, Y. The Corticotropin-Releasing Hormone Stimulation Test in White Coat Hypertension. *J. Clin. Endocrinol. Metab.* **2002**, *87*, 3672–3675. [CrossRef]
12. Niu, Z.; Zhang, W.; Yu, C.; Zhang, J.; Wen, Y. Recent Advances in Biological Sample Preparation Methods Coupled with Chromatography, Spectrometry and Electrochemistry Analysis Techniques. *TrAC Trends Anal. Chem.* **2018**, *102*, 123–146. [CrossRef]
13. Soltani Zarrin, P.; Ibne Jamal, F.; Roeckendorf, N.; Wenger, C. Development of a Portable Dielectric Biosensor for Rapid Detection of Viscosity Variations and Its In Vitro Evaluations Using Saliva Samples of COPD Patients and Healthy Control. *Healthcare* **2019**, *7*, 11. [CrossRef]
14. Petropoulos, K.; Piermarini, S.; Bernardini, S.; Palleschi, G.; Moscone, D. Development of a Disposable Biosensor for Lactate Monitoring in Saliva. *Sens. Actuators B Chem.* **2016**, *237*, 8–15. [CrossRef]
15. Roda, A.; Guardigli, M.; Calabria, D.; Calabretta, M.M.; Cevenini, L.; Michelini, E. A 3D-Printed Device for a Smartphone-Based Chemiluminescence Biosensor for Lactate in Oral Fluid and Sweat. *Analyst* **2014**, *139*, 6494–6501. [CrossRef] [PubMed]
16. Yao, Y.; Li, H.; Wang, D.; Liu, C.; Zhang, C. An Electrochemiluminescence Cloth-Based Biosensor with Smartphone-Based Imaging for Detection of Lactate in Saliva. *Analyst* **2017**, *142*, 3715–3724. [CrossRef]
17. Ahmed, A.; Rushworth, J.V.; Wright, J.D.; Millner, P.A. Novel Impedimetric Immunosensor for Detection of Pathogenic Bacteria Streptococcus Pyogenes in Human Saliva. *Anal. Chem.* **2013**, *85*, 12118–12125. [CrossRef]
18. Wang, R.; Lin, J.; Lassiter, K.; Srinivasan, B.; Lin, L.; Lu, H.; Tung, S.; Hargis, B.; Bottje, W.; Berghman, L.; et al. Evaluation Study of a Portable Impedance Biosensor for Detection of Avian Influenza Virus. *J. Virol. Methods* **2011**, *178*, 52–58. [CrossRef]
19. Hao, Z.; Pan, Y.; Shao, W.; Lin, Q.; Zhao, X. Graphene-Based Fully Integrated Portable Nanosensing System for on-Line Detection of Cytokine Biomarkers in Saliva. *Biosens. Bioelectron.* **2019**, *134*, 16–23. [CrossRef]
20. Ferguson, B.S.; Buchsbaum, S.F.; Wu, T.-T.; Hsieh, K.; Xiao, Y.; Sun, R.; Soh, H.T. Genetic Analysis of H1N1 Influenza Virus from Throat Swab Samples in a Microfluidic System for Point-of-Care Diagnostics. *J. Am. Chem. Soc.* **2011**, *133*, 9129–9135. [CrossRef]
21. Piermarini, S.; Volpe, G.; Federico, R.; Moscone, D.; Palleschi, G. Detection of Biogenic Amines in Human Saliva Using a Screen-Printed Biosensor. *Anal. Lett.* **2010**, *43*, 1310–1316. [CrossRef]
22. Stevens, R.C.; Soelberg, S.D.; Near, S.; Furlong, C.E. Detection of Cortisol in Saliva with a Flow-Filtered, Portable Surface Plasmon Resonance Biosensor System. *Anal. Chem.* **2008**, *80*, 6747–6751. [CrossRef]
23. Ma, X.; Chen, Z.; Zhou, J.; Weng, W.; Zheng, O.; Lin, Z.; Guo, L.; Qiu, B.; Chen, G. Aptamer-Based Portable Biosensor for Platelet-Derived Growth Factor-BB (PDGF-BB) with Personal Glucose Meter Readout. *Biosens. Bioelectron.* **2014**, *55*, 412–416. [PubMed]
24. Lu, Y.-P.; Huang, J.-W.; Lee, I.-N.; Weng, R.-C.; Lin, M.-Y.; Yang, J.-T.; Lin, C.-T. A Portable System to Monitor Saliva Conductivity for Dehydration Diagnosis and Kidney Healthcare. *Sci. Rep.* **2019**, *9*, 1–9. [CrossRef]
25. García-Carmona, L.; Martín, A.; Sempionatto, J.R.; Moreto, J.R.; González, M.C.; Wang, J.; Escarpa, A. Pacifier Biosensor: Toward Noninvasive Saliva Biomarker Monitoring. *Anal. Chem.* **2019**, *91*, 13883–13891.
26. CDC. Avian Influenza A Virus Infections in Humans. Available online: https://www.cdc.gov/flu/avianflu/avian-in-humans.htm (accessed on 10 January 2020).
27. Lee, J.; Choi, B.Y.; Jung, E. Metapopulation Model Using Commuting Flow for National Spread of the 2009 H1N1 Influenza Virus in the Republic of Korea. *J. Theor. Biol.* **2018**, *454*, 320–329. [CrossRef]
28. Scully, C. Halitosis. *BMJ Clin. Evid.* **2014**, *2014*, 1305. [CrossRef]
29. Bhide, A.; Muthukumar, S.; Saini, A.; Prasad, S. Simultaneous Lancet-Free Monitoring of Alcohol and Glucose from Low-Volumes of Perspired Human Sweat. *Sci. Rep.* **2018**, *8*, 1–11. [CrossRef]
30. He, W.; Wang, C.; Wang, H.; Jian, M.; Lu, W.; Liang, X.; Zhang, X.; Yang, F.; Zhang, Y. Integrated Textile Sensor Patch for Real-Time and Multiplex Sweat Analysis. *Sci. Adv.* **2019**, *5*, eaax0649.

31. Munje, R.D.; Muthukumar, S.; Jagannath, B.; Prasad, S. A New Paradigm in Sweat Based Wearable Diagnostics Biosensors Using Room Temperature Ionic Liquids (RTILs). *Sci. Rep.* **2017**, *7*, 1–12. [CrossRef]
32. Kinnamon, D.; Ghanta, R.; Lin, K.-C.; Muthukumar, S.; Prasad, S. Portable Biosensor for Monitoring Cortisol in Low-Volume Perspired Human Sweat. *Sci. Rep.* **2017**, *7*, 13312. [CrossRef]
33. Gamella, M.; Campuzano, S.; Manso, J.; Rivera GG de López-Colino, F.; Reviejo, A.J.; Pingarrón, J.M. A Novel Non-Invasive Electrochemical Biosensing Device for in Situ Determination of the Alcohol Content in Blood by Monitoring Ethanol in Sweat. *Anal. Chim. Acta* **2014**, *806*, 1–7.
34. Gao, W.; Emaminejad, S.; Nyein, H.Y.Y.; Challa, S.; Chen, K.; Peck, A.; Fahad, H.M.; Ota, H.; Shiraki, H.; Kiriya, D.; et al. Fully Integrated Wearable Sensor Arrays for Multiplexed in Situ Perspiration Analysis. *Nature* **2016**, *529*, 509–514. [CrossRef] [PubMed]
35. Zhou, S.; Gan, Y.; Kong, L.; Sun, J.; Liang, T.; Wang, X.; Wan, H.; Wang, P. A Novel Portable Biosensor Based on Aptamer Functionalized Gold Nanoparticles for Adenosine Detection. *Anal. Chim. Acta* **2020**, *1120*, 43–49. [CrossRef] [PubMed]
36. Soler, M.; Belushkin, A.; Cavallini, A.; Kebbi-Beghdadi, C.; Greub, G.; Altug, H. Multiplexed Nanoplasmonic Biosensor for One-Step Simultaneous Detection of Chlamydia Trachomatis and Neisseria Gonorrhoeae in Urine. *Biosens. Bioelectron.* **2017**, *94*, 560–567. [CrossRef]
37. Huang, C.Y.; Hsieh, C.H.; Chen, Y.L.; Lee, M.H.; Lin, C.F.; Tsai, H.H.; Juang, Y.Z.; Liu, B.D.; Lin, H.Y. Portable Potentiostatic Sensor Integrated with Neopterin-Imprinted Poly(Ethylene-Co-Vinyl Alcohol)-Based Electrode. *IET Nanobiotechnol.* **2011**, *5*, 126–131. [CrossRef]
38. Salehi, A.S.M.; Yang, S.O.; Earl, C.C.; Shakalli Tang, M.J.; Porter Hunt, J.; Smith, M.T.; Wood, D.W.; Bundy, B.C. Biosensing Estrogenic Endocrine Disruptors in Human Blood and Urine: A RAPID Cell-Free Protein Synthesis Approach. *Toxicol. Appl. Pharmacol.* **2018**, *345*, 19–25. [CrossRef]
39. Miyashita, M.; Ito, N.; Ikeda, S.; Murayama, T.; Oguma, K.; Kimura, J. Development of Urine Glucose Meter Based on Micro-Planer Amperometric Biosensor and Its Clinical Application for Self-Monitoring of Urine Glucose. *Biosens. Bioelectron.* **2009**, *24*, 1336–1340. [CrossRef]
40. Nikolelis, D.P.; Raftopoulou, G.; Chatzigeorgiou, P.; Nikoleli, G.-P.; Viras, K. Optical Portable Biosensors Based on Stabilized Lipid Membrane for the Rapid Detection of Doping Materials in Human Urine. *Sens. Actuators B Chem.* **2008**, *130*, 577–582. [CrossRef]
41. Dirkzwager, R.M.; Liang, S.; Tanner, J. Development of Aptamer-Based Point-of-Care Diagnostic Devices for Malaria Using Three-Dimensional Printing Rapid Prototyping. *ACS Sens.* **2016**, *1*, 420–426. [CrossRef]
42. Fraser, L.A.; Kinghorn, A.B.; Dirkzwager, R.M.; Liang, S.; Cheung, Y.-W.; Lim, B.; Shiu, S.C.-C.; Tang, M.S.L.; Andrew, D.; Manitta, J.; et al. A Portable Microfluidic Aptamer-Tethered Enzyme Capture (APTEC) Biosensor for Malaria Diagnosis. *Biosens. Bioelectron.* **2018**, *100*, 591–596. [CrossRef]
43. Afsahi, S.; Lerner, M.B.; Goldstein, J.M.; Lee, J.; Tang, X.; Bagarozzi, D.A.; Pan, D.; Locascio, L.; Walker, A.; Barron, F.; et al. Novel Graphene-Based Biosensor for Early Detection of Zika Virus Infection. *Biosens. Bioelectron.* **2018**, *100*, 85–88. [CrossRef]
44. Zaytseva, N.V.; Montagna, R.A.; Lee, E.M.; Baeumner, A.J. Multi-Analyte Single-Membrane Biosensor for the Serotype-Specific Detection of Dengue Virus. *Anal. Bioanal. Chem.* **2004**, *380*, 46–53. [CrossRef]
45. Wei, H.; Guo, Z.; Zhu, Z.; Tan, Y.; Du, Z.; Yang, R. Sensitive Detection of Antibody against Antigen F1 of Yersinia Pestis by an Antigen Sandwich Method Using a Portable Fiber Optic Biosensor. *Sens. Actuators B Chem.* **2007**, *127*, 525–530. [CrossRef]
46. Zou, Z.; Du, D.; Wang, J.; Smith, J.N.; Timchalk, C.; Li, Y.; Lin, Y. Quantum Dot-Based Immunochromatographic Fluorescent Biosensor for Biomonitoring Trichloropyridinol, a Biomarker of Exposure to Chlorpyrifos. *Anal. Chem.* **2010**, *82*, 5125–5133. [CrossRef]
47. Wang, L.; Lu, D.; Wang, J.; Du, D.; Zou, Z.; Wang, H.; Smith, J.N.; Timchalk, C.; Liu, F.; Lin, Y. A Novel Immunochromatographic Electrochemical Biosensor for Highly Sensitive and Selective Detection of Trichloropyridinol, a Biomarker of Exposure to Chlorpyrifos. *Biosens. Bioelectron.* **2011**, *26*, 2835–2840. [CrossRef]
48. Ming, J.; Fan, W.; Jiang, T.-F.; Wang, Y.-H.; Lv, Z.-H. Portable and Sensitive Detection of Copper(II) Ion Based on Personal Glucose Meters and a Ligation DNAzyme Releasing Strategy. *Sens. Actuators B Chem.* **2017**, *240*, 1091–1098. [CrossRef]

49. Sang, S.; Feng, Q.; Jian, A.; Li, H.; Ji, J.; Duan, Q.; Zhang, W.; Wang, T. Portable Microsystem Integrates Multifunctional Dielectrophoresis Manipulations and a Surface Stress Biosensor to Detect Red Blood Cells for Hemolytic Anemia. *Sci. Rep.* **2016**, *6*, 33626. [CrossRef]
50. Zhou, H.; Ran, G.; Masson, J.-F.; Wang, C.; Zhao, Y.; Song, Q. Novel Tungsten Phosphide Embedded Nitrogen-Doped Carbon Nanotubes: A Portable and Renewable Monitoring Platform for Anticancer Drug in Whole Blood. *Biosens. Bioelectron.* **2018**, *105*, 226–235. [CrossRef] [PubMed]
51. Davis, C.E.; Bogan, M.J.; Sankaran, S.; Molina, M.A.; Loyola, B.R.; Zhao, W.; Benner, W.H.; Schivo, M.; Farquar, G.R.; Kenyon, N.J.; et al. Analysis of Volatile and Non-Volatile Biomarkers in Human Breath Using Differential Mobility Spectrometry (DMS). *IEEE Sens. J.* **2010**, *10*, 114–122. [CrossRef]
52. Sempionatto, J.R.; Brazaca, L.C.; García-Carmona, L.; Bolat, G.; Campbell, A.S.; Martin, A.; Tang, G.; Shah, R.; Mishra, R.K.; Kim, J.; et al. Eyeglasses-Based Tear Biosensing System: Non-Invasive Detection of Alcohol, Vitamins and Glucose. *Biosens. Bioelectron.* **2019**, *137*, 161–170. [CrossRef]
53. Yao, H.; Shum, A.J.; Cowan, M.; Lähdesmäki, I.; Parviz, B.A. A Contact Lens with Embedded Sensor for Monitoring Tear Glucose Level. *Biosens. Bioelectron.* **2011**, *26*, 3290–3296. [CrossRef]
54. Chu, M.; Shirai, T.; Takahashi, D.; Arakawa, T.; Kudo, H.; Sano, K.; Sawada, S.; Yano, K.; Iwasaki, Y.; Akiyoshi, K.; et al. Biomedical Soft Contact-Lens Sensor for in Situ Ocular Biomonitoring of Tear Contents. *Biomed. Microdevices* **2011**, *13*, 603–611. [CrossRef]
55. Sreekumar, J.; France, N.; Taylor, S.; Matthews, T.; Turner, P.; Bliss, P.; Brook, A.H.; Watson, A. Diagnosis of Helicobacter Pylori by Carbon-13 Urea Breath Test Using a Portable Mass Spectrometer. *SAGE Open Med.* **2015**, *3*, 2050312115569565. [CrossRef]
56. Righettoni, M.; Tricoli, A.; Gass, S.; Schmid, A.; Amann, A.; Pratsinis, S.E. Breath Acetone Monitoring by Portable Si:WO3 Gas Sensors. *Anal. Chim. Acta* **2012**, *738*, 69–75. [CrossRef]
57. Bagchi, S.; SenGupta, S.; Mondal, S. Development and Characterization of Carbonic Anhydrase-Based CO_2 Biosensor for Primary Diagnosis of Respiratory Health. *IEEE Sens. J.* **2017**, *17*, 1384–1390. [CrossRef]
58. Strand, N.; Bhushan, A.; Schivo, M.; Kenyon, N.J.; Davis, C.E. Chemically Polymerized Polypyrrole for On-Chip Concentration of Volatile Breath Metabolites. *Sens. Actuators B Chem.* **2010**, *143*, 516–523. [CrossRef]
59. Yu, J.; Wang, S.; Ge, L.; Ge, S. A Novel Chemiluminescence Paper Microfluidic Biosensor Based on Enzymatic Reaction for Uric Acid Determination. *Biosens. Bioelectron.* **2011**, *26*, 3284–3289. [CrossRef]
60. Chuang, C.-H.; Chiang, Y.-Y. Bio-O-Pump: A Novel Portable Microfluidic Device Driven by Osmotic Pressure. *Sens. Actuators B Chem.* **2019**, *284*, 736–743. [CrossRef]

biosensors

MDPI

Communication

Automatic and Accurate Sleep Stage Classification via a Convolutional Deep Neural Network and Nanomembrane Electrodes

Kangkyu Kwon [1,2,†], Shinjae Kwon [2,3,†] and Woon-Hong Yeo [2,3,4,5,*]

1 School of Electrical and Computer Engineering, Georgia Institute of Technology, Atlanta, GA 30332, USA; kkwon49@gatech.edu
2 IEN Center for Human-Centric Interfaces and Engineering, Institute for Electronics and Nanotechnology, Georgia Institute of Technology, Atlanta, GA 30332, USA; skwon64@gatech.edu
3 George W. Woodruff School of Mechanical Engineering, Georgia Institute of Technology, Atlanta, GA 30332, USA
4 Wallace H. Coulter Department of Biomedical Engineering, Parker H. Petit Institute for Bioengineering and Biosciences, Georgia Institute of Technology, Atlanta, GA 30332, USA
5 Neural Engineering Center, Institute for Materials, Institute for Robotics and Intelligent Machines, Georgia Institute of Technology, Atlanta, GA 30332, USA
* Correspondence: whyeo@gatech.edu; Tel.: +1-404-385-5710; Fax: +1-404-894-1658
† These authors contributed equally to this work.

Abstract: Sleep stage classification is an essential process of diagnosing sleep disorders and related diseases. Automatic sleep stage classification using machine learning has been widely studied due to its higher efficiency compared with manual scoring. Typically, a few polysomnography data are selected as input signals, and human experts label the corresponding sleep stages manually. However, the manual process includes human error and inconsistency in the scoring and stage classification. Here, we present a convolutional neural network (CNN)-based classification method that offers highly accurate, automatic sleep stage detection, validated by a public dataset and new data measured by wearable nanomembrane dry electrodes. First, our study makes a training and validation model using a public dataset with two brain signal and two eye signal channels. Then, we validate this model with a new dataset measured by a set of nanomembrane electrodes. The result of the automatic sleep stage classification shows that our CNN model with multi-taper spectrogram pre-processing achieved 88.85% training accuracy on the validation dataset and 81.52% prediction accuracy on our laboratory dataset. These results validate the reliability of our classification method on the standard polysomnography dataset and the transferability of our CNN model for other datasets measured with the wearable electrodes.

Keywords: automatic sleep stage classification; convolutional neural network; nanomembrane electrode; multi-taper spectrogram

Citation: Kwon, K.; Kwon, S.; Yeo, W.-H. Automatic and Accurate Sleep Stage Classification via a Convolutional Deep Neural Network and Nanomembrane Electrodes. *Biosensors* **2022**, *12*, 155. https://doi.org/10.3390/bios12030155

Received: 13 December 2021
Accepted: 28 February 2022
Published: 2 March 2022

1. Introduction

An accurate sleep stage classification [1–3] plays a significant role in sleep quality monitoring and the diagnosis of disorders. The polysomnogram (PSG) is widely used in the diagnosis of obstructive sleep apnea (OSA) syndrome [4]. PSG is non-invasive and consists of a simultaneous recording of multiple physiological parameters related to sleep and sleep disorders. Standard polysomnography includes the measurement of various physiological signals such as an electroencephalogram (EEG), an electrooculogram (EOG), an electromyogram (EMG), and an electrocardiogram (ECG). Typically, a series of polysomnographic signals for a 30-second-long epoch is labeled as a certain sleep stage by an expert sleep scorer.

Compared to the manual scoring of sleep stages, automatic sleep stage classification serves as a more efficient way to evaluate a large amount of sleep data. Machine learning algorithms have been adopted in automatic sleep stage classification to increase classification efficiency and performance in recent years. Among them, conventional statistical machine learning algorithms, such as Support Vector Machine [1,5], Hidden Markov Model [6], k-nearest neighbors [7], and Random Forests [7] are adopted at the early stage. Recent progress of deep learning in computer vision, natural language processing, and robotics has advanced these methods to application in automatic sleep stage classification. A convolutional neural network (CNN) has been frequently employed for the task. The weight sharing mechanism at the convolutional layers forces the shift-invariance of the learned features and greatly reduces the model's complexity, consequently improving the model's generalization. Other network variants, such as Deep Belief Networks (DBNs), Auto-encoder, and Deep Neural Networks (DNNs), have also been explored. Moreover, Recurrent Neural Networks (RNNs), e.g., Long Short-Term Memory (LSTM), capable of sequential modeling, have been found to be efficient in capturing long-term sleep stage transitions. However, these methods still have limited accuracy in sleep stage classification as they have been trained and tested merely on a public dataset, without validation study with real lab datasets.

This work presents an automatic sleep stage classification model that could be applied to the public dataset, and that could also be applied to the classification of our laboratory datasets measured with a novel wearable system. In the public dataset from ISRUC used for this study [8], four channels of signals (two EEG and two EOG) were selected based on their proximity to the electrode locations of our new wearable system being tested. The four signals were preprocessed with various filters and a multi-taper spectral analysis was performed. They were then split into 30-second-long epochs and converted into spectrogram images to be used and tested with our newly developed CNN sleep stage classification model. This CNN model trained with a public dataset was then applied to our lab dataset measured with nanomembrane electrodes that were pre-processed with the same methods. A comparison study with a multi-taper spectrogram and band-pass-filtered raw signals showed the advantage of a multi-taper spectrogram in enhancing the transferability of the model. The final result of this study supports not only the performance of our new classification model on the standard PSG dataset, but also the model's transferability to a dataset measured with our novel system.

2. Materials and Methods

2.1. ISRUC Public Dataset

The ISRUC sleep dataset (Figure 1A) consists of complete overnight standard PSG recordings of 118 subjects with three health statuses (healthy, sick, and under-treatment). For this study, a total of 100 data from 100 subjects from subgroup 1 were used. ISRUC subgroup 1 included subjects aged between 20 and 85 years (51 on average), with 55 males and 45 females. The subjects were diagnosed with various sleep disorders. More details of individual subject information can be found in Khalighi et al. [8]. Each recording contained six EEG channels (i.e., C3-A2, C4-A1, F3-A2, O1-A2, O2-A1, and F4-A1), two EOG channels (i.e., LOC-A2 and ROC-A1), and three EMG channels (i.e., X1, X2, and X3) as well as an annotation file with detailed events. For this study, two of the EEG channels (F3-A2 and F4-A1) and both of the EOG channels (LOC-A2 and ROC-A1) were used. The recording rate was 200 Hz. In addition, each 30-second-long epoch was labeled with one of the five sleep stages (W, N1, N2, N3, R), as scored by two experts according to the American Academy of Sleep Medicine (AASM) rules [8].

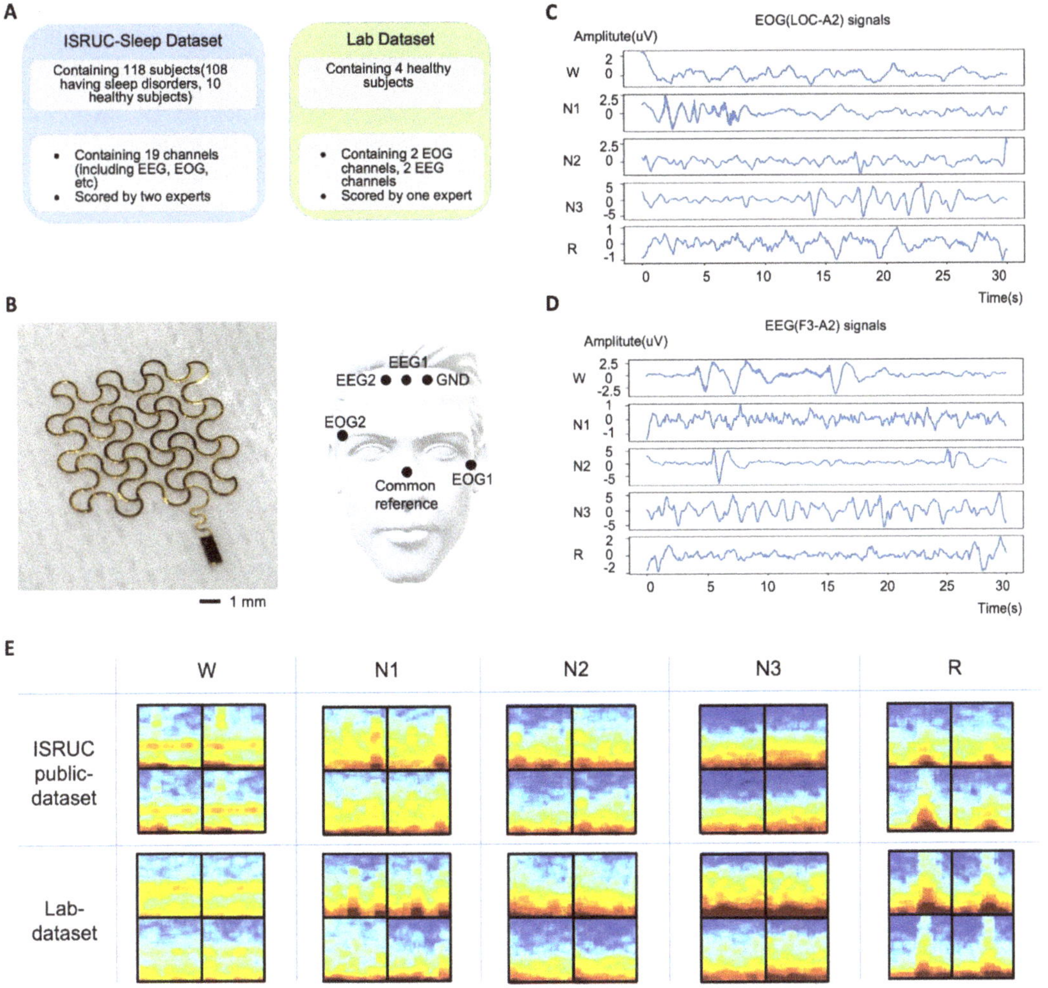

Figure 1. Overview of a public dataset (ISRUC) and the measured lab dataset. (**A**) Detailed information of both datasets. (**B**) Data recording system using nanomembrane bioelectrodes (left) and the sensor mounting locations (right) were the upper center of the forehead (EEG1 and EEG2) to measure two-channel EEG, one electrode on the lower-left corner of the left eye (EOG1) to measure two-channel EOG, and another electrode on the upper-right corner of the right eye (EOG2). (**C**) Measured EOG signals of five different sleep stages: W, N1, N2, N3, and R. (**D**) Measured EEG signals of five different sleep stages: W, N1, N2, N3, and R. (**E**) Examples of multi-taper spectrograms of both the ISRUC public and the lab datasets with five sleep stages. From top-to-bottom and left-to-right, the spectrograms show channels F3-A2, F4-A1, EOGL, and EOGR of the public dataset, and channels EEG1, EEG2, EOG1, and EOG2 of the lab dataset.

2.2. Measured Lab Dataset

The lab dataset used for this study was measured from four healthy male subjects aged between 24 and 27 years. A total of four data were collected, with one recording per subject. To measure our own dataset in the lab, we fabricated a set of nanomembrane, stretchable electrodes using a gold and polyimide (PI) composite, laminated on a silicone adhesive (Figure 1B). This fabrication utilized a microfabrication technique, including photolithography, developing, and etching for making stretchable patterns [9,10]. Afterward, the patterned electrode was transfer-printed onto a soft silicone elastomer for skin mounting [11,12]. For the two-channel EEG setup, two electrodes were placed near the upper center of the forehead (EEG1 and EEG2) to measure frontopolar EEG. For the two-channel EOG, one electrode was placed on the lower-left corner of the left eye (EOG1), and the other electrode was placed on the upper right corner of the right eye (EOG2). All the EEG and EOG channels were derived with a single common reference electrode placed on the bony area of the nose. In PSG, the mastoid is the most widely used common reference point, but the nose is also considered one of the inactive areas suitable as a common reference alternative to the mastoid. Some of the previous works related to EEG measurement adopted the nose as the reference on special occasions [13–16]. The nanomembrane dry electrode needs to be placed on clean skin without hair to measure signals with high quality, so the nose was selected as the common reference for this study. The ground electrode was placed on the forehead next to the EEG1 electrode. These electrode locations were chosen to develop a compact facial patch device for sleep monitoring in future studies.

A customized printed circuit board (PCB) with an nRF52 (Nordic Semiconductor, Trondheim, Norway) and an ADS 1299 (Texas Instruments, Dallas, TX, USA) was used to collect EEG and EOG signals at a sampling rate of 250 Hz and to transmit them to an Android mobile device via Bluetooth for data storage. The systems used to collect the lab datasets, the nanomembrane-based electrodes and the custom PCB with the nRF52 and ADS 1299 have been extensively studied and validated by comparison with well-established measurement systems by numerous related previous studies [17–21]. A set of example datasets in Figure 1C,D, measured by standard PSG setup and the wearable device, show EOG signals and EEG signals with different patterns based on sleep stages. Figure 1E shows representative multi-taper spectrograms of data measured by the standard PSG setup and the setup used for this study at each of the five sleep stages.

2.3. *Data Pre-Processing*

Rather than training an automatic classification model based on raw sleep data, the data pre-processing method was applied for better classification performance. In the ISRUC public dataset, preprocessing was already applied to eliminate undesired noise and DC offset, enhancing the signal quality and the signal-to-noise ratio. The filtering stage consisted of a notch filter to eliminate the 50 Hz powerline noise and a bandpass Butterworth filter with a lower cutoff of 0.3 Hz and a higher cutoff of 35 Hz for both the EEG and EOG channels. To maximize the performance and transferability of the classification model, the same bandpass filtering parameters were used for the lab dataset. The notch filter setting was adjusted to remove a 60 Hz, rather than 50 Hz, power line noise because the frequency of powerline noise varies based on the place of measurement. Moreover, to match the per-epoch data size to the public dataset, the lab dataset was down-sampled from 250 Hz to 200 Hz by interpolating the datapoints that matched the timepoints corresponding with the 200 Hz sampling rate.

2.4. *Input Dataset for Deep Learning*

EEG and EOG signals are commonly analyzed with time-frequency processing techniques or spectrograms, since they are frequently related to behavioral patterns [22]. CNN models are mainly applied to classify and recognize two-dimensional images due to their good compatibility and unprecedented ability to extract image features. As a result, there were many attempts to use spectrograms generated from EEG and EOG signals as the input dataset of a CNN [23–26]. The spectrogram used for this study was generated by multi-taper spectral analysis, which utilizes multiple taper functions to compute single-taper spectra for better resolution and reduced bias and variance compared to the traditional method. The default settings and parameters provided by Prerau et al. were used for generating spectrograms [27]. The frequency range of spectral analysis was set between 0 and 20 Hz. The time-half-bandwidth product was set to 5, and the number of tapers was set to 9. A window size of 5 s was used, with a step size of 1 s. The entire dataset was first converted into a multi-taper spectrogram, which was then segmented into a 30-second-long epoch. The size of the spectrogram matrix was 30 × 103 for each epoch. Since four data channels were used for this study, four spectrogram matrices were put together as a 60 × 206 matrix, which was then converted into a PNG image file sized 256 × 256 (Figure 2A). The same dataset was prepared with raw data for a comparison study to show the advantage of using a multi-taper spectrogram. The dataset with raw data was composed of bandpass-filtered raw data. The filtered data were then segmented into 30-second-long epochs of four channels, with a matrix size of 4 × 6000. Figure 2B is the flow diagram of how our training dataset (sampled from the ISRUC dataset) and testing dataset (sampled from the lab dataset) were processed.

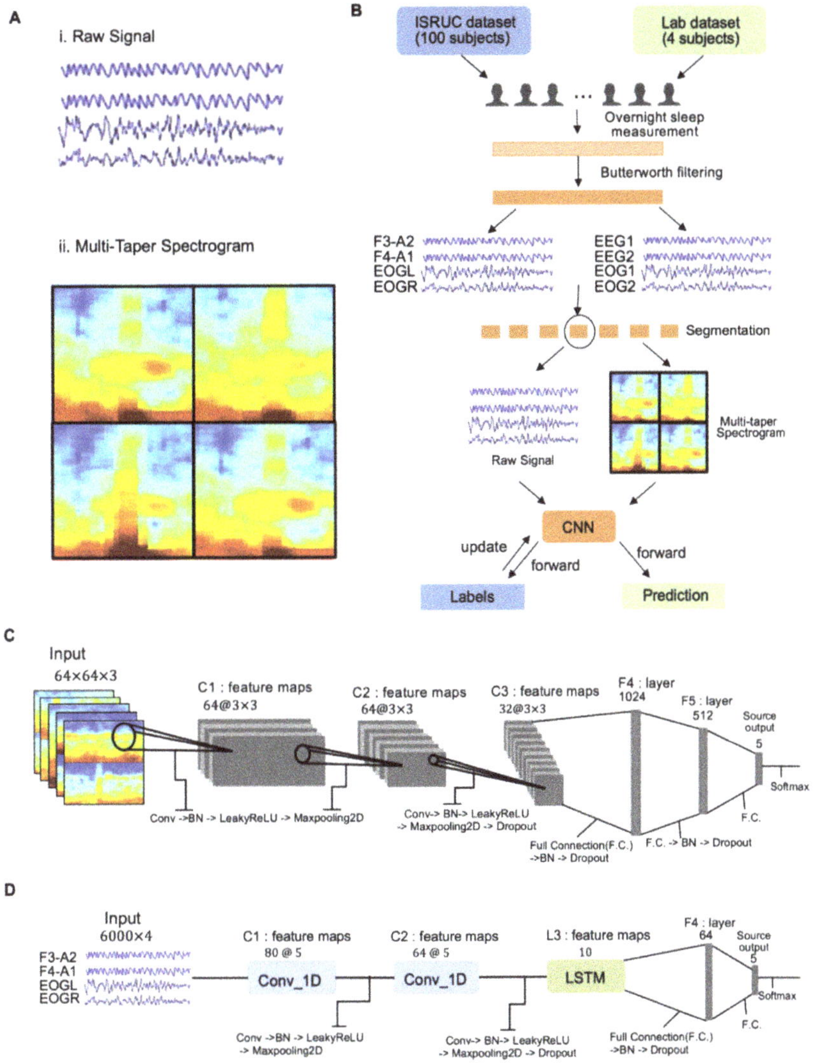

Figure 2. (**A**) Arrangement of four multi-taper spectrograms for deep learning dataset input. (**B**) Flow chart capturing data processing overview. (**C**,**D**) Proposed machine learning architectures for multi-taper spectrograms (**C**) and raw signals (**D**); in this figure, Conv: convolution, F.C.: fully connected layers, and BN: batch normalization.

2.5. CNN-Based Classifier

The architecture was developed by trial and error, drawing influence from earlier models [28,29]. Two models were created according to the form of input data: the CNN architecture in the case of image-based multi-taper spectrograms and the CNN + LSTM architecture in the case of time-based raw signal data. The sleep stage classification CNN architecture is described in Figure 2C,D. For the multi-taper spectrogram, the inputs of our CNN were 30-second-long spectrogram images (256 × 256 pixels) of 4 channels (two EEG and two EOG) connected together in a square. The spectrogram image was then resized to 64 × 64 and converted to a value between 0–1 using normalization. Since the color-image consisted of 3 channels (Red, Green, and Blue), every input matrix became a 3-dimensional matrix (64 × 64 × 3). The non-linear activation function employed was the Leaky Rectified Linear Unit (Leaky ReLU). ADAM (learning rate = 0.002) was utilized for the optimization of the CNN architecture. The batch size was set to 16 and the dropout deactivation rate was set to 0.5. Early stopping was used to prevent overfitting by randomly eliminating 20% of the data from the training set and utilizing it as a validation set at the start of the optimization phase. When the validation loss stopped improving, learning rate annealing was performed with a factor of 5. The training was terminated when two successive decays occurred with no network performance improvement on the validation set. A single convolutional cell (Conv_N) consisted of a convolutional layer, one layer of batch normalization, one layer of max pooling, and one layer of the Leaky ReLu function. The final output of the Deep Neural Network was a 5 × 1 vector. It was then passed through a softmax layer and finally outputted the predicted class (one of the five sleep stages). For the raw signals, the inputs of our CNN_LSTM were 30-second raw signal data of 4 channels (two EEG and two EOG) with an input size of 6000 × 4. The kernel layer was composed of two convolutional cells and one LSTM cell. Most of the set-ups were the same as those of the spectrogram CNN architecture, except structure, while the learning rate of ADAM was 0.001 and the batch size was set to 128.

3. Results and Discussion

3.1. Experimental Setup

In this section, we elaborate on the details of our experimental set-ups, outcomes, and the significance of the results. Figure 2 summarizes the overview of the automatic sleep stage classification process using a CNN model we developed. To evaluate the performance of the proposed CNN architecture, we designed two experiments: (1) training a CNN model that could correctly classify sleep stages and evaluate the performance with the ISRUC dataset, and (2) Using the trained CNN model to classify the sleep stages in the newly measured lab data. These two experiments were conducted on a laptop equipped with an Intel i7 processor (I7-9750H). To compare the transferability, both experiments were performed with two different types of input data: raw data and multi-taper spectrogram data.

In the first experiment, the first 100 subjects' data were selected in subgroup 1 of the ISRUC dataset. To enhance the accuracy and minimize the bias associated with our classification model, only the epochs where the two scorers agreed with each other were used. The epochs were then split into three parts: 60% of the dataset for training (42,094 epochs), 20% for validation (14,032 epochs), and 20% for the test (14,032 epochs). The number of epochs of each of the five classes for the three separate parts is listed in Table 1. For each training step, the weight of the CNN network parameters was updated based on the result of model training validation accuracy. Most of the hyperparameter values (learning rate, kernel size, and filter of each convolutional layer, and unit of each dropout) were selected by a random search method. In the end, we chose the model with the highest validation accuracy as our best model. The performance of this best model was evaluated based on the prediction accuracy of the test dataset.

Table 1. Number of epochs of each sleep stage for training, validation, and testing.

Input Type	Number of Epochs (ISRUC Public Dataset)														
	Training Set					Validation Set					Test Set				
	Aw	N1	N2	N3	R	Aw	N1	N2	N3	R	Aw	N1	N2	N3	R
Raw signal	10,968	3299	13,366	8264	6197	3591	1148	4570	2692	2031	3617	1065	4492	2739	2119
Spectrogram	11,013	3275	13,210	8189	6207	3568	1073	4729	2675	1987	3575	1144	4469	2791	2053

As a result, for the multi-taper spectrogram, CNN architecture, a (2,2) pool size of 2D-max pooling, 64 filters and a (3,3) kernel size were used on the first two 2D-convolutional layers and 32 filters and a (3,3) kernel size were used on the last 2D-convolutional layers. Moreover, in order, dense layers with the units 1024, 512 and 5 were used for the fully-connected layer. Batch normalization, first dropout (0.25), and second dropout (0.40) were utilized to prevent overfitting. For the raw-signal CNN + LSTM architecture, four pool sizes of 1D-max pooling, 80 filters, and three kernel sizes were used on the first 1D convolutional layers, and 32 filters and five kernel sizes were used on the last 1D-convolutional layers and unit 10 on the LSTM layers. Moreover, in order, dense layers with the units 64 and 5 were used for the fully-connected layer. Batch normalization and dropout (0.45) were utilized to prevent overfitting (Figure 2C,D).

In the second experiment, we evaluated the transferability of our trained CNN model on our lab dataset. We used the same model architecture as the first experiment. Our best model was used to predict sleep stages in the lab dataset, and this prediction performance was evaluated through comparison with the manual sleep stage scorings performed, based on AASM criteria, by one human expert with about one year of experience.

3.2. Performance Comparison with Other Works

The classification model was well-trained, based on the accuracy and loss of the training and validation graphs shown in Figure 3A,B. Table 2 summarizes the result of the first experiment. As a result of the first experiment with multi-taper spectrogram input data, our classification model's prediction of the 100 subjects showed 88.85% accuracy and a Cohen's kappa value of 0.854 with the consensus scores of the two expert scorers of the ISRUC dataset (Figure 3C). The classification results with raw data as input showed an accuracy of 87.05% and a Cohen's kappa value of 0.829.

Table 3 summarizes the result of the second experiment and enumerates the number of epochs of each sleep stage that were included in the lab dataset. As a result of the second experiment with the multi-taper spectrogram input data, an accuracy of 81.85% and a Cohen's kappa value of 0.734 could be achieved when the exact same classification model was used to predict the lab dataset measured with our own system (Figure 3D). The classification results with raw data as input showed an accuracy of 72.94% and a Cohen's kappa value of 0.608. The results of these experiments clearly show that, compared to using just raw signal, converting the signal to multi-taper spectrogram as the input data provides not only comparable or higher classification performance within the public dataset but also superior transferability of the trained model for the classification of another dataset. The average inter-scorer agreement on standard PSG data was usually reported between 82% and 89% [3]. In agreement with this reported value, the average agreement between the two expert scorers of the ISRUC dataset was calculated to be 82.00%, with a Cohen's kappa value of 0.766. The results of the second experiment (81.85%) fall very close to this expected inter-scorer reliability value, and this can show the potential of the effective transferability of our classification model into our lab-based custom system with high performance. The hypnograms in Figure 3E,F show the prediction results from the ISRUC and lab datasets, respectively.

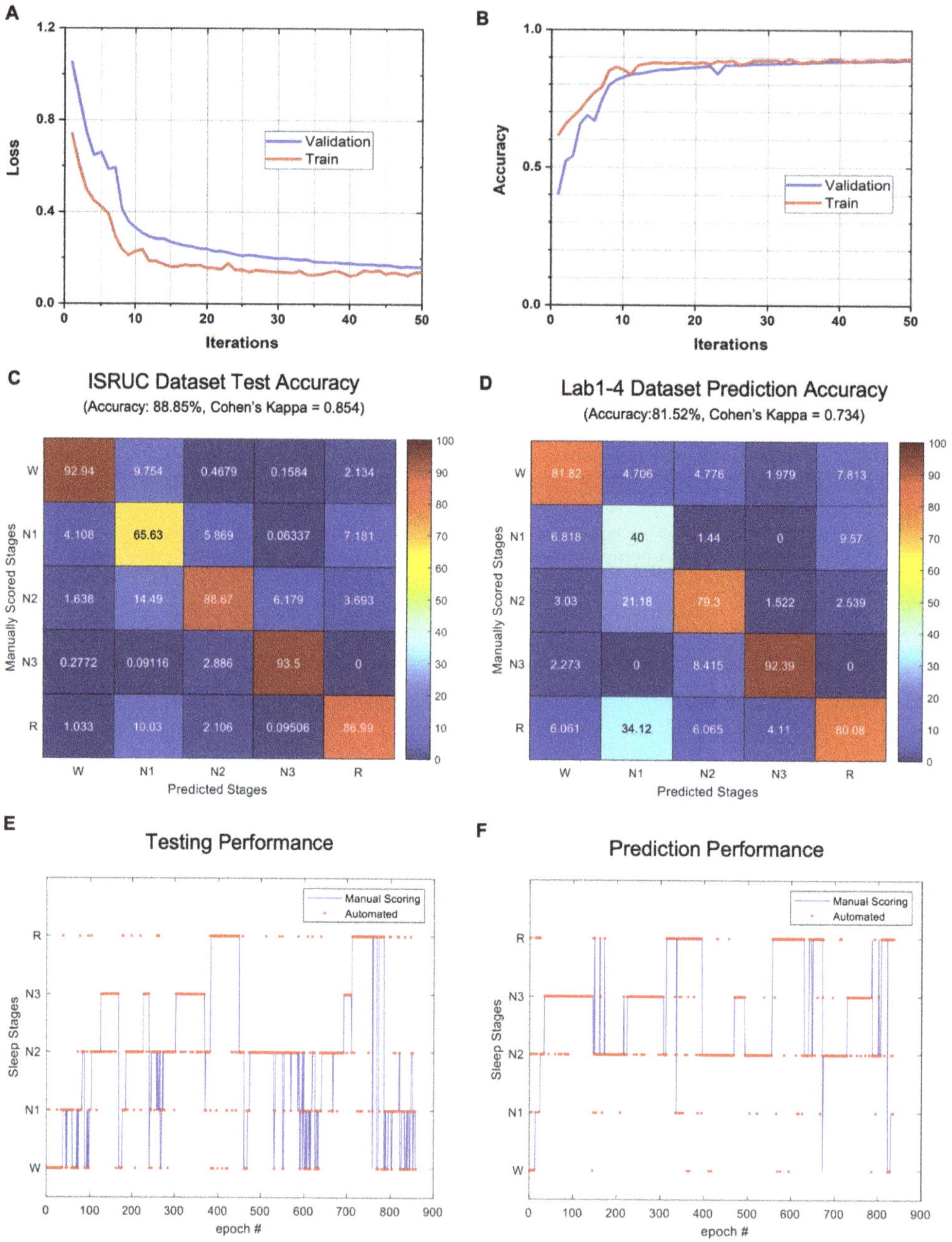

Figure 3. CNN classification results. (**A**) Loss curves of the training on the ISRUC dataset (red: loss on the training; blue: loss on the testing). (**B**) Accuracy curves of the training on the ISRUC dataset (red: accuracy on the training; blue: accuracy on the testing). (**C**) Confusion matrix with the public dataset (accuracy 88.85%, Cohen's kappa = 0.854). (**D**) Confusion matrix with lab dataset (accuracy 81.52%, Cohen's kappa = 0.734). (**E**,**F**) Hypnograms of prediction results from the ISRUC (**E**) and lab datasets (**F**).

Table 2. Public dataset based on classification models trained and tested with raw signals and multi-taper spectrograms.

Input Type	ISRUC Public Dataset	
	Test Accuracy	Cohen's Kappa
Raw signal	87.05%	0.829
Multi-taper spectrogram	88.85%	0.854

Table 3. Lab dataset prediction based on classification models trained and tested with raw signal and multi-taper spectrograms, and the combined number of epochs of each sleep stage.

Input Type	Lab Dataset		Number of Epochs (Lab Dataset)				
	Prediction Accuracy	Cohen's Kappa	Prediction Set				
			Aw	N1	N2	N3	R
Raw signal	72.94%	0.608	230	111	1091	721	554
Multi-taper spectrogram	81.52%	0.734	230	111	1091	721	554

Table 4 compares the performance of our CNN method in sleep stage classification with other prior works. To evaluate the performance of the sleep stage classification, there are multiple performance metrics being used in the field, including sensitivity, specificity, and F-measure. Among these metrics, the accuracy rate and Cohen's kappa coefficient are the most commonly used metrics [3], so these metrics are presented and used for comparison in this table. Most of the existing works focused on analyzing public sleep datasets, except for a few cases. Compared to the resulting accuracy and kappa values of these works, our work in the first experiment within the public dataset shows comparable performance. Among the prior works, the work from Bresch et al. presented a study similar to ours where a classification model was built from a public dataset (SIESTA) and transfer-tested to a private dataset [30]. Their results showed a kappa value of 0.760 in the public dataset and 0.703 in their private dataset. Compared to this work, our work shows improved performance with both the public and private datasets. Overall, this study shows the human-level performance of our CNN-based sleep classification model in scoring the standard PSG dataset and presents the potential of its effective transferability to other types of datasets, such as our own custom lab dataset with novel nanomembrane electrodes.

Although we could demonstrate transferability of the classification model from the public PSG dataset to a private dataset, the setup and results from the current study still possess some limitations that need to be considered for future studies. First, the public dataset used for this study, ISRUC subgroup 1, includes data from subjects with sleep disorders. Sleep patterns and signal characteristics of subjects with various sleep disorders are likely to be different from those of healthy subjects, and this aspect could have led to reduced performance when the classification model was applied to healthy subject data. Since this study was intended to build a model to classify data from healthy subjects, for future studies, the inclusion of data from a healthy population will be necessary and helpful to enhance the classification performance. Next, a small population of four subjects was used for the tested lab dataset to explore the potential of the transferability of the classification model and to compare the pre-processing methods for more effective transferability. To further validate the effectiveness of multi-taper spectrograms along with a CNN to build a more globally transferable classification model, a much larger number of subjects from various cohorts will need to be included in future studies.

Table 4. Comparison of sleep-stage classification performance with prior works.

Ref.	Year	Data Type	Input Data	Number of Subjects	Public Dataset Accuracy (%) /Kappa	Private Dataset Accuracy (%) /Kappa	Number of Channels	Classification Method
This work	2022	ISRUC and Lab dataset	Multi-taper spectrogram and Raw data	100	88.85/0.854 87.05/0.829	81.52/0.734 72.94/0.608	2 EEG, 2 EOG	CNN
[31]	1993	Private data	Extracted features	12	-	80.60/-	2 EEG, 1 EOG, 1 EMG	Multilayer Neural Network
[32]	2005	SIESTA	Extracted features	590	79.6/0.72	-	1 EEG, 2 EOG, 1 EMG	LDA, Decision tree
[5]	2014	Sleep-EDF	Extracted features	1	88.9/-	-	1 EEG	SVM
[33]	2016	Sleep-EDF	Raw data	20	74/0.65	-	1 EEG	CNN
[34]	2016	Sleep-EDF	Extracted features	20	78/-	-	1 EEG	Stacked Sparse Autoencoders
[35]	2017	Montreal archive	Extracted features	62	83.35/-	-	1 EEG	Mixed Neural Network
[36]	2017	Sleep-EDF & Montreal	Raw data	32	86.2/0.80	-	1 EEG	DeepSleepNET (CNN + LSTM)
[37]	2018	Montreal archive	Raw data	61	78/0.80	-	6 EEG, 2 EOG, 3 EMG	Multivariate Network
[38]	2018	Private dataset	Extracted features	76	-	-/0.8	1 EEG, 2 EOG	Random Forest, CNN, LSTM
[39]	2018	SHHS	Raw data	5728	87/0.81	-	1 EEG	CNN
[40]	2018	12 sleep centers	Raw data	1086	87/0.766	-	4 EEG, 2 EOG, 1 EMG	CNN
[7]	2018	ISRUC	Extracted features	100	75.29/-	-	6 EEG	Random Forest
[41]	2018	ISRUC	Raw data	116	92.2/-	-	6 EEG, 2 EOG, 3 EMG	CNN
[30]	2018	SIESTA/private data	Raw data	147	-/0.760	-/0.703	1 EEG, 2 EOG	RNN
[6]	2019	ISRUC	Extracted features	10	79.64/0.74	-	6 EEG	HMM
[42]	2019	Sleep-EDF	Raw data	61	91.22/-	-	1 EEG, 1 EOG	CNN
[43]	2019	Montreal archive	Extracted features	200	83.6/-	-	1 EEG, 1EOG, 1EMG	CNN
[44]	2020	ISRUC	Extracted features	10	81.65/0.76	-	1 EEG	IMBEFs
[45]	2020	Sleep-EDF	Raw data	100	85.52/-	-	2 EEG	CNN
[46]	2020	ISRUC	Raw data	294	81.8/0.72	-	2 EEG, 2 EOG, 1 EMG, 1 ECG	CNN + RNN

Moreover, despite the transferability of the classification model shown in this study, there was a clear reduction in accuracy when the model was tested on the lab dataset. This reduction in the accuracy came from the intrinsic differences between the two different measurement settings, such as subject population, electrode type, equipment, sampling rate, etc. These discrepancies resulted in slightly different spectral analysis signal characteristics and reduced classification performance. One of the critical differences was the electrode locations, especially the EEG electrodes on the forehead and the common reference electrode on the nose. Although the nose is considered to be a relatively inactive area, nose referencing still suffers from larger artifacts from facial muscle activity in both the EEG and EOG channels, and especially EOG artifacts in the EEG channels, due to its proximity to the eyes [47,48] In our lab system, the EEG electrodes were placed closer to the eyes on the forehead, and the reference was placed on the nose. With the measurement and reference electrode of each EEG channel placed on the top and bottom sides of the eyes, the vertical eye movement signals observed in the EEG channels were large, and they were also larger than those observed in our EOG channels. As shown in Figure 1E, the described discrepancy in the signals observed from the EEG and EOG channels of each system could be observed, with slightly different spectral characteristics at each stage potentially leading to a reduction in accuracy, most likely in stages N1, where slow eye movement (SEM) is present, and R, where rapid eye movement (REM) is present. In stages N1 and R of the public dataset, the EOG channels generally showed stronger activity observed in the lower frequency range, caused by SEM and REM, as compared to the EEG channels. On the other hand, in the lab datasets, the EEG channels often show comparable or stronger activity in the lower frequency range compared to the EOG channels, caused by strong vertical eye movement signals in the EEG channels and stronger horizontal eye movement signals observed in the EOG channels. In addition to the well-known difficulty in classifying N1, the number of N1 epochs used for both training the model and prediction of the lab dataset was much smaller compared to other stages, and this could have resulted in the misrepresentation of the model's classification performance of N1 with the numerical results obtained in this study [49,50]. These discrepancies between the systems and the smaller number of channels in our system could have led to less accurate scoring of the lab dataset, as it was not measured with the standard PSG setup used for proper scoring with AASM criteria, which resulted in larger uncertainty in the classification performance assessment. For future study, the use of both a standard setup and our novel lab-based setup is desired for more objective and fair classification performance assessment, comparison with expert scorings and inter-scorer reliability.

Furthermore, there were two factors that could have led to the overestimation of our classification model's performance within the public dataset: (1) using consensus epochs for the testing of the model, and (2) using all subjects' data throughout the training, validation, and testing without subject separation. Consensus epochs have clearer signal characteristics of corresponding sleep stages compared to the epochs without consensus, so using consensus epochs for the testing of model may have led to performance overestimation. For future studies, it would be preferred to use all epochs for performance evaluation, and compare the results with inter-scorer reliability. Moreover, due to signal characteristic variability from subject to subject, a more objective evaluation of the performance would be achieved by separating the epochs of certain subjects and keeping them independent for testing purposes alone. If the same subject's epochs used for training and validation are also used for testing, the testing performance could be higher than the result obtained when the model is used on another subject's data. For future studies, the use of the leave-one-subject-out method for the evaluation of the model would be preferred, for more objective evaluation and comparison with other works.

4. Conclusions

In this work, we presented an automatic sleep stage classification model that could achieve good performance on the public dataset and accurately predict the sleep stage on our own laboratory dataset. A set of nanomembrane electrodes and custom wireless circuits were used to record lab datasets with EEG and EOG from multiple subjects during their sleep. We developed a classification model based on CNN, which was utilized for training and validating the classifier model based on the ISRUC public dataset using two EEG (F3-A2, F4-A1) and two EOG (EOGL, EOGR) channels. Then we transferred our model to the classification of our experimental dataset, which was collected with the nanomembrane electrodes. Overall, the collective results show that our model had high performance on both the test dataset (accuracy = 88.85%, Cohen's kappa = 0.854) and on our lab dataset (accuracy = 81.85%, Cohen's kappa = 0.734). Future work will resolve the limitations of the current study discussed above and expand this research to include a larger group of sleep patients to measure data with the wearable system for automatic sleep stage classification.

Author Contributions: K.K., S.K. and W.-H.Y. conceived and designed the research; K.K. designed the machine learning algorithm; S.K. conducted the experimental study; K.K., S.K. and W.-H.Y. wrote the paper. All authors have read and agreed to the published version of the manuscript.

Funding: We acknowledge the support from the IEN Center for Human-Centric Interfaces and Engineering at Georgia Tech, and this study was partially supported by the Institute of Information and Communications Technology Planning and Evaluation (IITP) grant funded by the Korean government (MSIT) (2021-0-01517). The electronic devices used in this work were fabricated at the Institute for Electronics and Nanotechnology, a member of the National Nanotechnology Coordinated Infrastructure, which is supported by the National Science Foundation (grant ECCS-2025462).

Institutional Review Board Statement: The study was conducted according to the guidelines of the following the approved IRB protocol (#H20211) at the Georgia Institute of Technology.

Informed Consent Statement: Informed consent was obtained from all subjects involved in the study.

Data Availability Statement: The data presented in this study are available on request from the corresponding author.

Conflicts of Interest: Georgia Tech has a pending US patent application related to the work described here.

References

1. Rahman, M.M.; Bhuiyan, M.I.H.; Hassan, A.R. Sleep stage classification using single-channel EOG. *Comput. Biol. Med.* **2018**, *102*, 211–220. [CrossRef]
2. Kim, H.; Kwon, S.; Kwon, Y.-T.; Yeo, W.-H. Soft Wireless Bioelectronics and Differential Electrodermal Activity for Home Sleep Monitoring. *Sensors* **2021**, *21*, 354. [CrossRef] [PubMed]
3. Kwon, S.; Kim, H.; Yeo, W.-H. Recent advances in wearable sensors and portable electronics for sleep monitoring. *Iscience* **2021**, *24*, 102461. [CrossRef] [PubMed]
4. Armon, C. Polysomnography. *Medscape* **2020**, *31*, 281–297.
5. Zhu, G.; Li, Y.; Wen, P.P. Analysis and classification of sleep stages based on difference visibility graphs from a single-channel EEG signal. *IEEE J. Biomed. Health Inform.* **2014**, *18*, 1813–1821. [CrossRef]
6. Ghimatgar, H.; Kazemi, K.; Helfroush, M.S.; Aarabi, A. An automatic single-channel EEG-based sleep stage scoring method based on hidden Markov Model. *J. Neurosci. Methods* **2019**, *324*, 108320. [CrossRef]
7. Tzimourta, K.D.; Tsilimbaris, A.; Tzioukalia, K.; Tzallas, A.T.; Tsipouras, M.G.; Astrakas, L.G.; Giannakeas, N. EEG-based automatic sleep stage classification. *Biomed. J.* **2018**, *1*, 6.
8. Khalighi, S.; Sousa, T.; Santos, J.M.; Nunes, U. ISRUC-Sleep: A comprehensive public dataset for sleep researchers. *Comput. Methods Programs Biomed.* **2016**, *124*, 180–192. [CrossRef]
9. Lim, H.R.; Kim, H.S.; Qazi, R.; Kwon, Y.T.; Jeong, J.W.; Yeo, W.H. Advanced soft materials, sensor integrations, and applications of wearable flexible hybrid electronics in healthcare, energy, and environment. *Adv. Mater.* **2020**, *32*, 1901924. [CrossRef]
10. Herbert, R.; Kim, J.-H.; Kim, Y.S.; Lee, H.M.; Yeo, W.-H. Soft material-enabled, flexible hybrid electronics for medicine, healthcare, and human-machine interfaces. *Materials* **2018**, *11*, 187. [CrossRef]
11. Kwon, S.; Kwon, Y.-T.; Kim, Y.-S.; Lim, H.-R.; Mahmood, M.; Yeo, W.-H. Skin-conformal, soft material-enabled bioelectronic system with minimized motion artifacts for reliable health and performance monitoring of athletes. *Biosens. Bioelectron.* **2020**, *151*, 111981. [CrossRef] [PubMed]
12. Kim, Y.-S.; Mahmood, M.; Kwon, S.; Herbert, R.; Yeo, W.-H. Wireless Stretchable Hybrid Electronics for Smart, Connected, and Ambulatory Monitoring of Human Health. In *Proceedings of the Meeting Abstracts*; IOP Publishing: Bristol, UK, 2019; p. 2293.
13. George, N.; Jemel, B.; Fiori, N.; Renault, B. Face and shape repetition effects in humans: A spatio-temporal ERP study. *NeuroReport* **1997**, *8*, 1417–1422. [CrossRef] [PubMed]
14. Teplan, M. Fundamentals of EEG measurement. *Meas. Sci. Rev.* **2002**, *2*, 1–11.
15. Yao, D.; Qin, Y.; Hu, S.; Dong, L.; Vega, M.L.B.; Sosa, P.A.V. Which reference should we use for EEG and ERP practice? *Brain Topogr.* **2019**, *32*, 530–549. [CrossRef] [PubMed]
16. O'Regan, S.; Faul, S.; Marnane, W. Automatic detection of EEG artefacts arising from head movements. In Proceedings of the 2010 Annual International Conference of the IEEE Engineering in Medicine and Biology, Buenos Aires, Argentina, 31 August–4 September 2010; pp. 6353–6356.

17. Norton, J.J.; Lee, D.S.; Lee, J.W.; Lee, W.; Kwon, O.; Won, P.; Jung, S.-Y.; Cheng, H.; Jeong, J.-W.; Akce, A. Soft, curved electrode systems capable of integration on the auricle as a persistent brain–computer interface. *Proc. Natl. Acad. Sci. USA* **2015**, *112*, 3920–3925. [CrossRef]
18. Mahmood, M.; Mzurikwao, D.; Kim, Y.-S.; Lee, Y.; Mishra, S.; Herbert, R.; Duarte, A.; Ang, C.S.; Yeo, W.-H. Fully portable and wireless universal brain–machine interfaces enabled by flexible scalp electronics and deep learning algorithm. *Nat. Mach. Intell.* **2019**, *1*, 412–422. [CrossRef]
19. Tian, L.; Zimmerman, B.; Akhtar, A.; Yu, K.J.; Moore, M.; Wu, J.; Larsen, R.J.; Lee, J.W.; Li, J.; Liu, Y. Large-area MRI-compatible epidermal electronic interfaces for prosthetic control and cognitive monitoring. *Nat. Biomed. Eng.* **2019**, *3*, 194–205. [CrossRef]
20. Mahmood, M.; Kwon, S.; Berkmen, G.K.; Kim, Y.-S.; Scorr, L.; Jinnah, H.; Yeo, W.-H. Soft nanomembrane sensors and flexible hybrid bioelectronics for wireless quantification of blepharospasm. *IEEE Trans. Biomed. Eng.* **2020**, *67*, 3094–3100. [CrossRef]
21. Zavanelli, N.; Kim, H.; Kim, J.; Herbert, R.; Mahmood, M.; Kim, Y.-S.; Kwon, S.; Bolus, N.B.; Torstrick, F.B.; Lee, C.S. At-home wireless monitoring of acute hemodynamic disturbances to detect sleep apnea and sleep stages via a soft sternal patch. *Sci. Adv.* **2021**, *7*, eabl4146. [CrossRef]
22. Kandel, E.R.; Schwartz, J.H.; Jessell, T.M.; Siegelbaum, S.; Hudspeth, A.J.; Mack, S. *Principles of Neural Science*; McGraw-Hill: New York, NY, USA, 2000; Volume 4.
23. Vrbancic, G.; Podgorelec, V. Automatic classification of motor impairment neural disorders from EEG signals using deep convolutional neural networks. *Elektron. Ir Elektrotechnika* **2018**, *24*, 3–7. [CrossRef]
24. Kuanar, S.; Athitsos, V.; Pradhan, N.; Mishra, A.; Rao, K.R. Cognitive analysis of working memory load from EEG, by a deep recurrent neural network. In Proceedings of the 2018 IEEE International Conference on Acoustics, Speech and Signal Processing (ICASSP), Calgary, AB, Canada, 15–20 April 2018; pp. 2576–2580.
25. Vilamala, A.; Madsen, K.H.; Hansen, L.K. Deep convolutional neural networks for interpretable analysis of EEG sleep stage scoring. In Proceedings of the 2017 IEEE 27th international workshop on machine learning for signal processing (MLSP), Tokyo, Japan, 25–28 September 2017; pp. 1–6.
26. Jiao, Z.; Gao, X.; Wang, Y.; Li, J.; Xu, H. Deep convolutional neural networks for mental load classification based on EEG data. *Pattern Recognit.* **2018**, *76*, 582–595. [CrossRef]
27. Prerau, M.J.; Brown, R.E.; Bianchi, M.T.; Ellenbogen, J.M.; Purdon, P.L. Sleep neurophysiological dynamics through the lens of multitaper spectral analysis. *Physiology* **2017**, *32*, 60–92. [CrossRef] [PubMed]
28. Kwon, Y.-T.; Kim, Y.-S.; Kwon, S.; Mahmood, M.; Lim, H.-R.; Park, S.-W.; Kang, S.-O.; Choi, J.J.; Herbert, R.; Jang, Y.C. All-printed nanomembrane wireless bioelectronics using a biocompatible solderable graphene for multimodal human-machine interfaces. *Nat. Commun.* **2020**, *11*, 1–11. [CrossRef] [PubMed]
29. Jeong, J.W.; Yeo, W.H.; Akhtar, A.; Norton, J.J.; Kwack, Y.J.; Li, S.; Jung, S.Y.; Su, Y.; Lee, W.; Xia, J. Materials and optimized designs for human-machine interfaces via epidermal electronics. *Adv. Mater.* **2013**, *25*, 6839–6846. [CrossRef] [PubMed]
30. Bresch, E.; Großekathöfer, U.; Garcia-Molina, G. Recurrent deep neural networks for real-time sleep stage classification from single channel EEG. *Front. Comput. Neurosci.* **2018**, *12*, 85. [CrossRef]
31. Schaltenbrand, N.; Lengelle, R.; Macher, J.-P. Neural network model: Application to automatic analysis of human sleep. *Comput. Biomed. Res.* **1993**, *26*, 157–171. [CrossRef]
32. Anderer, P.; Gruber, G.; Parapatics, S.; Woertz, M.; Miazhynskaia, T.; Klösch, G.; Saletu, B.; Zeitlhofer, J.; Barbanoj, M.J.; Danker-Hopfe, H. An E-health solution for automatic sleep classification according to Rechtschaffen and Kales: Validation study of the Somnolyzer 24 × 7 utilizing the Siesta database. *Neuropsychobiology* **2005**, *51*, 115–133. [CrossRef]
33. Tsinalis, O.; Matthews, P.M.; Guo, Y.; Zafeiriou, S. Automatic sleep stage scoring with single-channel EEG using convolutional neural networks. *arXiv* **2016**, arXiv:1610.01683.
34. Tsinalis, O.; Matthews, P.M.; Guo, Y. Automatic sleep stage scoring using time-frequency analysis and stacked sparse autoencoders. *Ann. Biomed. Eng.* **2016**, *44*, 1587–1597. [CrossRef]
35. Dong, H.; Supratak, A.; Pan, W.; Wu, C.; Matthews, P.M.; Guo, Y. Mixed neural network approach for temporal sleep stage classification. *IEEE Trans. Neural Syst. Rehabil. Eng.* **2017**, *26*, 324–333. [CrossRef]
36. Supratak, A.; Dong, H.; Wu, C.; Guo, Y. DeepSleepNet: A model for automatic sleep stage scoring based on raw single-channel EEG. *IEEE Trans. Neural Syst. Rehabil. Eng.* **2017**, *25*, 1998–2008. [CrossRef] [PubMed]
37. Chambon, S.; Galtier, M.N.; Arnal, P.J.; Wainrib, G.; Gramfort, A. A deep learning architecture for temporal sleep stage classification using multivariate and multimodal time series. *IEEE Trans. Neural Syst. Rehabil. Eng.* **2018**, *26*, 758–769. [CrossRef] [PubMed]
38. Malafeev, A.; Laptev, D.; Bauer, S.; Omlin, X.; Wierzbicka, A.; Wichniak, A.; Jernajczyk, W.; Riener, R.; Buhmann, J.; Achermann, P. Automatic human sleep stage scoring using deep neural networks. *Front. Neurosci.* **2018**, *12*, 781. [CrossRef] [PubMed]
39. Sors, A.; Bonnet, S.; Mirek, S.; Vercueil, L.; Payen, J.-F. A convolutional neural network for sleep stage scoring from raw single-channel EEG. *Biomed. Signal Process. Control* **2018**, *42*, 107–114. [CrossRef]
40. Stephansen, J.B.; Olesen, A.N.; Olsen, M.; Ambati, A.; Leary, E.B.; Moore, H.E.; Carrillo, O.; Lin, L.; Han, F.; Yan, H. Neural network analysis of sleep stages enables efficient diagnosis of narcolepsy. *Nat. Commun.* **2018**, *9*, 1–15. [CrossRef]
41. Cui, Z.; Zheng, X.; Shao, X.; Cui, L. Automatic sleep stage classification based on convolutional neural network and fine-grained segments. *Complexity* **2018**, *2018*. [CrossRef]

42. Yildirim, O.; Baloglu, U.B.; Acharya, U.R. A deep learning model for automated sleep stages classification using PSG signals. *Int. J. Environ. Res. Public Health* **2019**, *16*, 599. [CrossRef]
43. Phan, H.; Andreotti, F.; Cooray, N.; Chén, O.Y.; De Vos, M. Joint classification and prediction CNN framework for automatic sleep stage classification. *IEEE Trans. Biomed. Eng.* **2018**, *66*, 1285–1296. [CrossRef]
44. Shen, H.; Ran, F.; Xu, M.; Guez, A.; Li, A.; Guo, A. An Automatic Sleep Stage Classification Algorithm Using Improved Model Based Essence Features. *Sensors* **2020**, *20*, 4677. [CrossRef]
45. Lee, T.; Hwang, J.; Lee, H. Trier: Template-guided neural networks for robust and interpretable sleep stage identification from eeg recordings. *arXiv* **2020**, arXiv:2009.05407.
46. Zhang, X.; Xu, M.; Li, Y.; Su, M.; Xu, Z.; Wang, C.; Kang, D.; Li, H.; Mu, X.; Ding, X. Automated multi-model deep neural network for sleep stage scoring with unfiltered clinical data. *Sleep Breath.* **2020**, *24*, 581–590. [CrossRef] [PubMed]
47. Essl, M.; Rappelsberger, P. EEG cohererence and reference signals: Experimental results and mathematical explanations. *Med. Biol. Eng. Comput.* **1998**, *36*, 399–406. [CrossRef] [PubMed]
48. Trujillo, L.T.; Peterson, M.A.; Kaszniak, A.W.; Allen, J.J. EEG phase synchrony differences across visual perception conditions may depend on recording and analysis methods. *Clin. Neurophysiol.* **2005**, *116*, 172–189. [CrossRef] [PubMed]
49. Mousavi, S.; Afghah, F.; Acharya, U.R. SleepEEGNet: Automated sleep stage scoring with sequence to sequence deep learning approach. *PLoS ONE* **2019**, *14*, e0216456. [CrossRef] [PubMed]
50. Melek, M.; Manshouri, N.; Kayikcioglu, T. An automatic EEG-based sleep staging system with introducing NAoSP and NAoGP as new metrics for sleep staging systems. *Cogn. Neurodynamics* **2021**, *15*, 405–423. [CrossRef]

biosensors

MDPI

Review

Adaptive Triboelectric Nanogenerators for Long-Term Self-Treatment: A Review

Zequan Zhao [1], Yin Lu [1], Yajun Mi [1], Jiajing Meng [1], Xueqing Wang [1], Xia Cao [2,3,*] and Ning Wang [1,2,*]

[1] Center for Green Innovation, School of Mathematics and Physics, University of Science and Technology Beijing, Beijing 100083, China
[2] Beijing Institute of Nanoenergy and Nanosystems, Chinese Academy of Sciences, Beijing 100083, China
[3] School of Chemistry and Biological Engineering, University of Science and Technology Beijing, Beijing 100083, China
* Correspondence: caoxia@ustb.edu.cn (X.C.); wangning@ustb.edu.cn (N.W.)

Abstract: Triboelectric nanogenerators (TENGs) were initially invented as an innovative energy−harvesting technology for scavenging mechanical energy from our bodies or the ambient environment. Through adaptive customization design, TENGs have also become a promising player in the self-powered wearable medical market for improving physical fitness and sustaining a healthy lifestyle. In addition to simultaneously harvesting our body's mechanical energy and actively detecting our physiological parameters and metabolic status, TENGs can also provide personalized medical treatment solutions in a self-powered modality. This review aims to cover the recent advances in TENG-based electronics in clinical applications, beginning from the basic working principles of TENGs and their general operation modes, continuing to the harvesting of bioenergy from the human body, and arriving at their adaptive design toward applications in chronic disease diagnosis and long-term clinical treatment. Considering the highly personalized usage scenarios, special attention is paid to customized modules that are based on TENGs and support complex medical treatments, where sustainability, biodegradability, compliance, and bio-friendliness may be critical for the operation of clinical systems. While this review provides a comprehensive understanding of TENG-based clinical devices that aims to reach a high level of technological readiness, the challenges and shortcomings of TENG-based clinical devices are also highlighted, with the expectation of providing a useful reference for the further development of such customized healthcare systems and the transfer of their technical capabilities into real-life patient care.

Keywords: triboelectric nanogenerator; self-powered device; adaptivity; clinical treatment; self-diagnosis

Citation: Zhao, Z.; Lu, Y.; Mi, Y.; Meng, J.; Wang, X.; Cao, X.; Wang, N. Adaptive Triboelectric Nanogenerators for Long-Term Self-Treatment: A Review. *Biosensors* **2022**, *12*, 1127. https://doi.org/10.3390/bios12121127

Received: 9 November 2022
Accepted: 1 December 2022
Published: 5 December 2022

1. Introduction

Since their initial invention in 2012, the triboelectric nanogenerators (TENGs) have attracted extensive attention due to their tremendous potential in the fields of energy harvesting and active sensing. Currently, TENGs are undergoing rapid progress in a variety of other fields, such as green energy, molecular detection, health care, and gesture recognition, due to characteristics that make them exceptional for application in self-powered electronic systems, where TENGs can act as both power sources and as smart sensors, including as dynamic force sensors and chemical sensors, with intrinsic sensitivity toward chemical reactions at the triboelectric interface [1,2]. As a result, TENGs could possibly become a part of people's daily lives in the form of either power accessories or active sensors, or, in some cases, both [3].

In the field of health care and clinical treatment, bio−friendly TENGs can be worn directly on or implanted into the body, and thus can be used to observe and analyze the patient's physiological parameters and metabolic status, and can even be used to treat diseases with the support of various information technologies, such as wireless connection, cloud services, and information storage [4]. With advantages that include simple operation and easy miniaturization, TENGs can be adaptively designed and seamlessly embedded into intelligent systems for the scavenging of mechanical energy from either the ambient environment or the human body, thus endowing the system with features such as sustainability, wearability, and portability. As a result, the application of TENGs in the field of clinical treatment would help to meet the requirement for clinical devices with predictive, personalized, and participatory characteristics, making it possible to simultaneously detect physiological signals, maintain sustainable operation, and provide continuous exercise guidance while harvesting bioenergy, thus achieving in vivo, accurate and intelligent self-treatment and self-monitoring [5,6].

In addition to enabling the measurement of clinically relevant parameters and showing the health status of individuals [7–16], TENGs can complement traditional power sources, which are generally fabricated using toxic chemicals and have limited capacity. The introduction of TENGs into the operation and implementation of the above-mentioned systems could alleviate the dependence on power sources and sensor technology, thus increasing wireless mobility, interactivity, and intelligence [17–22]. TENGs can be especially helpful in the treatment of chronic stubborn disorders, in which rapid recovery often fails to be achieved. In these cases, long-term follow-up is the most effective approach for improving prognosis, including long-term collection and analysis of body data, along with continuous personalized treatment. Depending on the patient's disease type and needs, treatment may unavoidably involve flexible and highly customized biomedical equipment requiring sustainable operation [23].

Therefore, this review aims to cover the advances in TENGs and TENG-based wearable sensor technology (Figure 1), which present enormous opportunities for their deployment in health care [24–27], especially in connected health care and long-term personalized treatment, in the context of which TENGs can provide both high-quality, real-time measurement of personal health parameters as well as a long-lasting power source [28]. In addition to discussing the current application of TENG-based wearable devices in health care, including daily health and safety monitoring and the use of TENGs in clinical practice and treatment, we also emphasize their current shortcomings and suggest directions for further research.

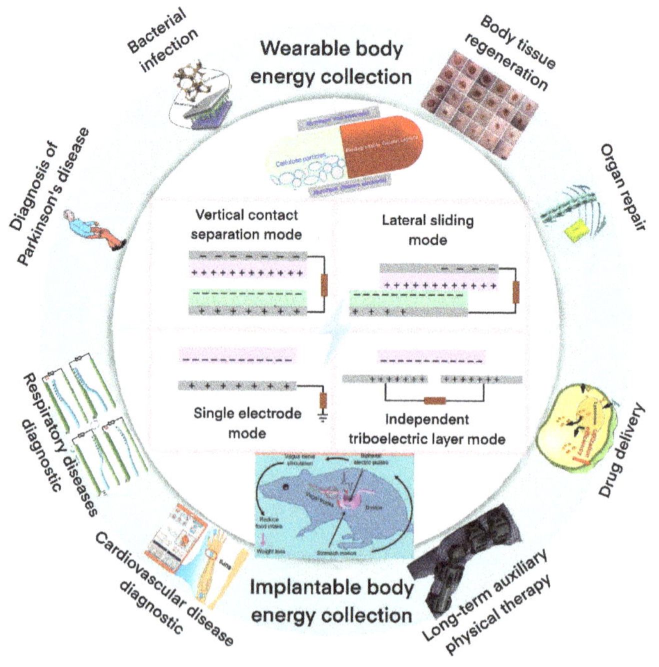

Figure 1. Triboelectric nanogenerators for long-term self-treatment and self-diagnosis.

2. Biological Energy Collection

Considering their personalized usage scenarios, TENG-based devices will be able to support more complex functional modules in order to meet the needs of different groups of users, requiring TENGs with higher power output. The key to solving this problem is to expand the methods of biological energy collection, thus improving efficiency [29–33].

2.1. Working Principle of TENG

TENGs mainly use the triboelectric effect and electrostatic induction coupling to convert biomechanical energy into electrical energy to power medical equipment. Theoretically, when two materials with different degrees of electronegativity come into contact, electrons will flow between them. When they are separated, due to the electrostatic induction effect, electrons will flow to the external load. Upon repetition of the above process, the TENG will output alternating current [34]. On this basis, TENGs can be divided into four working modes (Figure 2): vertical contact-separation mode [35], lateral sliding mode [36], single-electrode mode [37], and independent triboelectric layer mode [38].

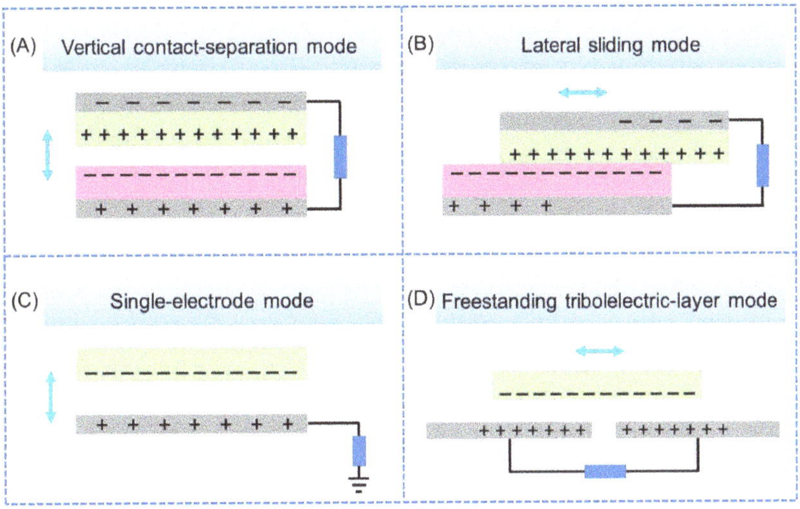

Figure 2. (**A**) Vertical contact-separation mode. (**B**) Lateral sliding mode. (**C**) Single-electrode mode. (**D**) Freestanding triboelectric-layer mode. Reprinted with permission from [39]. 2020, copyright John Wiley and Sons.

Vertical contact-separation (CS) mode: When two objects with different degrees of electronegativity are in vertical contact, electrons are exchanged at the contact surface. Then, when two objects are separated, due to there being an equal number of opposite charges between them, electrostatic induction leads to a potential difference between the electrodes attached to them, generating electric current when connecting through the wires, and then the potential difference gradually disappears. When the two separated objects come into contact again, the opposite potential difference is generated between the two electrodes again, thus generating opposite currents through the wires. With the repetition of contact-separation cycles, alternating current is output.

Lateral sliding (LS) mode: The principle of lateral sliding is similar to that of the vertical Contact-separation mode, except that the relative displacement is changed from vertical to horizontal. Alternating current is output as a result of repeated displacement in the horizontal direction.

Single-electrode (SE) mode: This is the simplest mode in terms of structure. The method takes the earth as an electrode and generates a potential difference between the metal electrode and the earth through electrostatic induction, thus producing current.

Independent triboelectric layer (FT) mode: FT mode involves placing the charged object between two electrodes, which are attached to the dielectric layer. When the charged object moves between the two electrodes, the potential difference between the electrodes changes, thus generating current.

Theoretically, due to the low requirements of TENG power generation, a variety of friction layer materials and electrode materials are available to choose from. The TENG can then be designed according to the personalized needs of patients.

2.2. *Wearable Body Energy Collection*

TENGs can be customized to a certain extent according to the energy collection requirements due to the possibility of selecting diverse raw materials and their loose structural design requirements. Therefore, appropriate materials and shapes can be selected for the production of TENGs through the process of adaptive design in order to be able to collect the bioenergy dispersed in the human body and to maintain a certain degree of biological friendliness [40]. Saqib et al. proposed a TENG that was able to obtain energy from omnidirectional movements in the human body (Figure 3a [41]) The TENG was made by placing cellulose-based particles in rapidly degradable gelatin capsules. Small cellulose particles (~6 μ m) were used as friction anode materials, and gelatin capsules were used as friction cathode layers. When tested, the power harvested by the TENG ranged from 5.488 to 70 μW, with a maximum energy conversion efficiency of 74.35%. Due to the advantages of all-around energy collection, the TENG had a wider energy collection channel, which was able to perform energy collection under complex motion while maintaining a high energy collection efficiency.

Park and others ingeniously used the electric charge generated by friction in the human body to make simple aluminum electrode triboelectric nanogenerators (Figure 3b) [42]. The system collects the frictional electric energy between the sole and the ground through the electrostatic induction of aluminum electrodes.In addition, the power generated in each step is enough to instantly light 100 commercial light-emitting diodes (LEDs). Although this aluminum electrode TENG has the advantages of easy fabrication, its simple structure also leads to it having unsatisfactory energy conversion efficiency. Zhu et al. integrated TENGs into a mask via 3D printing, and produced breath-driven TENGs (Figure 3c) [43]. The TENG generates electrical signals corresponding to the breath airflow and extracts personal information during breathing. This 3D-printed TENG has the advantage of it being easy to perform shape customization and meet the personalized needs of different people.

Wang's team developed a new TENG using conductive elastic sponges (ES-TENG) [44]. This soft and special structure has great flexibility, and the adaptive deformation of the sponge enables it to collect kinetic energy from tumbling motions of different amplitudes from different surfaces of flexible objects, thus effectively improving the efficiency of energy collection. In addition, as a result of its adaptive design, this TENG can be easily installed on the body in order to be able to collect energy from multi-angle body movement.

Compared with traditional power generation methods, the collection of human motion energy using wearable devices avoids bloated power design and has the advantages of small size, flexibility, stability, etc.

2.3. *Implantable Body Energy Collection*

For implantable medical devices, there is a risk of exposure due to wounds and rejection by the human immune system. This makes it necessary to control the number of operations and the biological safety of medical equipment. The use of TENGs for the collection of biological energy from the human body can guarantee the long-term operation of the implanted medical device, thereby reducing the number of surgeries required to change batteries. In addition, the extensive selection of raw materials usable for TENGs provides multiple channels for biological safety [45–48]. Zhao et al. developed a TENG [49] that could be used to obtain energy from the beating of the heart. The TENG was used to generate a new environmentally friendly in situ gap through the evaporation of distilled water in which it was soaked (Figure 4a), which was then used to manufacture a no-spacer triboelectric nanogenerator (NSTENG). This unique manufacturing method ensures biological safety and avoids pollution in the body. In addition, when installed on a rat heart, it was also able to monitor normal heart movement, with the accuracy of the heart rate measurements reaching as high as 99.73%. Implantable TENGs provide the possibility of developing self-powered heart detection instrument in the future.

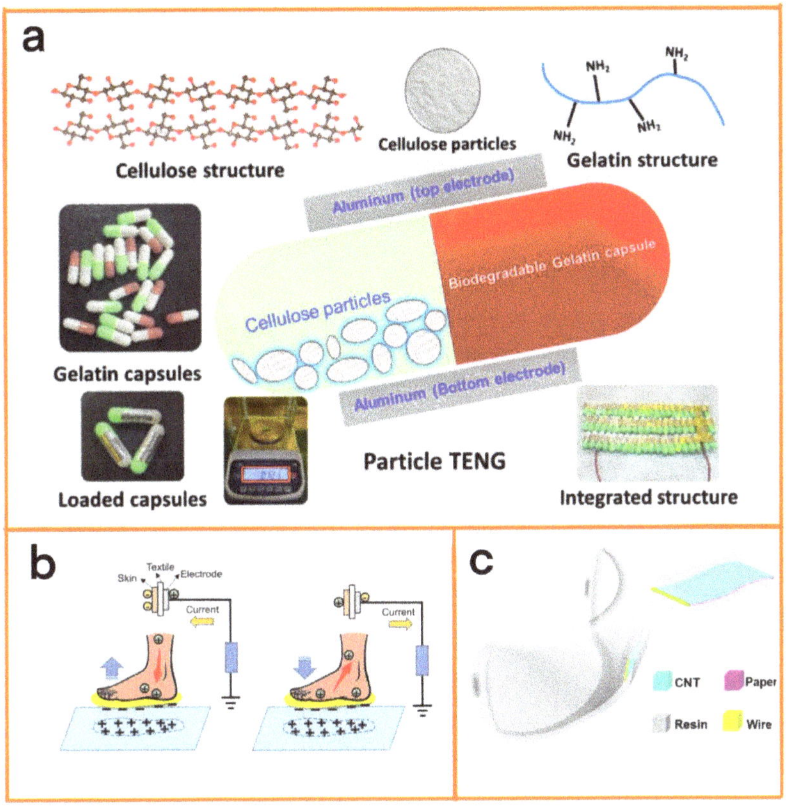

Figure 3. (**a**) Design scheme and schematic diagram of the rapid degradation of P-TENGs showing the tiny cellulose particles and gelatin capsules. Reprinted with permission from [41]. 2022, Elsevier. (**b**) Schematic diagram of the working mechanism of the single-electrode mode triboelectric system. Reprinted with permission from [42]. 2019, Elsevier. (**c**) Structure diagram of the 3D-printed breath-driven TENG. Reprinted with permission from [43]. 2022, Springer Nature.

Yao et al. introduced a vagus nerve stimulation system that generates electricity through gastric peristalsis (Figure 4c) [50]. The system includes a flexible, biocompatible nanogenerator attached to the surface of the stomach. This generates biphasic electrical pulses in response to gastric peristalsis, which can also be used to control the weight of rats by stimulating the vagus nerve to reduce food intake (Figure 4b).

In 2018, Liu et al. proposed a new endocardial pressure monitoring technology based on implantable TENG, which used inductively coupled plasma and corona discharge to conduct triboelectric treatment on polytetrafluoroethylene film, so that its output increased to 6.2 V. To improve biological safety, flexible PDMS with biocompatibility and blood compatibility was selected for the packaging of the device, with a size of 1.0 cm × 1.5 cm × 0.1 cm. In addition, the device could also be used to monitor cardiovascular diseases such as ventricular premature beat and ventricular fibrillation by detecting the ventricular EP of pigs [51].

Shi et al. proposed a TENG that was able to generate electricity through subcutaneous muscle movement (M-TENG) [52]. The system has a straightforward structure, including only one electrode. Immersing it in the body makes it possible to convert biological activity into electrical energy. For example, a 1.5 cm × 2 cm titanium alloy film was implanted between the skin and muscle layers on the back of the rabbit, and the titanium alloy film was connected to the LED bulb through wires. Then, the rhythmic flashing of the LED bulb could be observed when the rabbit moved (Figure 4d). Different power generation methods and raw materials affect the output of TENG. We can compare different TENG outputs to find out the suitable device (Table 1).

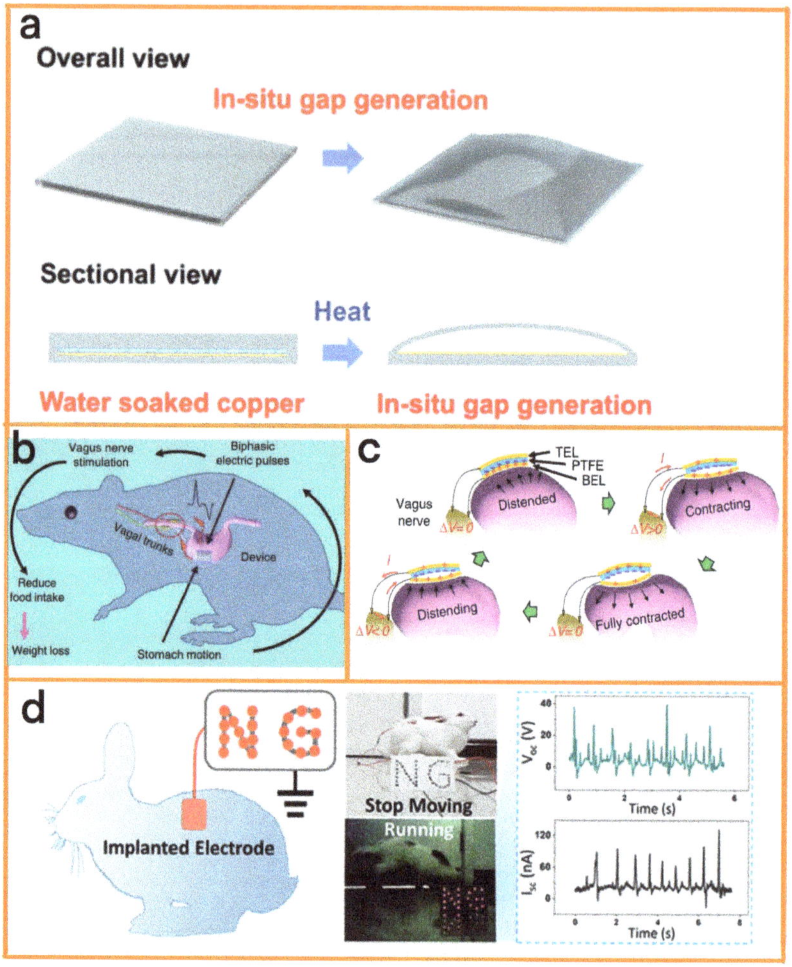

Figure 4. (**a**) Schematic diagram briefly showing the in situ air gap generation of NSTENG. Reprinted with permission from [49]. 2021, Elsevier. (**b**) Working principle of the relevant vagus nerve stimulation system, schematically showing the generation of two-phase electrical signals and the path of vagus nerve stimulation. (**c**) Schematic diagram of the power generation principle of the vagus nerve stimulation device at different gastric motility stages. Reprinted with permission from [50]. 2018, nature. (**d**) LED bulbs lit by BISS implanted in rabbits and the open circuit voltage and short circuit current of BISS during operation. Reprinted with permission from [52]. 2019, ACS.

Table 1. Summary of parameters of wearable and implantable TENGs.

Date	Positions	Sizes [cm²]	Materials	Energy Sources	Outputs	Applications	Working Modes
2022 [41]	Wearable	None	Cellulose particles	Particle vibration	70 μW	Electricity generation	Contact-separation
2019 [42]	Foot	2 × 2	Al	Walk	1.67 μW	Electricity generation	Contact-separation
2022 [43]	Nose	None	CNT, Wire	Breathing	150 V	Respiratory monitoring	Contact-separation
2021 [44]	Wearable	4 × 4	Sponge, PANI	Vibration	280 μW	Electricity generation	Contact-separation
2021 [49]	Heart, rat	1.2 × 1.2	Ecoflex	Heart beating	51.74 nA	Biomedical monitoring	Contact-separation
2018 [50]	Stomach, rat	1 × 2	PDMS, PI	Stomach Peristalsis	40 μW	Nerve stimulation	Contact-separation
2019 [51]	Muscle, rabbit	1.5 × 2	Titanium	Muscle vibration	80 nA	Biomedical monitoring	Contact-separation
2018 [52]	Heart, pig	1.0 × 1.5	Al, PTFE PDMS	Heart beating	6.2 V	EP monitoring	Contact-separation

3. Real-Time Medical Diagnostic Equipment

The vast majority of diseases cause a gradual deterioration in the patient over time, and the rapid detection and treatment of diseases in their early stages can not only greatly reduce the investment in medical treatment required for patients, but also effectively reduce the severity of sequelae. TENG-based real-time medical monitoring equipment can provide a variety of physiological data measurements of the human body over a long time. And the equipment has different outputs with different raw materials and testing positions (Table 2). Through terminal data analysis and processing, diseases can be quickly diagnosed, and personalized treatment plans can be provided for patients, effectively improving the use of medical resources.

3.1. Diagnostic Equipment for Cardiovascular Disease

As a disease of the circulatory system, cardiovascular disease includes heart disease and vascular disease. The main diagnostic methods for heart disease include invasive and non−invasive examinations [53]. Invasive tests, including cardiovascular endoscopy, endomyocardial biopsy, and other studies, which may cause trauma to patients, come with certain risks. Noninvasive investigations, including ECG and echocardiography, are not traumatic, but have low diagnostic value and diagnosis cannot be performed in real time over a long time. Therefore, finding new diagnosis methods is key to solving these problems.

3.1.1. Blood Pressure Diagnosis

Blood pressure detection is a key means of diagnosing cardiovascular diseases. Effective long-term collection blood pressure data could help to analyze personal health changes, thus assisting in determining the causes of diseases. Doctors are able to analyze patients' comprehensive physical conditions on the basis of long-term data, and provide constructive suggestions with the aim of providing patients with personalized medical care. TENG-based blood pressure monitoring instruments are not only characterized by the use of lightweight and safe raw materials, they are also able to guarantee the long-term stable operation of the instrument because of its self-powered characteristics. Ran et al. developed a cuff-free, self-powered continuous blood pressure monitoring system. The system was based on a new double sandwich structure (a copper electrode sandwiched between two layers of silicone rubber and cardboard is added at the outermost layer to provide support) (Figure 5a) [54]. Using the adaptive design described above, this system was able to achieve a sensitivity of 0.89 V/kPa, and a response time of 32 ms; this sensor was easily able to capture blood vessel signals, and could be used for long-term and efficient real−time blood pressure diagnosis.

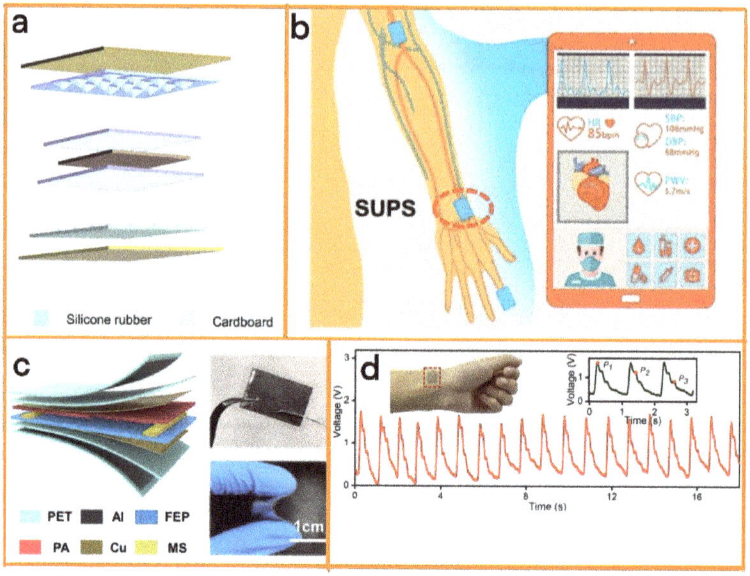

Figure 5. (**a**) Triboelectric nanogenerator sensor with a double sandwich structure. Reprinted with permission from [54]. 2022, Nano Research. (**b**) Integrated description of SUPS for non-invasive multi-index pulse monitoring. (**c**) Schematic diagram of the structure of SUPS. Optical photo of the built SUPS. Reprinted with permission from [55]. 2021, Elsevier. (**d**) FPS test radial pulse wave. Reprinted with permission from [56]. 2022, Elsevier.

3.1.2. Pulse Diagnosis

Real−time pulse diagnosis can be used to provide doctors with continuous information on the pulse rhythm information of patients. On the basis of the analysis of this information, clues can be found as early as possible of certain cardiovascular diseases, such as atrial fibrillation, supraventricular tachycardia, premature beats, etc., and they can be treated in a timely fashion. At the same time, long-term pulse information can indicate direction for doctors to follow in analyzing the heart rhythms of patients, thus providing strong support for the further personalization of the treatment of patients. Xu et al. designed a self-powered sensitive ultra-pulse sensor (SUPS) that could be used to conduct long-term non-invasive real-time cardiovascular monitoring (Figure 5c) [55]. The device uses an FEP film consisting of a nanowire array and a Polyamide (PA) film with a fiber structure as the triboelectric layer, copper foil as the electrode, with the addition of a melamine sponge with a porous structure as an interlayer between the triboelectric layers. As a result of the adaptive design described above, SUPS showed excellent sensing performance, including a super sensitivity of 10.29 nA/kPa, a low detection limit of 5 mg, and a rapid response time of 30 ms. It can be used to monitor cardiovascular systems in a long-term, stable and accurate manner, and is expected to be used in the diagnosis and prevention of cardiovascular diseases (Figure 5b).

Wang and his team proposed a flexible pressure sensor (FPS) for measuring the pulse of the cutaneous artery (Figure 5d) [56]. PTFE, copper powder, and conductive double-sided adhesive were used to perform detection following the TENG principle, and this was demonstrated to be suitable for the diagnosis of cardiovascular disease. This device was produced by means of a convenient coating operation, by which a copper powder layer with a natural microstructure with a 500-nanometer scale was formed on a conductive double-sided adhesive. This hierarchical microstructure was composed of copper powder, making the FPS sensitive to weak pressure signals; the FPS had a high sensitivity of 1.65 V/kPa, and was able to accurately detect arteries over a long period of time, thus making it useful for the diagnosis of cardiovascular diseases.

3.2. Diagnostic Equipment for Respiratory Diseases

Presently, a variety of methods can be employed for the diagnosis of respiratory diseases, including imaging diagnosis and endoscopy [57–59]. However, these conventional detection methods are not able to transmit the progress of disease in real time in cases of long-term diseases such as chronic rhinitis and pharyngitis. This leads to doctors being unable to quickly change treatment strategies, which affects the efficiency of treatment. In addition, the costly and time-consuming nature of testing equipment also affects patients' quality of life to varying degrees. New breath detection devices based on TENGs could find easy application for long-term operation due to their being self-powered and stable. In addition, because of their small size, light weight, and other advantages, they can be customized to a certain extent depending on the individual needs of patients, thus minimizing their impact on the lives of patients. For example, Zhang and his team proposed a TENG for use in the self—powered detection of exhaled gas and disease diagnosis (Figure 6a) [60]. The TENG was made of Ti_3C_2Tx MXene/amino functionalized multi-wall carbon nanotubes (MXene/NH_2-MWCNTs). It was driven by respiration, and could be used to determine the type of respiration on the basis of voltage changes in order to diagnose respiratory disease. Furthermore, on the basis of the long-term respiratory data collected, the physical condition of the patient and disease progression can be analyzed in detail. Additionally, since MXene/NH_2-MWCNTs are sensitive to formaldehyde gas, the device is also able to accurately detect formaldehyde gas in exhaled gas, which could play an important role in the determination of air safety.

3.2.1. Diagnosis of Diseases Caused by Infection with Gram-Positive Bacteria

Gram—positive bacteria such as Staphylococcus aureus can cause a series of diseases, such as upper respiratory tract infection, suppurative tonsillitis, bronchitis, pneumonia, and skin and surgical incision infections. They pose a significant challenge to human medical treatment. In addition, most bacterial infections cause a deterioration in the patient over time. Early detection and treatment can reduce wastage of medical resources and effectively reduce the severity of sequelae. Considering that routine invasive testing increases the risk of multiple infections in patients, it is urgently necessary to find non—invasive and efficient detection methods, including surface-enhanced Raman spectroscopy (SERS) and highly sensitive detection methods using TENGs.

Ma and his team, using Au@Ag NPs/slide as an enhanced substrate, constructed an aptamer-based SERS method for detecting Staphylococcus aureus. The ROX-aptamer of *S. aureus* was modified on the surface of Au@Ag NPs/slide by means of electrostatic interaction [61]. Because the aptamer is able to specifically bind to Staphylococcus aureus, it will cause the rox-aptamer to fall off the substrate surface, thus reducing the SERS signal intensity of the substrate. Then, the target bacteria can be successfully detected by analyzing the signal changes of SERS.

In this regard, Wang et al. developed a TENG especially for detecting Gram-positive bacteria in solution in order to be able to diagnose relevant diseases in time [62]. The system immobilized polyamine and vancomycin on the etched surface of ITO glass and recognized Gram-positive bacteria by means of vancomycin bacterial wall interaction (Figure 6b). Guanidine-functionalized multi-wall carbon nanotubes (CNT Arg) were used as signal amplification materials. Then, the system was able to specifically detect Gram-positive bacteria in solution by measuring the voltage change in the biosensor (Figure 6c). This equipment could be used to observe Gram-positive bacteria stably over a long time, and can be applied for the diagnosis of diseases resulting from infection with Gram-positive bacteria or for the determination of water quality in the future.

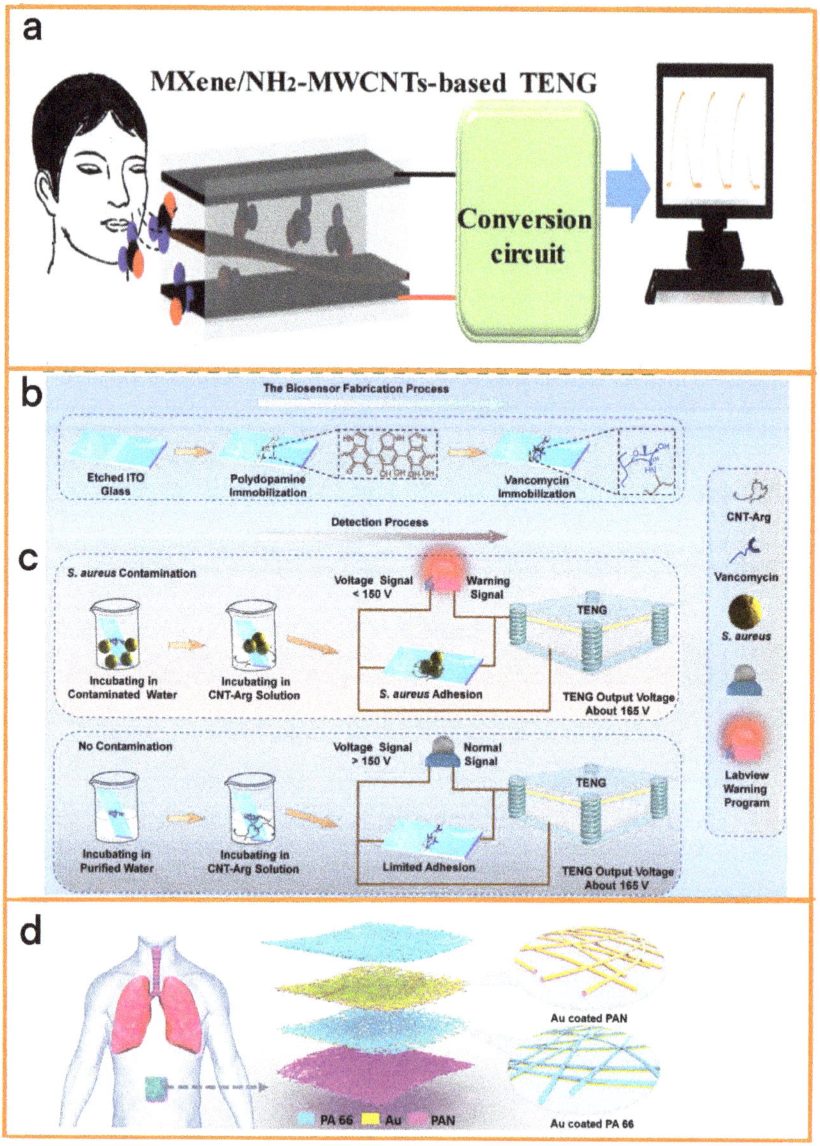

Figure 6. (**a**) Application diagram of MXene/NH2−MWCNTs-based TENG. Reprinted with permission from [60]. 2022, Elsevier. (**b**) The preparation process of ITO-Van, which is able to specifically capture Staphylococcus aureus, including the immobilization of dopamine and vancomycin on the etched surface of ITO glass. (**c**) Schematic diagram of staphylococcus aureus detection using a self-powered biosensor system. In the process of detecting Staphylococcus aureus, a liquid environment is assumed, and a vertical contact-separation TENG is used as the voltage signal source. Reprinted with permission from [62]. 2022, Elsevier. (**d**) SANES attached to the abdominal surface used in a respiratory monitoring application scenario; SANES schematic diagram; and an enlarged view of PAN nanofiber film and PA 66 nanofiber film coated with an Au electrode layer. Reprinted with permission from [63]. 2021, Elsevier.

Table 2. Summary of TENG parameters.

Date	Positions	Sizes [cm²]	Materials	Energy Sources	Outputs	Applications	Working Modes
2022 [54]	Pulse	5 × 5	Cu, Silicone rubber	Pulse vibration	0.89 V/kPa	Pulse monitoring	Contact-separation
2021 [55]	Pulse	None	FEP, PA, Cu, PET	Pulse vibration	10.29 nA/kPa	Pulse monitoring	Contact-separation
2022 [56]	Pulse	1.8 × 1.6	PTFE, Cu	Pulse vibration	1.65 V/kPa	Pulse monitoring	Contact-separation
2022 [60]	Nose	5 × 2	MXene	Respiratory drive	27 μW	Respiratory monitoring	Contact-separation
2022 [62]	Solution	2 × 0.5	ITO	Vibration	165 V	Bacterial detection	Contact-separation
2021 [63]	Nose	4 × 4	Polyacrylonitrile, Polyamide 66	Respiratory drive	420 v	OSAHS diagnostics	Contact-separation
2021 [64]	Wearable	31 × 3	Catechol, Chitosan, Diatom	Movement	29.8 mW/m²	Parkinson diagnosis	Contact-separation
2021 [65]	Wearable	4 × 3.5	Ecoflex, Al	Movement	2 V	Parkinson diagnosis	Contact-separation

3.2.2. Diagnosis of Obstructive Sleep Apnea-Hypopnea Syndrome

Obstructive sleep apnea-hypopnea syndrome (OSAHS) affects about 1 billion people worldwide. This disease can cause repeated upper airway collapse during sleep, further leading to intermittent hypoxia, sleep disorders, and even cerebrovascular diseases. At the same time, most OSAHS remains diagnosed. To solve this problem, Peng et al. prepared a respirable electronic skin (SANES) based on TENGs for real-time respiratory monitoring and diagnosis of OSAHS [63]. It was prepared using gold as an electrode, multilayer polyacrylonitrile, and "polyamide 66" nanofiber as positive and negative friction electrodes (Figure 6d); the highest pressure sensitivity obtained was 0.217 kPa^{-1}, and it also showed good air permeability. Therefore, the electronic skin was able to achieve accurate breath detection. At the same time, the team further developed a self−powered diagnostic system for the assessment of OSAHS severity. The automatic diagnostic system was able to diagnose OSAHS in real time, effectively prevent the occurrence of OSAHS, and improve sleep quality.

3.3. *Diagnosis of Parkinson's Disease*

Parkinson's disease is a common degenerative disease of the elderly nervous system that leads to motor disorders in patients. At present, doctors mainly rely on careful observation to assess the development of the disease. Therefore, Kim et al. synthesized a highly stretchable and self-healing hydrogel TENG with natural biomaterials (catechol chitosan was mixed with pill-shaped diatom frustules with sizes of 20–50 μm) [64] (Figure 7a) that had an instantaneous power density of 29.8 mW/m^2. The TENG obtains energy from human motion and combines it with the M-type Kapton film to form a self-powered tremor sensor. The sensor was able to diagnose and monitor Parkinson's disease through the measurement of the low-frequency motion of patients in combination with machine learning algorithms (Figure 7b). The individual needs of different patients can be met by changing the appearance structure. At the same time, Yuce et al. developed a self-powered TENG for diagnosis of Parkinson's disease [65]. This nanogenerator was made of flexible materials, and through customization was able to meet the need for patients to be able to wear it for a long time. It consisted of a 4 cm × 3.5 cm dielectric and 2 mm × 3 mm aluminum electrodes. When the patient's hand bends, the system generates voltage due to the change in the relative position of the dielectric material and the aluminum electrode. This sensor can be used to evaluate the patient's condition, and can be worn for long-term monitoring due to its self-powering characteristics.

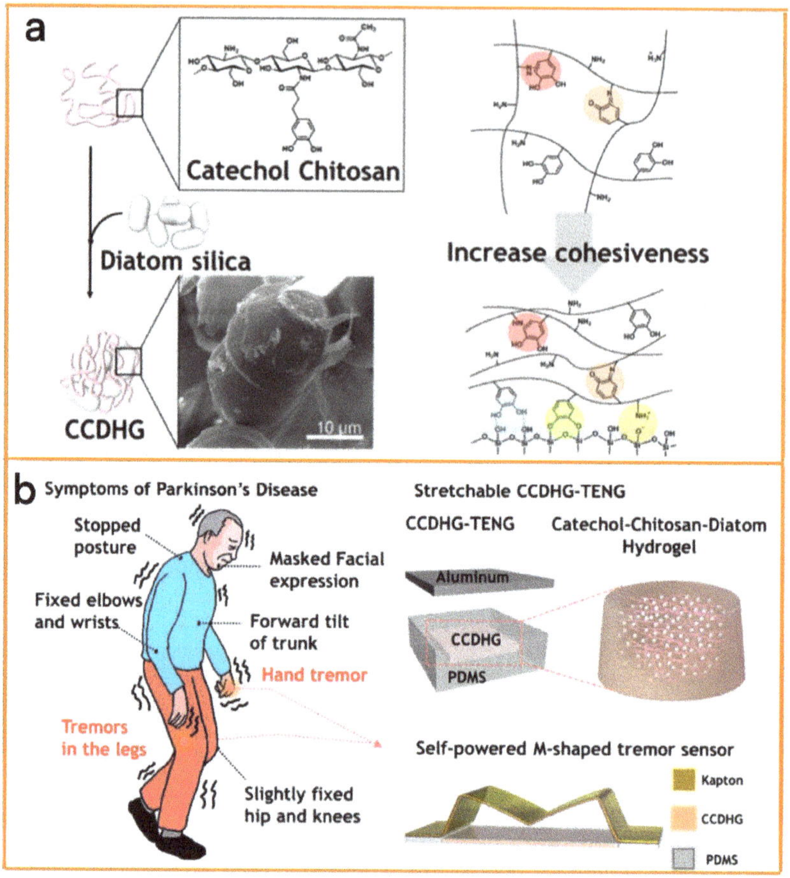

Figure 7. (**a**) Preparation method of catechol chitosan diatom hydrogel, and the mechanism of enhancing the cohesion of catechol chitosan diatom hydrogel. Optical image. (**b**) Typical symptoms of Parkinson's disease. Schematic diagram of catechol chitosan diatom hydrogel triboelectric nanogenerator and vibration sensor. Reprinted with permission from [64] 2021, Elsevier.

4. Long-Term Self-Treatment Equipment

Compared with acute diseases that can be effectively treated in a short time, rapid recovery often cannot be achieved for stubborn chronic diseases. In these cases, long-term customized treatment in accordance with the needs of patients is an effective way of solving this problem, but this inevitably involves the use of flexible and highly customized biomedical equipment. Biomedical equipment based on TENGs has a comparative advantage in terms of customization due to its self-powered character and flexible appearance. At the same time, the wide selection of raw materials from which TENGs can be produced also give them more room for development in terms of biodegradability, compliance, biological friendliness, and different energy collection methods and outputs (Table 3).

4.1. Body Tissue Regeneration

Self-powered flexible equipment can find wide application in various fields, and multifunctionality is always highly appreciated because it provides the advantages of miniaturization, higher integration, and lower power consumption.

4.1.1. Nerve Tissue Regeneration

Peripheral nerve injury is one of the common causes of disability, and it often requires a long duration of regular treatment to recover, even requiring treatment via serious nerve anastomosis surgery. Nerve stimulation devices based on TENGs can provide long-term and stable electrical stimulation, effectively promoting nerve regeneration and increasing the efficiency of treatment in combination with traditional treatment methods, and the high degree of possible customization of TENGs means that they can be adapted to the different injury conditions of different patients, thus reducing the discomfort of patients during the healing process [66–68]. Therefore, Zhou et al. developed an implanted sciatic nerve stimulation system (ISR-NES) that was able to effectively promote the regeneration of the sciatic nerve [69]. The system's Contact-separation triboelectric nanogenerator (Cs TENG) spontaneously generated a biphasic electric pulse in response to respiratory and body movement. Then, the electric pulse stimulated the injured sciatic nerve through the cuff electrode in order to repair it (Figure 8a). PDMS and polyamide 6 (PA6) films were selected as the friction layer of the TENG, and aluminum foil was pasted on the back of the two friction layers as the conductive layer. Because the vibration amplitude generated by the breathing of rats is small, it is difficult to collect energy using ordinary TENGs; therefore, the sensitivity of the TENG was improved using the spacing structure through adaptive design: the dielectric films of the two friction layers were stacked face to face, a surface charge with the opposite sign forms on the two contact surfaces, an air gap is formed in the middle during separation, and an induced potential difference is formed between the two electrodes. By menas of the above design, the output of the TENG was successfully improved. Due to the flexibility of the raw materials used, the system demonstrated high customizability and a stable power supply. In the future, it will be able to meet the personalized needs of patients and provide them with targeted long-term treatment.

Tactile loss is one of the more common outcomes of peripheral nerve injury. Implantable nerve prostheses represent a promising direction, but these still possess some disadvantages, including the complexity of their use scenarios and the requirement of bloated external power supplies. Therefore, to solve this problem, Shlomy et al. proposed triboelectric nanogenerators (TENG-IT) with simple structures that were self-powered, biocompatible, and highly customizable for tactile restoration [70]. PDMS, nylon (Ny), and cellulose acetate butyrate (CAB), which has the advantages of flexibility and biocompatibility, were selected as friction layers in this device, with PDMS being a negative layer, and Ny and CAB being positive layers. The device was implanted under human skin in order to convert pressure into potential, which was transmitted to healthy sensory nerves through cuff electrodes (Figure 8b). As a therapeutic device intended for long-term implantation, the personalized design enabled by its simple structure can result in the improvement of a patient's quality of life to a certain extent.

4.1.2. Connective Tissue Regeneration

Due to the limited osteogenic capacity of bone marrow mesenchymal stem cells (BMSCs) in elderly patients, treating elderly patients in need of bone repair has always been a challenging medical problem. Here, Wang et al. performed bone repair by means of the mechanical action of body−driven wearable triboelectric nanogenerators (WP-TENG) and piezoelectric ceramics (Figure 9a) [71]. To improve the friction performance of the equipment, nylon sheets were selected as the base material; soft foam was attached to the nylon to increase the friction, polytetrafluoroethylene (PTFE) film and aluminum foil were used as positive and negative friction layers, and two copper foils were attached to the back of the two friction layers as electrodes. The peak current reached 30 μA, and a good recovery effect on elderly bone marrow mesenchymal stem cells was demonstrated. WP−TENGs can also be customized, and can be produced in different shapes and sizes to meet the personalized needs of elderly patients, improving their quality of life when undergoing long-term treatment.

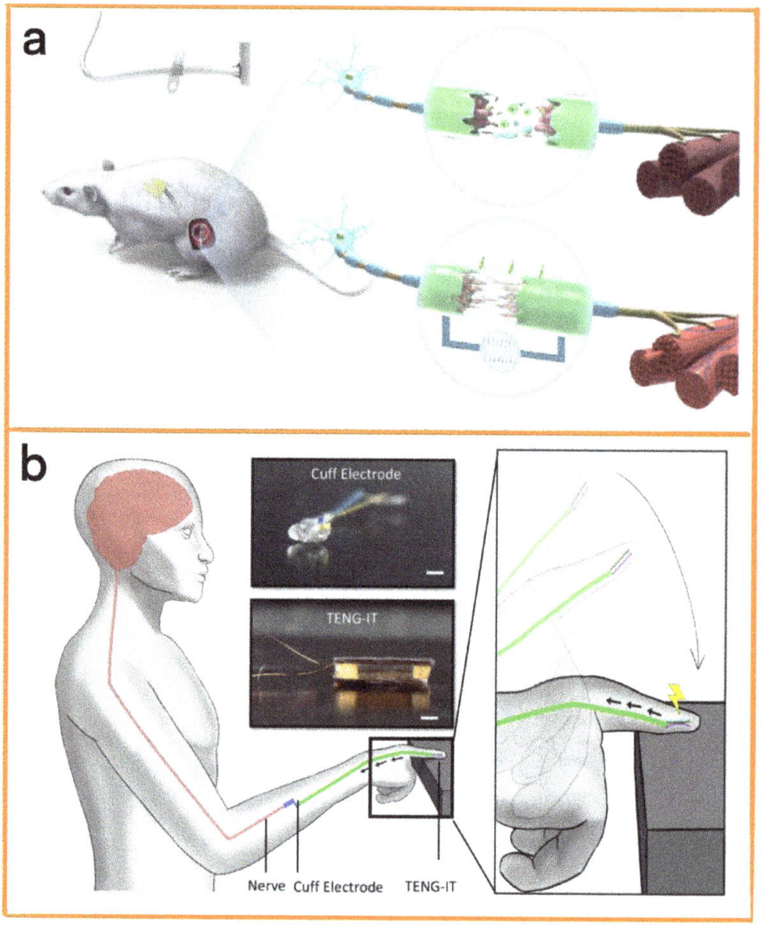

Figure 8. (**a**) Schematic diagram of electrode implant solution. Cut the skin, and introduce an electric stimulation cuff on the left sciatic nerve of the rats. Place Cs TENG as an energy collector at the waist of the rat, and connect the electrode with the encapsulated platinum wire to ensure that the damaged area is located between the two electrodes. Reprinted with permission from [69]. 2022, John Wiley and Sons. (**b**) Use of TENG-IT to restore touch. TENG-IT is implanted under the skin (desensitized fingers). Reprinted with permission from [70]. 2021, ACS.

With advances in society and science, alopecia has become an increasingly common modern disease [72,73]. Unlike acute illnesses that can take effect quickly in a short period of time, alopecia often requires long-term treatment. Here, Yao et al. designed a wearable electrical stimulation device (M-ESD) activated by body movement [74] to promote hair regeneration. Its working principle is the improvement of the secretion of growth factors in blood vessels through electrical stimulation (Figure 9b), thereby relieving hair keratin disorder and increasing the number of hair follicles. The M-ESD consisted of two modules: a TENG with an electric pulse generator function and a pair of interlaced electrodes. This TENG had two friction layers that were connected by a soft Ecoflex belt. Because Ecoflex allows arbitrary tension, bending, and torsion within the ~900% strain limit, the TENG was able to perform omnidirectional energy collection as a result of the adaptive design described above.

4.1.3. Muscle Tissue Function Repair

Loss of muscle function can lead to many diseases, including stroke, spinal cord injury, and multiple sclerosis [75,76]. Electrical stimulation has positive effects when treating this disease. However, the long treatment cycles can be inconvenient for patients. To coordinate the relationship between the treatment cycle and quality of life, flexible and stable biomedical equipment that is able to meet the individual needs of patients is essential. Wang et al. developed a neural stimulation system that used stacked TENGs as the power supply (Figure 9c) [77]. This system had the characteristics of small size, customizability, etc., and could easily be applied for long-term treatment. The TENGs were made of PET sheets folded into a zigzag structure. This special structure stored energy in the form of elastic properties, and the surface of each PET sheet was attached to an aluminum film as an electrode. At the same time, to improve the efficiency of power generation and meet the electrical demand over a long course of treatment, polytetrafluoroethylene film (PTFE) with high electronegativity was attached to the top of some of the aluminum films as a friction layer. The system used a new flexible multi-channel intramuscular electrode as a universal neural interface. Efficient muscle stimulation was successfully achieved using the TENGs. On this basis, it is expected that this system could be used in cases of loss of muscle function to help patients recover their ability to exercise.

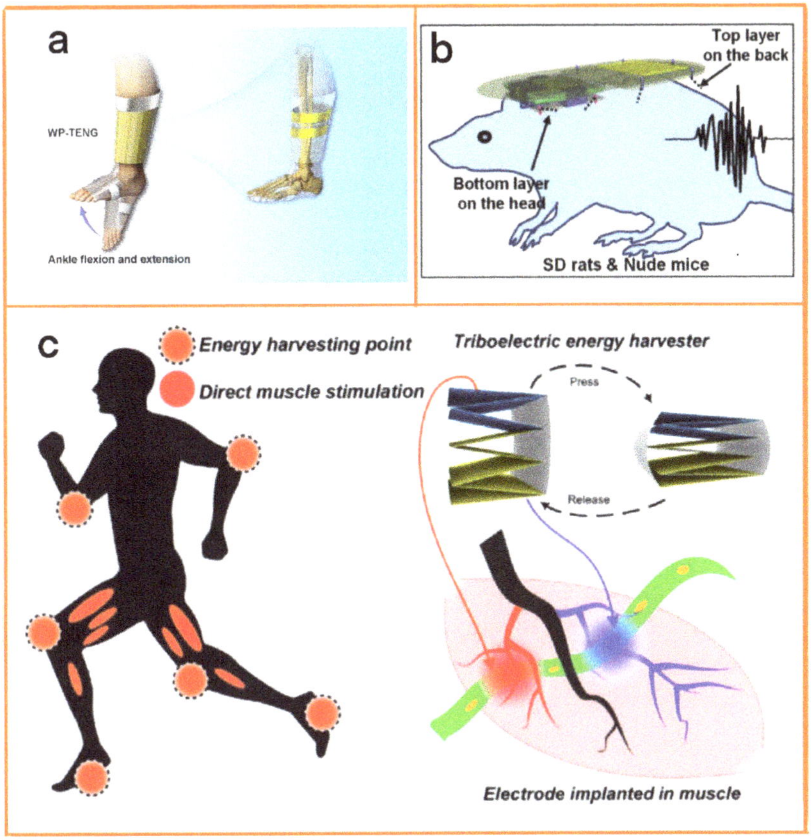

Figure 9. (**a**) Human limb movement activates the WP−TENG to achieve bone repair. Reprinted with permission from [71]. 2022, John Wiley and Sons. (**b**) Schematic diagram of M-ESD system for hair regeneration. Reprinted with permission from [74]. 2019, ACS. (**c**) Electrical muscle stimulation powered by TENGs. Reprinted with permission from [77]. 2019, ACS.

4.2. Organ Treatment

Organs include not only the heart, liver, and lungs, but also the outermost organ of the human body: the skin. At present, the treatment of minor internal organs and skin injuries is heavily dependent on the patient's self-healing, with severe cases requiring surgical treatment, ligation, hemostasis, and drug control. However, the rise of electric stimulation therapy presents another option for organ repair. At the same time, biomedical equipment based on TENGs are characterized by their flexibility and self-powered nature, can provide effective treatment over long periods of time, and can be customized to a certain extent according to a patient's individual circumstances, thus providing an effective route for personalized treatment of organs.

4.2.1. Cardiac Treatment

The heart is the center of the blood circulatory system, and plays a vital role in our body. In addition, compared with conventional acute diseases, it often takes longer for initial results to be achieved in heart−related diseases, resulting in the treatment process having higher biosafety requirements [78–80]. Therefore, Jiang et al. developed triboelectric nanogenerators (BN TENGs) that can be fully bio-absorbed for the treatment of bradycardia and arrhythmia using natural materials [81]. The friction layer of the equipment was made of cellulose, chitin, rice paper (RP), silk fibroin (SF), and egg white (EW), and ultra−thin Mg film was used as the electrode. To improve the power generation efficiency, the surface of the friction layer was treated using inductively coupled plasma reactive ion etching (ICP), thus increasing the contact area. Finally, SF film was used as the encapsulation layer. Importantly, this material has been proven to be degradable, and produced no obvious infection symptoms after implantation into rats (Figure 10b). Due to the use of natural materials and the high plasticity of the device, it is able to meet the individual needs of patients, and it thoroughly degrades and is absorbed by the body after the completion of its functions, thus improving biological safety (Figure 10a).

4.2.2. Skin or Wound Healing

As the outermost organ of the human body, the skin is much more likely to be injured than other organs. Wound healing is a long-term process, and the position and size of the wound is fraught with uncontrollability. It is therefore necessary that the corresponding healing equipment be able to be operated over long periods of time and be customizable in order to meet the different needs of different patients. Therefore, Sharma et al. proposed an interactive wound dressing based on TENGs [82] that provided an electrical stimulation environment for patients, accelerating wound healing (Figure 10c). The dressing consisted of carbonized polydopamine/polydopamine/polyacrylamide and was paired with polyvinylidene fluoride (PVDF) film. Therefore, the dressing exhibited mechanical strength and plasticity similar to that of muscle, and could be used in various scenarios. Since the hydrogel also provides a moist and effective wound environment, the TENG can help repair wounds that have difficulty healing under the effects of electrical stimulation, such as diabetic foot ulcers.

Du et al. designed a single-electrode working mode skin patch [83] that used electrical stimulation and photothermal heating to promote wound healing (Figure 10d). Polypyrrole/Pluronic F127 hydrogel was used as an electrolyte. In such hydrogel electrolyte designs, PPy endows the electrolyte with good conductivity and excellent photothermal conversion performance, while F127 endows the electrolyte with low modulus, continuity, and shape adaptability. In addition, the process of treatment using the skin patch could also be combined with photothermal heating technology to provide a suitable temperature for wound healing.

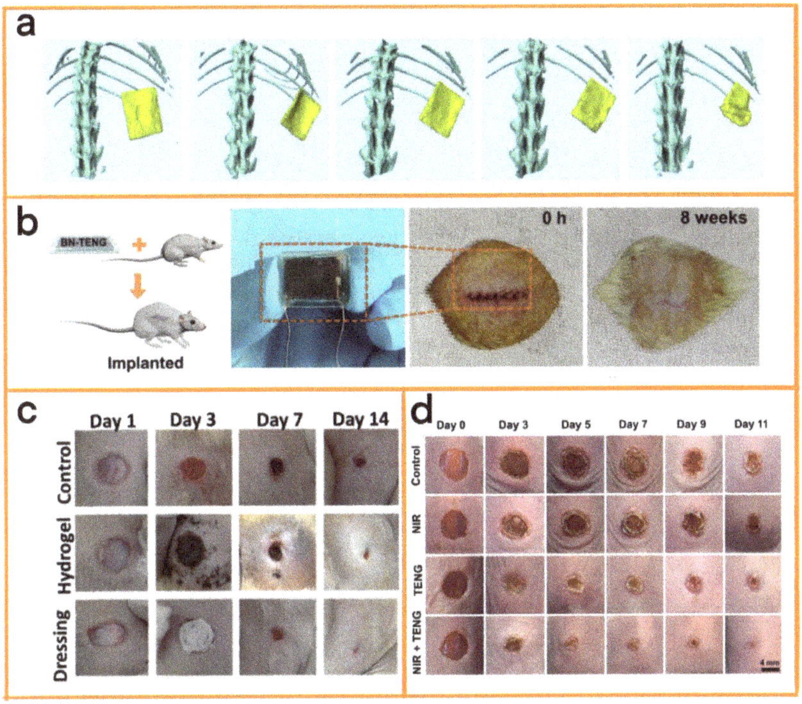

Figure 10. (**a**) Biodegradation in rats. (**b**) BN-TENG implantation: pictures of BN-TENG and the change in state at the site of implantation after suture. Reprinted with permission from [81]. 2018, John Wiley and Sons. (**c**) Representative images of wounds on days 1, 3, 7, and 14. Reprinted with permission from [82]. 2022, Elsevier. (**d**) Images of skin wounds from different treatment groups taken on days 0, 3, 5, 7, 9, and 11. Reprinted with permission from [83]. 2022, Elsevier.

4.3. Bacterial Infection

4.3.1. Long-Term Bacterial Eradication

The continuous and effective elimination of bacteria over longer periods of time is one of the main ways of fighting bacterial infection. Thanks to its flexibility and self-powered nature, TENG-based sterilization equipment can be customized for placement in areas with a high incidence of bacterial infection in order to block pathways of bacterial infection, and can be used to maintain sterile conditions in humans through the selection of materials with good biocompatibility. In this context, Lin et al. developed an edible battery with good biocompatibility (Figure 11a) [84]. The battery was made of a hydrogel and was powered using a self-charging TENG. The TENG consisted of a tooth-like polyethylene terephthalate (PET), and the PET was uniformly covered with a Pt film. In addition, to increase its biocompatibility, the top of the Pt was also covered in PTFE and a chitosan/glycerol film. The device generated a maximum voltage of 300 mV and was able to kill or eliminate 90% of bacteria (including Escherichia coli) within 30 min. Therefore, the battery could be used to fight against drug—resistant bacteria in the stomach and intestines. This battery shows great potential, and can be easily applied in the long-term treatment of gastrointestinal bacterial infection.

Feng et al. prepared a TENG with high power output that was able to achieve a sterilization efficiency of 98% [85]. The friction layer of the TENG consisted of a fluorinated polyurethane (F-PU) layer with a surface micronucleus prepared using maskless direct image lithography (DIL) technology and trichlorosilane (FOTS) steam (Figure 11b).

Compared with TENGs with a flat structure, the developed TENG achieved an increase in output power of 400%, and the sterilization efficiency obtained was 98%.

Huo et al. also developed a new disinfection system for bacteria and viruses [86]. The disinfection system consisted of a supercoiling–mediated rotational triboelectric nanogenerator (S-TENG), a power management system with a rectifier, and a disinfection filter for the inactivation of microorganisms in water. In order to improve the efficiency of power generation, the S-TENG was constructed using six butyl melamine formaldehyde (CCTO-BMF) friction layers doped with $CaCu_3Ti_4O_{12}$ particles, and was able to achieve an ultra-fast speed of 7500 rpm for driving a new oxidation-assisted electroporation mechanism (Figure 11c). Thanks to its ultra–high rotation speed, it was able to simultaneously realize a nanowire-enhanced local electric field and the generation of oxidative species, inactivating 99.9999% of microorganisms at a high flux of 15,000 L h^{-1} m^{-2}. This rapid, efficient and stable method for the long-term disinfection and sterilization of viruses meets the requirements of emergency water disinfection and the sterilization of portable medical equipment in areas with power shortages.

4.3.2. Anti-Inflammatory Treatment of Sepsis

Bacterial infection is one of the essential sources of disease [87–89]. With the abuse of antibiotics and the emergence of various drug-resistant bacteria, the development of new targeted treatment methods is an urgent need. In this context, Chen et al. designed a vagus nerve stimulator based on an implantable high-performance hydrogel nanogenerator (HENG) [90]. The nanogenerator was based on a polyacrylamide/graphene conductive hydrogel, and generates alternating current through ultrasonic-induced vibration at the conductive hydrogel/electrolyte interface. Without the use of an auxiliary rectifier, the subcutaneous implanted HENG can be used directly as a wireless nerve stimulator, and the current density and waveform can be programmed with the use of external ultrasonic pulses to inhibit the release of pro-inflammatory cytokines for the long-term anti–inflammatory treatment of sepsis (Figure 11d).

4.4. Long-Term Auxiliary Physical Therapy

4.4.1. Adjuvant Treatment of Hearing Impairment

With the development of TENGs, physical auxiliary treatment of hearing impairment has also taken a new direction. Thanks to the flexibility and self-powering characteristics of TENGs, physical auxiliary equipment based on TENGs can be customized in terms of shape and materials depending on the personal needs of patients. Zhou et al. designed a TENG-based symbol-to-speech translation glove to help people with language disabilities carry out long-term physical therapy [91]. The sensing unit of the glove was composed of conductive yarn wound on the rubber fiber. A plurality of sensing units formed a scalable sensor array (YSSA) (Figure 12a). Due to its helical structure, the TENG is able to meet the individual needs of different patients, and can be woven into different shapes. At the same time, by means of a machine learning algorithm, the sign language recognition rate of the YSSA was improved to 98.63%, and it was possible to achieve real-time conversion of sign language into language. Yuce et al. designed an eye movement sensor based on TENGs for the long-term physical auxiliary treatment of paralyzed people [92]. The TENG, which was integrated into the human–computer interface, detected eyelash movement by identifying the direct triboelectric interaction between hair and silicone to help paralyzed people communicate. In addition, due to the plasticity of the raw materials, the device is also able to meet the personalized needs of different patients through designs using different shapes, thus improving the long-term wearing comfort for patients.

4.4.2. Adjuvant Treatment of Knee Osteoarthritis

Due to the increasing aging of the world's population, diseases of the elderly are becoming more common. Knee osteoarthritis is one of the most common diseases among the elderly, and can be treated using total knee arthroplasty (TKA). To improve the patient's quality of life after surgery, Luo et al. proposed a portable self-evaluation stent for the rehabilitation of TKA patients (Figure 12c) [93]. The friction layer of the TENG consists of Kapton film, with a thickness of about 50 μm. In addition, the whole TENG sensor was produced using Printed Circuit Board (PCB) technology, making it suitable for use in prolonged auxiliary physical therapy. The system can be used to detect the knee bending angle and isometric muscle strength of patients over a long period of time, and to conduct targeted treatment of patients on the basis of data analysis (Figure 12b).

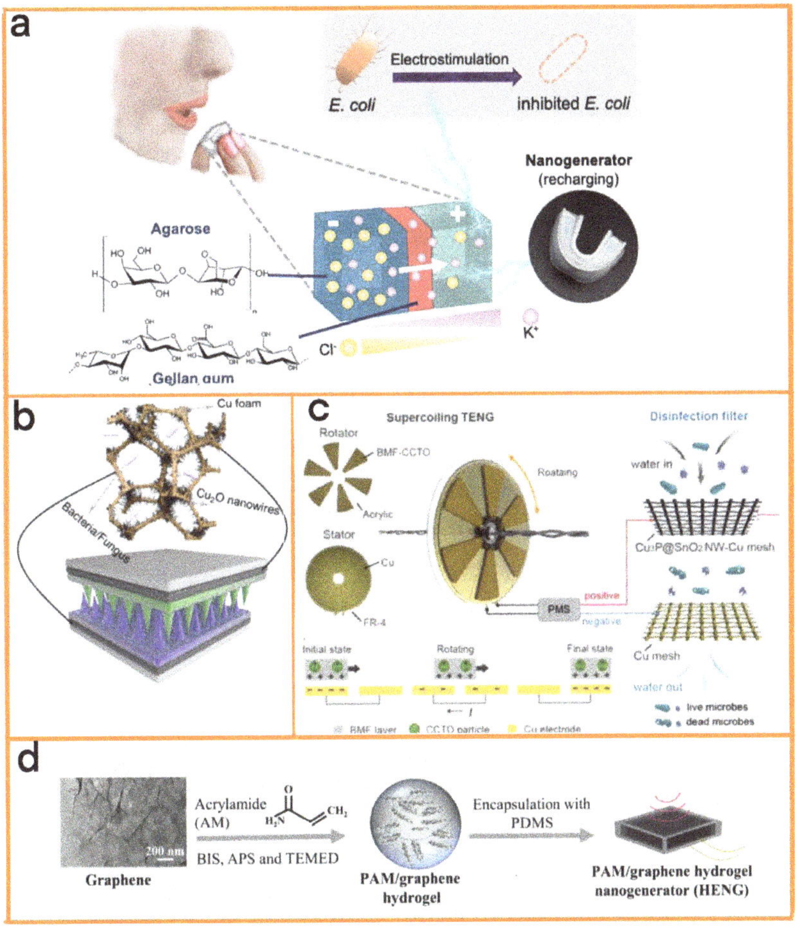

Figure 11. (**a**) Schematic diagram of a cube polysaccharide battery composed of the soft natural hydrogel. Reprinted with permission from [84]. 2021, Elsevier. (**b**) Schematic diagram of sterilization system. Cu_2O and Staphylococcus aureus. Reprinted with permission from [85]. 2022, Elsevier. (**c**) Schematic diagram of S-TENG disinfection system, including an S-TENG, a power management system (PMS) with rectifier, and a disinfection filter for inactivating microorganisms in water. Reprinted with permission from [86]. 2022, John Wiley and Sons. (**d**) The schematic diagram of ultrasonic-driven vagus nerve electrical stimulation based on implanted soft HENG and the manufacturing process of HENG. Reprinted with permission from [90]. 2022, Elsevier.

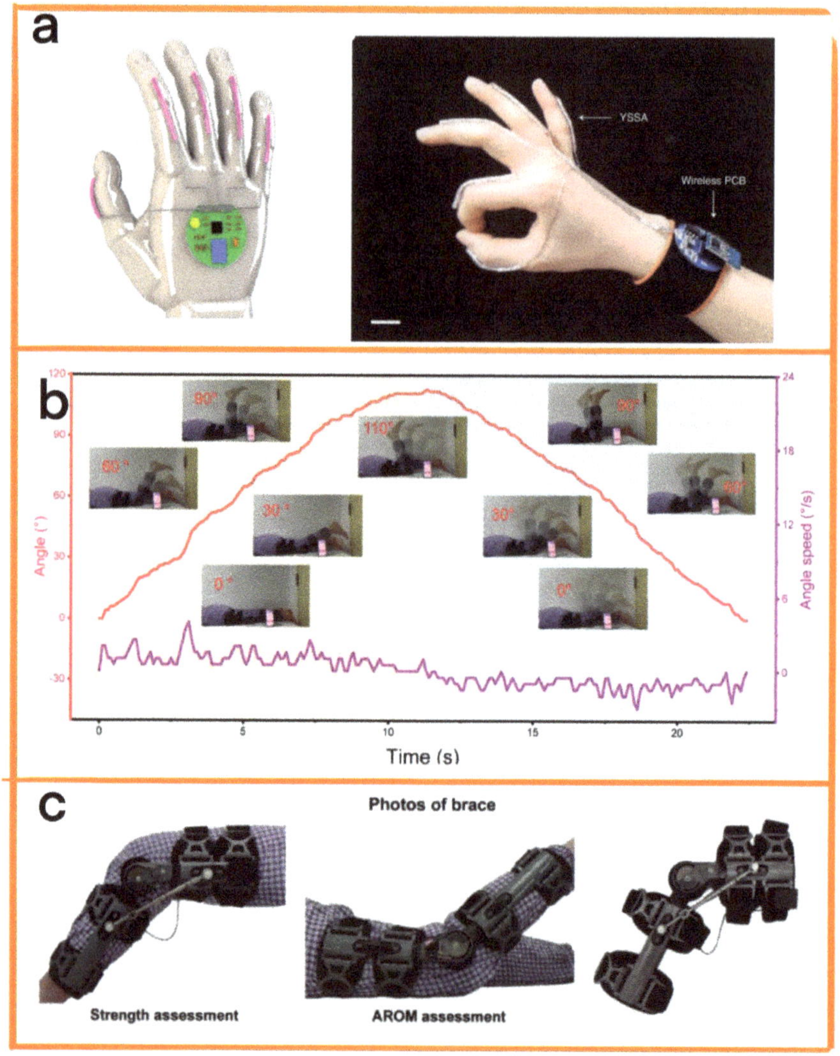

Figure 12. (**a**) Schematic diagram of a wearable sign language voice translation system. Reprinted with permission from [91]. 2020, Elsevier. (**b**) Real−time angle signal, angle speed, and photos within the range of motion. (**c**) Schematic diagram of rehabilitation brace system. Reprinted with permission from [93]. 2022, Elsevier.

4.5. Drug Delivery

When treating long-term diseases such as cancer, an accurate drug delivery system is essential to reduce side effects and improve treatment efficiency. To this end, Chen et al. designed a self-powered disc-shaped TENG (D-TENG) [94]. The disc-shaped TENG used PVDF and PA as friction layers, and Cr/Ag electrodes were attached to the bottom of the PVDF. As a result of its special disc-shaped design, it was able to obtain energy from the surrounding environment through rotation, and contained a pair of gold electrodes that could be used to electrically stimulate cells in the electrodes. Upon electrical stimulation of cancer cells by the drug delivery system, the chemotherapy drug doxorubicin (DOX) was significantly absorbed by the cancer cells (Figure 13a). Therefore, the use of new TENG devices for the precise treatment of some long-term diseases shows broad prospects.

Table 3. Summar of TENG treatment parameters.

Date	Positions	Sizes [cm^2]	Materials	Energy Sources	Outputs	Applications	Working Modes
2022 [69]	Sciatic nerve, rat	3.5 × 2.5	PDMS, PA6	Respiratory drive	0.13 μA	Nerve repair	Contact-separation
2021 [70]	Finger	0.5 × 0.5	PMDS, Ny, CAB	Tactile pressure	2.5 V	Tactile recovery	Contact-separation
2022 [71]	Bone	None	PTFE, Al	Movement	30 μA	Bone repair	Lateral sliding
2019 [74]	Head, rat	2 × 2	PET, PTFE	Movement	430 mV	Hair regeneration	Lateral sliding
2019 [77]	Muscle	10 × 10	PTFE, PET	Movement	95 μW	Muscle repair	Contact-separation
2018 [81]	Heart	1 × 2	Celllose, Chitin, RP, SF, and EW	None	0.6 μA	Heart disease treatment	Contact-separation
2022 [82]	Wound	None	PDA, PVDF	Press	42 mV	Wound repair	Contact-separation
2022 [83]	Wound	4 × 4	PPy	Press	33 mW m^{-2}	Wound repair	Contact-separation
2021 [84]	Stomach	10	PET, PTFE, Pt	Micro vibration	185 mV	Sterilization	Contact-separation
2022 [85]	None	5 × 5	Fluornated Polyurethane	Press	22 μA	Sterilization	Contact-separation
2022 [86]	Solution	None	CCTO-BMF, Cu, Acrylic	Gravity	322 μA	Sterilization	Contact-separation
2021 [90]	Subcutaneous, rat	1.5 × 1.5	Polyacrylamide, Graphene	Ultrasonic drive	1.6 mA	Anti inflammatory Treatment of sepsis	Contact-separation
2020 [91]	Hand	None	Polyester, PDMS	Hand movement	2.47 V	Auxiliary physical Therapy	Contact-separation
2022 [93]	Knee	None	Kapton, Cu	Movement	35 V	Treatment of knee osteoarthritis	Contact-separation
2022 [94]	Internal environment	None	PVDF, PA Cr/Ag electrode	Micro vibration	3.7 μA	Promote drug absorption	Lateral sliding
2020 [95]	Internal environment	None	PDMS, PET, PVA	Micro vibration	165.6 μA	Drug transportation	Contact-separation

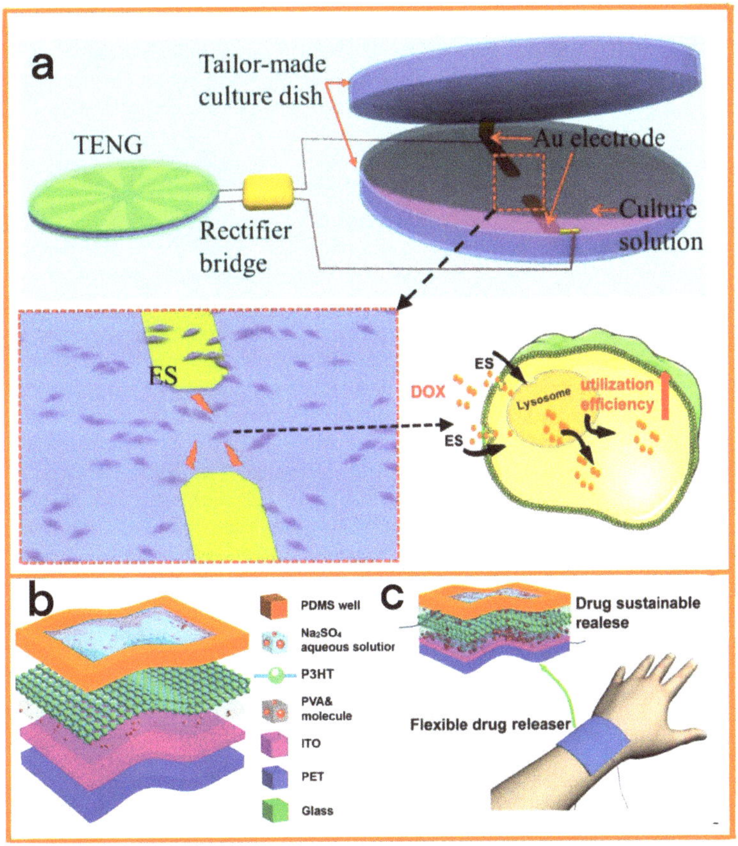

Figure 13. (**a**) Diagram of the equipment and schematic diagram of the co-culture of cells and DOX after electrical stimulation. Reprinted with permission from [94]. 2022, Frontiers. (**b**) Structural diagram of this TENG. (**c**) Schematic diagram of the sustainable release of salicylic acid. Reprinted with permission from [95]. 2020, John Wiley and Sons.

Liu et al. also designed a self-powered drug delivery device (FDRD) [95]. The device integrated three TENG units, each consisting of multi-layer flexible structures (Figure 13b) that effectively collect disordered biological energy from the environment, providing electrical power for the device. At the same time, the device monitors the flow of small molecules (such as salicylic acid, which has exfoliating, bactericidal, and anti-inflammatory effects) out of the FDRD in real time (Figure 13c), and provides vital data support for the long-term personalized treatment of patients by recording and analyzing the flow rate of small molecules.

5. Conclusions and Perspectives

In the current paper, recent advances in TENG-based medical equipment for the diagnosis and long-term treatment of disease have been concisely introduced, and the corresponding design strategies, including design concepts, operation principles, and the problems and solutions of the designs, have been described in detail. For better understanding, the developed self-powered multifunctional systems described under the categories of bioenergy collection, real-time diagnosis, and long-term treatment. In addition to power enhancement measures, TENGs have also been developed with flexible structures so that they can be integrated with other electronics to achieve a perfect fit to skin or can be implanted. Meanwhile, TENGs can also be constructed using different raw materials to improve their biological safety and antibacterial performance and reduce discomfort to the body.

However, currently, having reached a stage beyond exploratory research, there are huge obstacles to achieving practical application of TENG-based clinical systems that persist due to the well-defined test environments in labs. Some of these shortcomings may arise from the systems, while some shortcomings lie in TENGs themselves.

5.1. TENG Energy Collection

5.1.1. Increased Output Power

When considering clinical applications, there are three main ways of improving the power output of devices: modifying the surface of the friction layer, choosing a biocompatible friction layer with a high surface charge, and changing the overall structure of the TENG.

Techniques for achieving the surface modification of the friction layer can be categorized into chemical and physical methods, whereby chemical processes involve the grafting of chemical groups to assist in electron transmission, while physical methods primarily employ modeling, laser engraving, plasma processing, etc., to change the surface contact area of the friction layer. The correct combination of the two approaches can be used to improve the output power.

For the long-term power supply of medical devices, in the future, it will be necessary to focus on finding materials with higher friction electronegativity and pay attention to the biological safety of new materials. When modifying the surface of the friction layer, it is necessary to find surface structures that can be adapted to the human body's internal environment in order to reduce rejection. The overall structure of TENGs is also an essential factor affecting triboelectricity and biocompatibility. Additionally, the design of structures that can achieve greater integration with the human body, that are more comfortable to wear, and that are more in line with physical laws is also a major future research direction.

5.1.2. Stability

It is essential to maintain a stable power supply in the treatment of long-term diseases. Most TENGs generate electricity through continuous contact between layers. Therefore, the corresponding loss in the friction layer is significant. Therefore, in order to reduce this loss and improve the service life and stability of TENGs, attention should be paid in the future to the identification of wear-resistant materials or new friction methods with low rates of loss.

In addition, some TENGs and medical devices need to be integrated into the human internal environment. Therefore, the need to improve the service life of TENGs in the human internal environment should be taken into account. Thus, in the future, acid- and alkali-resistant materials should be employed, or existing materials should be modified in order to improve their acid and alkali resistance. Secondly, waterproof coatings could also be added to the materials in order to reduce the impact of humid environments on the efficiency of power generation using TENGs. When using TENGs for medical diagnosis, various complex minor disturbances in the human body can seriously affect the stability of the devices. Therefore, in the future, interference could be reduced or eliminated by adding filter circuits.

5.2. *TENGs for Diagnosis*

5.2.1. Wireless Data Transmission

For long-term monitoring of diseases, it is necessary to continuously collect relevant data for further analysis. Currently, due to the relatively bulky nature of traditional cables, wireless transmission is mostly used. However, wireless communication is highly dependent on the chip, and its energy consumption is relatively high, which affects the stability of the device. Therefore, a future research direction would be a focus on the selection of more energy-efficient wireless transmission methods, such as by using the electrostatic induction effect to drive nearby coils via TENGs to achieve signal transmission. However, due to the significant internal resistance of TENGs, the transmission effect of this technology is not ideal. Therefore, in the future, the internal resistance of TENGs could be improved, making it possible to use TENG drive coils for signal transmission.

5.2.2. Higher Sensitivity

With the continuous development of modern medicine, greater sensitivity is required for the diagnosis of some diseases. To improve the sensitivity of devices in the future, more sensitive materials can be developed, and interference from the environment can be reduced by employing multiple groups of filter circuits. At the same time, accurate structural customization is also an important method of reducing errors in the systems. For example, overall structural error can be reduced through the use of high-precision 3D printing or laser etching.

5.2.3. Comfortability

Since diagnostic equipment needs to be worn for a long time, its comfort is of great importance. In this regard, new methods and materials should be explored to improve the comfort of the equipment. For example, the use of improved raw materials such as natural fibers such as cotton, silk, hemp, and cotton silk can achieve properties such as air permeability and hydrophobicity. It is widely known that a high degree of customizability will lead to an enhanced degree of fitting between the device and the skin. Similarly, from the perspective of overall design and aesthetics, personalized design of the appearance can be carried out in combination with clinical experiments to enhance practicability.

5.3. *TENG for Treatment*

5.3.1. Biosafety

Output power is not the only indicator of TENG in long-term treatment. Biosafety is very important for improving treatment quality for patients and reducing pain and side effects. Currently, the mainstream option is for biocompatible encapsulation materials in order to avoid human contact with the TENG equipment. However, due to the complex structure of the human body, encapsulation materials cannot guarantee that leakage will not occur, especially in the case of implantable treatment equipment. Human bodily fluids can flow into TENG equipment, affecting its normal functioning, while also resulting in a human rejection reaction. Therefore, it is important to carefully select the raw materials and optimize the structure of the packaging layer to improve environmental tolerance. In addition, assessment of long-term biosafety should be carried out with respect to manufacturing methods and raw materials in order to reduce the occurrence of accidents.

5.3.2. Multifunctionality

For medical devices that need to be worn for a long time, increasing the number of functionalities of TENGs is of great significance for improving patients' quality of life. For example, the integration of power supply, sensing, treatment, and other functions could be considered in these devices. This could lead to optimization of the volume of the equipment and reduce unnecessary time wastage, as well as being more convenient and straightforward. However, due to the requirements of convenience, space in such equipment is relatively limited, so seamlessly integrating these functions in practical application remains a challenge. Secondly, with the increasing integration of processes, such treatment equipment will require the supply of larger amounts of power, and it will also be necessary to improve the output power of TENGs. By achieving miniaturization, integrated multifunctional treatment devices would undoubtedly be of great help in the long-term treatment of disease.

5.3.3. Degradability

One of the advantages of degradable technology is that device removal surgery, which may lead to secondary infection, does not need to be carried out. Therefore, the risk of infection due to long-term treatment with implantable devices can be significantly reduced. Still, due to the complexity of the human environment, the output performance and degradability of TENGs need to be carefully balanced, and blindly pursuing degradability may result in a decrease in the service life of the TENG. Based on the current research, there are a number of natural materials that are good options, including cellulose, chitin, etc., as they can be absorbed by the human body, thus reducing unnecessary side effects. However, systematic research is still needed regarding their chemical properties, and finding the optimal balance between degradation time and output performance is still a big challenge.

Author Contributions: Z.Z.: investigation, writing—original draft and editing, conceptualization. Y.L.: resources, supervision, conceptualization, validation. Y.M.: resources, supervision, conceptualization, validation. J.M.: resources, supervision, conceptualization, validation. X.W.: resources, supervision, conceptualization, validation. X.C.: resources, supervision, conceptualization, validation. N.W.: resources, supervision, conceptualization, validation. All authors have read and agreed to the published version of the manuscript.

Funding: This work was financially supported by the National Natural Science Foundation of China (NSFC Nos. 51873020), and the Fundamental Research Funds for the Central Universities (No. FRF-MP-20-38). Patents have been filed to protect the reported inventions.

Institutional Review Board Statement: Not applicable.

Informed Consent Statement: Not applicable.

Data Availability Statement: Data available on request from the authors.

Conflicts of Interest: The authors declare no conflict of interest.

References

1. Chen, X.; Xie, X.; Liu, Y.; Zhao, C.; Wen, M.; Wen, Z. Advances in Healthcare Electronics Enabled by Triboelectric Nanogenerators. *Adv. Funct. Mater.* **2020**, *30*, 2004673. [CrossRef]
2. Parandeh, S.; Etemadi, N.; Kharaziha, M.; Chen, G.; Nashalian, A.; Xiao, X.; Chen, J. Advances in Triboelectric Nanogenerators for Self-Powered Regenerative Medicine. *Adv. Funct. Mater.* **2021**, *31*, 2105169. [CrossRef]
3. Salauddin, M.; Rana, S.S.; Sharifuzzaman, M.; Lee, S.H.; Zahed, M.A.; Do Shin, Y.; Seonu, S.; Song, H.S.; Bhatta, T.; Park, J.Y. Laser-Carbonized MXene/ZiF-67 Nanocomposite as an Intermediate Layer for Boosting the Output Performance of Fabric-Based Triboelectric Nanogenerator. *Nano Energy* **2022**, *100*, 107462. [CrossRef]
4. Chang, C.-W.; Lin, Y.-B.; Chen, J.-C. Reporting Mechanisms for Internet of Things. *Mob. Netw. Appl.* **2022**, *27*, 118–123. [CrossRef]
5. Wang, T.; Li, S.; Tao, X.; Yan, Q.; Wang, X.; Chen, Y.; Huang, F.; Li, H.; Chen, X.; Bian, Z. Fully Biodegradable Water-Soluble Triboelectric Nanogenerator for Human Physiological Monitoring. *Nano Energy* **2022**, *93*, 106787. [CrossRef]
6. Zhao, T.; Fu, Y.; Sun, C.; Zhao, X.; Jiao, C.; Du, A.; Wang, Q.; Mao, Y.; Liu, B. Wearable Biosensors for Real-Time Sweat Analysis and Body Motion Capture Based on Stretchable Fiber-Based Triboelectric Nanogenerators. *Biosens. Bioelectron.* **2022**, *205*, 114115. [CrossRef]

7. Zhu, G.; Ren, P.; Hu, J.; Yang, J.; Jia, Y.; Chen, Z.; Ren, F.; Gao, J. Flexible and Anisotropic Strain Sensors with the Asymmetrical Cross-Conducting Network for Versatile Bio-Mechanical Signal Recognition. *ACS Appl. Mater. Interfaces* **2021**, *13*, 44925–44934. [CrossRef]
8. Zhu, G.-J.; Ren, P.-G.; Wang, J.; Duan, Q.; Ren, F.; Xia, W.-M.; Yan, D.-X. A Highly Sensitive and Broad-Range Pressure Sensor Based on Polyurethane Mesodome Arrays Embedded with Silver Nanowires. *ACS Appl. Mater. Interfaces* **2020**, *12*, 19988–19999. [CrossRef]
9. Zhao, Z.; Lu, Y.; Mi, Y.; Meng, J.; Cao, X.; Wang, N. Structural Flexibility in Triboelectric Nanogenerators: A Review on the Adaptive Design for Self-Powered Systems. *Micromachines* **2022**, *13*, 1586. [CrossRef]
10. Yin, F. Stretchable and Helically Structured Fiber Nanogenerator for Multifunctional. *Nano Energy* **2022**, *11*, 107588.
11. Ye, C.; Liu, D.; Peng, X.; Jiang, Y.; Cheng, R.; Ning, C.; Sheng, F.; Zhang, Y.; Dong, K.; Wang, Z.L. A Hydrophobic Self-Repairing Power Textile for Effective Water Droplet Energy Harvesting. *ACS Nano* **2021**, *15*, 18172–18181. [CrossRef] [PubMed]
12. Yang, D.; Ni, Y.; Kong, X.; Li, S.; Chen, X.; Zhang, L.; Wang, Z.L. Self-Healing and Elastic Triboelectric Nanogenerators for Muscle Motion Monitoring and Photothermal Treatment. *ACS Nano* **2021**, *15*, 14653–14661. [CrossRef] [PubMed]
13. Wu, Y.; Li, Y.; Zou, Y.; Rao, W.; Gai, Y.; Xue, J.; Wu, L.; Qu, X.; Liu, Y.; Xu, G.; et al. A Multi-Mode Triboelectric Nanogenerator for Energy Harvesting and Biomedical Monitoring. *Nano Energy* **2022**, *92*, 106715. [CrossRef]
14. Wu, Y.; Dai, X.; Sun, Z.; Zhu, S.; Xiong, L.; Liang, Q.; Wong, M.-C.; Huang, L.-B.; Qin, Q.; Hao, J. Highly Integrated, Scalable Manufacturing and Stretchable Conductive Core/Shell Fibers for Strain Sensing and Self-Powered Smart Textiles. *Nano Energy* **2022**, *98*, 107240. [CrossRef]
15. Wu, H.; Yang, G.; Zhu, K.; Liu, S.; Guo, W.; Jiang, Z.; Li, Z. Materials, Devices, and Systems of On-Skin Electrodes for Electrophysiological Monitoring and Human–Machine Interfaces. *Adv. Sci.* **2021**, *8*, 2001938. [CrossRef]
16. Wang, J.; He, J.; Ma, L.; Yao, Y.; Zhu, X.; Peng, L.; Liu, X.; Li, K.; Qu, M. A Humidity-Resistant, Stretchable and Wearable Textile-Based Triboelectric Nanogenerator for Mechanical Energy Harvesting and Multifunctional Self-Powered Haptic Sensing. *Chem. Eng. J.* **2021**, *423*, 130200. [CrossRef]
17. Zhang, L.; Duan, Q.; Meng, X.; Jin, K.; Xu, J.; Sun, J.; Wang, Q. Experimental Investigation on Intermittent Spray Cooling and Toxic Hazards of Lithium-Ion Battery Thermal Runaway. *Energy Convers. Manag.* **2022**, *252*, 115091. [CrossRef]
18. Siczek, K. The Toxicity of Secondary Lithium-Sulfur Batteries Components. *Batteries* **2020**, *6*, 45. [CrossRef]
19. Qiao, Y.; Wang, S.; Gao, F.; Li, X.; Fan, M.; Yang, R. Toxicity Analysis of Second Use Lithium-Ion Battery Separator and Electrolyte. *Polym. Test.* **2020**, *81*, 106175. [CrossRef]
20. Khan, M.S.; Javed, M.; Rehman, M.T.; Urooj, M.; Ahmad, M.I. Heavy Metal Pollution and Risk Assessment by the Battery of Toxicity Tests. *Sci. Rep.* **2020**, *10*, 16593. [CrossRef]
21. Gao, Z.; Yu, H.; Li, M.; Li, X.; Lei, J.; He, D.; Wu, G.; Fu, Y.; Chen, Q.; Shi, H. A Battery of Baseline Toxicity Bioassays Directed Evaluation of Plastic Leachates—Towards the Establishment of Bioanalytical Monitoring Tools for Plastics. *Sci. Total Environ.* **2022**, *828*, 154387. [CrossRef] [PubMed]
22. Arefi-Oskoui, S.; Khataee, A.; Ucun, O.K.; Kobya, M.; Hanci, T.Ö.; Arslan-Alaton, I. Toxicity Evaluation of Bulk and Nanosheet MoS_2 Catalysts Using Battery Bioassays. *Chemosphere* **2021**, *268*, 128822. [CrossRef] [PubMed]
23. Dale, M.T.; Elkins, M.R. Chronic Disease. *J. Physiother.* **2021**, *67*, 84–86. [CrossRef] [PubMed]
24. Xiao, X.; Chen, G.; Libanori, A.; Chen, J. Wearable Triboelectric Nanogenerators for Therapeutics. *Trends Chem.* **2021**, *3*, 279–290. [CrossRef]
25. Xia, X.; Liu, Q.; Zhu, Y.; Zi, Y. Recent Advances of Triboelectric Nanogenerator Based Applications in Biomedical Systems. *EcoMat* **2020**, *2*, e12049. [CrossRef]
26. Meng, K.; Zhao, S.; Zhou, Y.; Wu, Y.; Zhang, S.; He, Q.; Wang, X.; Zhou, Z.; Fan, W.; Tan, X.; et al. A Wireless Textile-Based Sensor System for Self-Powered Personalized Health Care. *Matter* **2020**, *2*, 896–907. [CrossRef]
27. Shen, S.; Xiao, X.; Xiao, X.; Chen, J. Triboelectric Nanogenerators for Self-Powered Breath Monitoring. *ACS Appl. Energy Mater.* **2022**, *5*, 3952–3965. [CrossRef]
28. Kou, H.; Wang, H.; Cheng, R.; Liao, Y.; Shi, X.; Luo, J.; Li, D.; Wang, Z.L. Smart Pillow Based on Flexible and Breathable Triboelectric Nanogenerator Arrays for Head Movement Monitoring during Sleep. *ACS Appl. Mater. Interfaces* **2022**, *14*, 23998–24007. [CrossRef] [PubMed]
29. Mariello, M.; Scarpa, E.; Algieri, L.; Guido, F.; Mastronardi, V.M.; Qualtieri, A.; De Vittorio, M. Novel Flexible Triboelectric Nanogenerator Based on Metallized Porous PDMS and Parylene C. *Energies* **2020**, *13*, 1625. [CrossRef]
30. Lu, Z.; Jia, C.; Yang, X.; Zhu, Y.; Sun, F.; Zhao, T.; Zhang, S.; Mao, Y. A Flexible TENG Based on Micro-Structure Film for Speed Skating Techniques Monitoring and Biomechanical Energy Harvesting. *Nanomaterials* **2022**, *12*, 1576. [CrossRef]
31. Li, W.; Lu, L.; Kottapalli, A.G.P.; Pei, Y. Bioinspired Sweat-Resistant Wearable Triboelectric Nanogenerator for Movement Monitoring during Exercise. *Nano Energy* **2022**, *95*, 107018. [CrossRef]
32. Li, M.; Xu, B.; Li, Z.; Gao, Y.; Yang, Y.; Huang, X. Toward 3D Double-Electrode Textile Triboelectric Nanogenerators for Wearable Biomechanical Energy Harvesting and Sensing. *Chem. Eng. J.* **2022**, *450*, 137491. [CrossRef]
33. Li, L.; Chen, Y.-T.; Hsiao, Y.-C.; Lai, Y.-C. Mycena Chlorophos-Inspired Autoluminescent Triboelectric Fiber for Wearable Energy Harvesting, Self-Powered Sensing, and as Human–Device Interfaces. *Nano Energy* **2022**, *94*, 106944. [CrossRef]
34. Wang, Z.L. Self-Powered Nanosensors and Nanosystems. *Adv. Mater.* **2012**, *24*, 280–285. [CrossRef] [PubMed]

35. Liu, S.; Wang, H.; He, T.; Dong, S.; Lee, C. Switchable Textile-Triboelectric Nanogenerators (S-TENGs) for Continuous Profile Sensing Application without Environmental Interferences. *Nano Energy* **2020**, *69*, 104462. [CrossRef]
36. Ji, S.; Fu, T.; Hu, Y. Effect of Surface Texture on the Output Performance of Lateral Sliding-Mode Triboelectric Nanogenerator. *J. Phys. Conf. Ser.* **2020**, *1549*, 042095. [CrossRef]
37. Manjari Padhan, A.; Hajra, S.; Sahu, M.; Nayak, S.; Joon Kim, H.; Alagarsamy, P. Single-Electrode Mode TENG Using Ferromagnetic NiO−Ti Based Nanocomposite for Effective Energy Harvesting. *Mater. Lett.* **2022**, *312*, 131644. [CrossRef]
38. Opportunities and Challenges in Triboelectric Nanogenerator (TENG) Based Sustainable Energy Generation Technologies: A Mini-Review. *Chem. Eng. J. Adv.* **2022**, *9*, 100237. [CrossRef]
39. Zhao, L.; Li, H.; Meng, J.; Li, Z. The Recent Advances in Self-powered Medical Information Sensors. *InfoMat* **2020**, *2*, 212–234. [CrossRef]
40. Chen, H.; Zhang, S.; Zou, Y.; Zhang, C.; Zheng, B.; Huang, C.; Zhang, B.; Xing, C.; Xu, Y.; Wang, J. Performance-Enhanced Flexible Triboelectric Nanogenerator Based on Gold Chloride-Doped Graphene. *ACS Appl. Electron. Mater.* **2020**, *2*, 1106–1112. [CrossRef]
41. Saqib, Q.M.; Shaukat, R.A.; Chougale, M.Y.; Khan, M.U.; Kim, J.; Bae, J. Particle Triboelectric Nanogenerator (P-TENG). *Nano Energy* **2022**, *100*, 107475. [CrossRef]
42. Park, J.H.; Wu, C.; Sung, S.; Kim, T.W. Ingenious Use of Natural Triboelectrification on the Human Body for Versatile Applications in Walking Energy Harvesting and Body Action Monitoring. *Nano Energy* **2019**, *57*, 872–878. [CrossRef]
43. Zhu, P.; Zhang, B.; Wang, H.; Wu, Y.; Cao, H.; He, L.; Li, C.; Luo, X.; Li, X.; Mao, Y. 3D Printed Triboelectric Nanogenerator as Self-Powered Human-Machine Interactive Sensor for Breathing-Based Language Expression. *Nano Res.* **2022**, *15*, 7460–7467. [CrossRef]
44. Liu, Y.; Zheng, Y.; Wu, Z.; Zhang, L.; Sun, W.; Li, T.; Wang, D.; Zhou, F. Conductive Elastic Sponge-Based Triboelectric Nanogenerator (TENG) for Effective Random Mechanical Energy Harvesting and Ammonia Sensing. *Nano Energy* **2021**, *79*, 105422. [CrossRef]
45. Halappanavar, S.; Nymark, P.; Krug, H.F.; Clift, M.J.D.; Rothen-Rutishauser, B.; Vogel, U. Non-Animal Strategies for Toxicity Assessment of Nanoscale Materials: Role of Adverse Outcome Pathways in the Selection of Endpoints. *Small* **2021**, *17*, 2007628. [CrossRef]
46. Mukherjee, S.; Rananaware, P.; Brahmkhatri, V.; Mishra, M. Polyvinylpyrrolidone-Curcumin Nanoconjugate as a Biocompatible, Non-Toxic Material for Biological Applications. *J. Clust. Sci.* **2022**, 1–20. [CrossRef]
47. Pierau, L.; Elian, C.; Akimoto, J.; Ito, Y.; Caillol, S.; Versace, D.-L. Bio-Sourced Monomers and Cationic Photopolymerization–The Green Combination towards Eco-Friendly and Non-Toxic Materials. *Prog. Polym. Sci.* **2022**, *127*, 101517. [CrossRef]
48. Zeiner, M.; Juranović Cindrić, I. Review–Trace Determination of Potentially Toxic Elements in (Medicinal) Plant Materials. *Anal. Methods* **2017**, *9*, 1550–1574. [CrossRef]
49. Zhao, D.; Zhuo, J.; Chen, Z.; Wu, J.; Ma, R.; Zhang, X.; Zhang, Y.; Wang, X.; Wei, X.; Liu, L.; et al. Eco-Friendly in-Situ Gap Generation of No-Spacer Triboelectric Nanogenerator for Monitoring Cardiovascular Activities. *Nano Energy* **2021**, *90*, 106580. [CrossRef]
50. Yao, G.; Kang, L.; Li, J.; Long, Y.; Wei, H.; Ferreira, C.A.; Jeffery, J.J.; Lin, Y.; Cai, W.; Wang, X. Effective Weight Control via an Implanted Self-Powered Vagus Nerve Stimulation Device. *Nat. Commun.* **2018**, *9*, 5349. [CrossRef]
51. Liu, Z.; Ma, Y.; Ouyang, H.; Shi, B.; Li, N.; Jiang, D.; Xie, F.; Qu, D.; Zou, Y.; Huang, Y.; et al. Transcatheter Self-Powered Ultrasensitive Endocardial Pressure Sensor. *Adv. Funct. Mater.* **2019**, *29*, 1807560. [CrossRef]
52. Shi, B.; Liu, Z.; Zheng, Q.; Meng, J.; Ouyang, H.; Zou, Y.; Jiang, D.; Qu, X.; Yu, M.; Zhao, L.; et al. Body-Integrated Self-Powered System for Wearable and Implantable Applications. *ACS Nano* **2019**, *13*, 6017–6024. [CrossRef]
53. Lorenzo, E.; Evangelista, L.S. Disparities in Cardiovascular Disease: Examining the Social Determinants of Health. *Eur. J. Cardiovasc. Nurs.* **2022**, *21*, 187–189. [CrossRef] [PubMed]
54. Ran, X.; Luo, F.; Lin, Z.; Zhu, Z.; Liu, C.; Chen, B. Blood Pressure Monitoring via Double Sandwich-Structured Triboelectric Sensors and Deep Learning Models. *Nano Res.* **2022**, *15*, 5500–5509. [CrossRef]
55. Xu, L.; Zhang, Z.; Gao, F.; Zhao, X.; Xun, X.; Kang, Z.; Liao, Q.; Zhang, Y. Self-Powered Ultrasensitive Pulse Sensors for Noninvasive Multi-Indicators Cardiovascular Monitoring. *Nano Energy* **2021**, *81*, 105614. [CrossRef]
56. Wang, X.; Feng, Z.; Xia, Y.; Zhang, G.; Wang, L.; Chen, L.; Wu, Y.; Yang, J.; Wang, Z.L. Flexible Pressure Sensor for High-Precision Measurement of Epidermal Arterial Pulse. *Nano Energy* **2022**, *102*, 107710. [CrossRef]
57. Zou, X.H. Advances in Pathogen Diagnosis of Respiratory Infection Diseases in 2021. *Chin. J. Tuberc. Respir. Dis.* **2022**, *45*, 78–82. [CrossRef]
58. Wang, Y.; Xu, H.; Dong, Z.; Wang, Z.; Yang, Z.; Yu, X.; Chang, L. Micro/Nano Biomedical Devices for Point-of-Care Diagnosis of Infectious Respiratory Diseases. *Med. Nov. Technol. Devices* **2022**, *14*, 100116. [CrossRef]
59. Fernández, L.R.; Hernández, R.G.; Guerediaga, I.S.; Gato, J.M.; Fanjul, J.R.; Bilbao, V.A.; Quintela, P.A.; Ojembarrena, A.A. Usefulness of Lung Ultrasound in the Diagnosis and Follow-up of Respiratory Diseases in Neonates. *An. Pediatría Engl. Ed.* **2022**, *96*, 252.e1–252.e13. [CrossRef]
60. Wang, D.; Zhang, D.; Chen, X.; Zhang, H.; Tang, M.; Wang, J. Multifunctional Respiration-Driven Triboelectric Nanogenerator for Self-Powered Detection of Formaldehyde in Exhaled Gas and Respiratory Behavior. *Nano Energy* **2022**, *102*, 107711. [CrossRef]
61. Ma, X.; Xu, S.; Li, L.; Wang, Z. A Novel SERS Method for the Detection of Staphylococcus Aureus without Immobilization Based on Au@Ag NPs/Slide Substrate. *Spectrochim. Acta. A. Mol. Biomol. Spectrosc.* **2023**, *284*, 121757. [CrossRef] [PubMed]

62. Wang, C.; Wang, P.; Chen, J.; Zhu, L.; Zhang, D.; Wan, Y.; Ai, S. Self-Powered Biosensing System Driven by Triboelectric Nanogenerator for Specific Detection of Gram-Positive Bacteria. *Nano Energy* **2022**, *93*, 106828. [CrossRef]
63. Peng, X.; Dong, K.; Ning, C.; Cheng, R.; Yi, J.; Zhang, Y.; Sheng, F.; Wu, Z.; Wang, Z.L. All-Nanofiber Self-Powered Skin-Interfaced Real-Time Respiratory Monitoring System for Obstructive Sleep Apnea-Hypopnea Syndrome Diagnosing. *Adv. Funct. Mater.* **2021**, *31*, 2103559. [CrossRef]
64. Kim, J.-N.; Lee, J.; Lee, H.; Oh, I.-K. Stretchable and Self-Healable Catechol-Chitosan-Diatom Hydrogel for Triboelectric Generator and Self-Powered Tremor Sensor Targeting at Parkinson Disease. *Nano Energy* **2021**, *82*, 105705. [CrossRef]
65. Vera Anaya, D.; Yuce, M.R. Stretchable Triboelectric Sensor for Measurement of the Forearm Muscles Movements and Fingers Motion for Parkinson's Disease Assessment and Assisting Technologies. *Med. Devices Sens.* **2021**, *4*, e10154. [CrossRef]
66. Chu, X.-L.; Song, X.-Z.; Li, Q.; Li, Y.-R.; He, F.; Gu, X.-S.; Ming, D. Basic Mechanisms of Peripheral Nerve Injury and Treatment via Electrical Stimulation. *Neural Regen. Res.* **2022**, *17*, 2185. [CrossRef]
67. Cintron-Colon, A.; Almeida-Alves, G.; VanGyseghem, J.; Spitsbergen, J. GDNF to the Rescue: GDNF Delivery Effects on Motor Neurons and Nerves, and Muscle Re-Innervation after Peripheral Nerve Injuries. *Neural Regen. Res.* **2022**, *17*, 748. [CrossRef]
68. Li, C.; Liu, S.-Y.; Pi, W.; Zhang, P.-X. Cortical Plasticity and Nerve Regeneration after Peripheral Nerve Injury. *Neural Regen. Res.* **2021**, *16*, 1518. [CrossRef]
69. Zhou, M.; Huang, M.; Zhong, H.; Xing, C.; An, Y.; Zhu, R.; Jia, Z.; Qu, H.; Zhu, S.; Liu, S.; et al. Contact Separation Triboelectric Nanogenerator Based Neural Interfacing for Effective Sciatic Nerve Restoration. *Adv. Funct. Mater.* **2022**, *32*, 2200269. [CrossRef]
70. Shlomy, I.; Divald, S.; Tadmor, K.; Leichtmann-Bardoogo, Y.; Arami, A.; Maoz, B.M. Restoring Tactile Sensation Using a Triboelectric Nanogenerator. *ACS Nano* **2021**, *15*, 11087–11098. [CrossRef]
71. Wang, B.; Li, G.; Zhu, Q.; Liu, W.; Ke, W.; Hua, W.; Zhou, Y.; Zeng, X.; Sun, X.; Wen, Z.; et al. Bone Repairment via Mechanosensation of Piezo1 Using Wearable Pulsed Triboelectric Nanogenerator. *Small* **2022**, *18*, 2201056. [CrossRef]
72. Heymann, W.R. The Inflammatory Component of Androgenetic Alopecia. *J. Am. Acad. Dermatol.* **2022**, *86*, 301–302. [CrossRef]
73. Satcher, K.G.; Schoch, J.J.; Walker, A. Alopecia in Hereditary Mucoepithelial Dysplasia. *J. Cutan. Pathol.* **2022**, *49*, 103–105. [CrossRef] [PubMed]
74. Yao, G.; Jiang, D.; Li, J.; Kang, L.; Chen, S.; Long, Y.; Wang, Y.; Huang, P.; Lin, Y.; Cai, W.; et al. Self-Activated Electrical Stimulation for Effective Hair Regeneration via a Wearable Omnidirectional Pulse Generator. *ACS Nano* **2019**, *13*, 12345–12356. [CrossRef]
75. Cung, S.; Pyle, L.; Nadeau, K.; Dabelea, D.; Cree-Green, M.; Davis, S.M. In-Vivo Skeletal Muscle Mitochondrial Function in Klinefelter Syndrome. *J. Investig. Med.* **2022**, *70*, 104–107. [CrossRef] [PubMed]
76. Dassios, T.; Vervenioti, A.; Dimitriou, G. Respiratory Muscle Function in the Newborn: A Narrative Review. *Pediatr. Res.* **2022**, *91*, 795–803. [CrossRef] [PubMed]
77. Wang, J.; Wang, H.; Thakor, N.V.; Lee, C. Self-Powered Direct Muscle Stimulation Using a Triboelectric Nanogenerator (TENG) Integrated with a Flexible Multiple-Channel Intramuscular Electrode. *ACS Nano* **2019**, *13*, 3589–3599. [CrossRef]
78. Azarine, A.; Scalbert, F.; Garçon, P. Cardiac Functional Imaging. *Presse Médicale* **2022**, *51*, 104119. [CrossRef]
79. Lu, Z.; Jiang, Z.; Tang, J.; Lin, C.; Zhang, H. Functions and Origins of Cardiac Fat. *FEBS J.* **2022**, *2*, febs.16388. [CrossRef]
80. Weisel, R.D. Tissue Engineering to Restore Cardiac Function. *Engineering* **2022**, *13*, 13–17. [CrossRef]
81. Jiang, W.; Li, H.; Liu, Z.; Li, Z.; Tian, J.; Shi, B.; Zou, Y.; Ouyang, H.; Zhao, C.; Zhao, L.; et al. Fully Bioabsorbable Natural-Materials-Based Triboelectric Nanogenerators. *Adv. Mater.* **2018**, *30*, 1801895. [CrossRef] [PubMed]
82. Sharma, A.; Panwar, V.; Mondal, B.; Prasher, D.; Bera, M.K.; Thomas, J.; Kumar, A.; Kamboj, N.; Mandal, D.; Ghosh, D. Electrical Stimulation Induced by a Piezo-Driven Triboelectric Nanogenerator and Electroactive Hydrogel Composite, Accelerate Wound Repair. *Nano Energy* **2022**, *99*, 107419. [CrossRef]
83. Du, S.; Suo, H.; Xie, G.; Lyu, Q.; Mo, M.; Xie, Z.; Zhou, N.; Zhang, L.; Tao, J.; Zhu, J. Self-Powered and Photothermal Electronic Skin Patches for Accelerating Wound Healing. *Nano Energy* **2022**, *93*, 106906. [CrossRef]
84. Lin, Z.-H.; Hsu, W.-S.; Preet, A.; Yeh, L.-H.; Chen, Y.-H.; Pao, Y.-P.; Lin, S.-F.; Lee, S.; Fan, J.-C.; Wang, L.; et al. Ingestible Polysaccharide Battery Coupled with a Self-Charging Nanogenerator for Controllable Disinfection System. *Nano Energy* **2021**, *79*, 105440. [CrossRef]
85. Feng, H.; Li, H.; Xu, J.; Yin, Y.; Cao, J.; Yu, R.; Wang, B.; Li, R.; Zhu, G. Triboelectric Nanogenerator Based on Direct Image Lithography and Surface Fluorination for Biomechanical Energy Harvesting and Self-Powered Sterilization. *Nano Energy* **2022**, *98*, 107279. [CrossRef]
86. Huo, Z.; Lee, D.; Jeong, J.; Kim, Y.; Kim, J.; Suh, I.; Xiong, P.; Kim, S. Microbial Disinfection with Supercoiling Capacitive Triboelectric Nanogenerator. *Adv. Energy Mater.* **2022**, *12*, 2103680. [CrossRef]
87. Kaplan, R.L.; Cruz, A.T.; Freedman, S.B.; Smith, K.; Freeman, J.; Lane, R.D.; Michelson, K.A.; Marble, R.D.; Middelberg, L.K.; Bergmann, K.R.; et al. Omphalitis and Concurrent Serious Bacterial Infection. *Pediatrics* **2022**, *149*, e2021054189. [CrossRef]
88. Vannata, B.; Pirosa, M.C.; Bertoni, F.; Rossi, D.; Zucca, E. Bacterial Infection-Driven Lymphomagenesis. *Curr. Opin. Oncol.* **2022**, *34*, 454–463. [CrossRef]
89. Ashby, T.; Staiano, P.; Najjar, N.; Louis, M. Bacterial Pneumonia Infection in Pregnancy. *Best Pract. Res. Clin. Obstet. Gynaecol.* 2022. *in press*. [CrossRef]
90. Chen, P.; Wang, Q.; Wan, X.; Yang, M.; Liu, C.; Xu, C.; Hu, B.; Feng, J.; Luo, Z. Wireless Electrical Stimulation of the Vagus Nerves by Ultrasound-Responsive Programmable Hydrogel Nanogenerators for Anti-Inflammatory Therapy in Sepsis. *Nano Energy* **2021**, *89*, 106327. [CrossRef]
91. Zhou, Z.; Chen, K.; Li, X.; Zhang, S.; Wu, Y.; Zhou, Y.; Meng, K.; Sun, C.; He, Q.; Fan, W.; et al. Sign-to-Speech Translation Using Machine-Learning-Assisted Stretchable Sensor Arrays. *Nat. Electron.* **2020**, *3*, 571–578. [CrossRef]

92. Vera Anaya, D.F.; Yuce, M.R. A Hands-Free Human-Computer-Interface Platform for Paralyzed Patients Using a TENG-Based Eyelash Motion Sensor. In Proceedings of the 2020 42nd Annual International Conference of the IEEE Engineering in Medicine & Biology Society (EMBC); IEEE: Montreal, QC, Canada, July, 2020; pp. 4567–4570.
93. Luo, J.; Li, Y.; He, M.; Wang, Z.; Li, C.; Liu, D.; An, J.; Xie, W.; He, Y.; Xiao, W.; et al. Rehabilitation of Total Knee Arthroplasty by Integrating Conjoint Isometric Myodynamia and Real-Time Rotation Sensing System. *Adv. Sci.* **2022**, *9*, 2105219. [CrossRef] [PubMed]
94. Chen, Q.; Deng, W.; He, J.; Cheng, L.; Ren, P.-G.; Xu, Y. Enhancing Drug Utilization Efficiency via Dish-Structured Triboelectric Nanogenerator. *Front. Bioeng. Biotechnol.* **2022**, *10*, 950146. [CrossRef]
95. Liu, G.; Xu, S.; Liu, Y.; Gao, Y.; Tong, T.; Qi, Y.; Zhang, C. Flexible Drug Release Device Powered by Triboelectric Nanogenerator. *Adv. Funct. Mater.* **2020**, *30*, 1909886. [CrossRef]

biosensors

MDPI

Article

A Portable and Flexible Self-Powered Multifunctional Sensor for Real-Time Monitoring in Swimming

Yupeng Mao [1], Yongsheng Zhu [1], Tianming Zhao [1,2,3], Changjun Jia [1], Meiyue Bian [1], Xinxing Li [4], Yuanguo Liu [5] and Baodan Liu [1,2,*]

1 Physical Education Department, Northeastern University, Shenyang 110819, China; maoyupeng@pe.neu.edu.cn (Y.M.); 2001276@stu.neu.edu.cn (Y.Z.); zhaotm@stumail.neu.edu.cn (T.Z.); 2071367@stu.neu.edu.cn (C.J.); 2001264@stu.neu.edu.cn (M.B.)
2 Foshan Graduate School, Northeastern University, Foshan 528300, China
3 College of Sciences, Northeastern University, Shenyang 110819, China
4 Health and Exercise Science Laboratory, Institute of Sport Science, Seoul National University, Seoul 08826, Korea; shinsunglee2021@snu.ac.kr
5 Sports Training Institute, Shenyang Sport University, Shenyang 110102, China; liuyg@syty.edu.cn
* Correspondence: liubaodan@mail.neu.edu.cn

Abstract: A portable and flexible self-powered biosensor based on ZnO nanowire arrays (ZnO NWs) and flexible PET substrate has been designed and fabricated for real-time monitoring in swimming. Based on the piezoelectric effect of polar ZnO NWs, the fabricated biosensor can work in both air and water without any external power supply. In addition, the biosensor can be easily attached to the surface of the skin to precisely monitor the motion state such as joint moving angle and frequency during swimming. The constant output piezoelectric signal in different relative humidity levels enables actual application in different sports, including swimming. Therefore, the biosensor can be utilized to monitor swimming strokes by attaching it on the surface of the skin. Finally, a wireless transmitting application is demonstrated by implanting the biosensor in vivo to detect angiogenesis. This portable and flexible self-powered biosensor system exhibits broad application prospects in sport monitoring, human–computer interaction and wireless sport big data.

Keywords: biosensor; ZnO NWs; piezoelectric effect; self-powered; real-time monitoring

Citation: Mao, Y.; Zhu, Y.; Zhao, T.; Jia, C.; Bian, M.; Li, X.; Liu, Y.; Liu, B. A Portable and Flexible Self-Powered Multifunctional Sensor for Real-Time Monitoring in Swimming. *Biosensors* **2021**, *11*, 147. https://doi.org/10.3390/bios11050147

Received: 31 March 2021
Accepted: 5 May 2021
Published: 8 May 2021

1. Introduction

Flexible biosensors have received extensive attention in the field of clinical medicine and exercise rehabilitation, and more advanced nanomaterials have been used to monitor human health-related actions [1–6]. Physical exercises can not only prevent diseases, but also assist physical rehabilitation. Among the various sports, swimming can obviously improve cardiopulmonary function and further promote muscle formation. Moreover, swimming is also a self-help skill for humans and the most popular event in the Olympic games. In a swimming competition, athletes need to use their own high-quality skills under the condition of saving the most energy, which enables swimmers to extend the effective stroke time to achieve the best competition performance [7–11]. In swimming training, heart rate detection as a common and effective method is always used to monitor the energy consumption. The force produced by the coordination of arms and legs drives the swimmer forward quickly. The coordination involves the changes in joint angle of the whole body and the time to coordinate the forces (frequency) in the process of swimming [12,13]. Therefore, it is indispensable to monitor the joint angle of the body, motion frequency and the changes in heart rate for promoting the development of swimming skills.

Currently, the methods of swimming skill monitoring include kinematic analysis [9,13], dynamic analysis [14,15] and electromyography (EMG) analysis [16,17]. Among them, kinematic analysis mainly relies on video recording to observe the changes in swimming skills (joint angle and frequency). Dynamic analysis mostly uses joint instruments to test the force of each part on land, while EMG analysis tests the electrical signal of muscles. However, these regular monitoring methods also encounter some inevitable bottlenecks in the process of continuous development. For example, multiple cameras need to be arranged in water and underwater to collect the motion angle and frequency information in kinetic analysis [18,19] and skill in swimming needs multi-joint coordination. In this process, the position and direction of the joints are constantly changing. In order to observe their motion state, it may be necessary to arrange multi-point cameras to capture them. Therefore, monitoring is difficult and the cost is high. The lengthy recording with multiple cameras also leads to high power consumption and increases the difficulty of testing. The dynamic and EMG tests on land are also composed of multiple devices, which are very huge and cannot be used in water, increasing the complexity in dynamic swimming and making it impossible to achieve portable applications. In recent years, there have been many studies on portable human motion monitoring sensors, most of which were carried out in air [20,21]. The application of water sensors involves studies monitoring water quality [22,23]. Therefore, it is extremely urgent to develop portable, self-powered and efficient hydrophilic biosensors that are not limited by batteries and volume to precisely and quickly monitor exercise skills and heart rate changes in the future [24–30].

In this work, we report the design and integration of a self-powered, flexible biosensor based on ZnO nanowire arrays (NWs) with inter-digital electrodes. Based on the piezoelectric effect of polar ZnO, the biosensor can harvest the mechanical energy coming from body activity to drive the biosensor to monitor the motion process in air and water. In this way, the motion information and swimming skills such as the change in joint angle and motion frequency can be monitored in real time. Moreover, this study also simulates a sensor that can be attached to the big artery to detect the change in heart rate and the signals can be further transmitted based on conventional wireless technology. Therefore, the developed work and related technology of the biosensor show significant application prospects in sport monitoring, human–computer interaction and infinite sport big data.

2. Experimental

2.1. Fabrication of Self-Powered Biosensor

First, the ZnO NWs were synthesized on a PET substrate by a simple hydrothermal method, as reported in our previous work [29–34]. A 2.2 mL ammonia solution was gradually added to a 38 mL solution containing 0.8 g zinc nitrate and heated at 93 °C for 24 h. Then, the obtained vertical ZnO NWs were transferred to flexible PET substrate. Thirdly, a photolithography process and electron beam evaporation process were used to deposit the Ti electrode on both sides of ZnO NWs. The thickness of the photoresist and Ti electrodes was ~2 μm and ~200 μm, respectively. Typically, the length of ZnO NWs was more than ~10 μm to fully cover the electrode pairs (5 μm).

2.2. Characterization and Measurement

The morphology of the ZnO NWs was studied by a scanning electron microscope (SEM, JEOL JSM-6700F). The crystalline phase of ZnO NWs was characterized by X-ray diffraction (XRD, D/max 2550 V, CuKa radiation). It should be pointed out that the biosensor was placed in an open container for standard measurements and the performance on human skin was finally tested in a swimming pool. A low-noise preamplifier (Model SR560, Stanford Research Systems) was used to measure the piezoelectric output.

3. Results and Discussion

Figure 1 shows the experiment design, potential scenario and the schematic fabrication process of a self-powered biosensor in swimming monitoring. The fabrication process of the biosensor and the details of the electrode and ZnO NWs are shown in Figure 1d. Firstly, the length of vertically aligned ZnO is controlled in the range of 5–15 μm by a hydrothermal method to make sure that it can fully cover the neighboring electrodes. As schematically illustrated in Figure 1a, the flexible self-powered biosensor can be easily attached to the tester's joint in in vivo monitoring. Due to the piezoelectric effect of polar ZnO NWs, the biosensor can convert motion energy (produced by the human body in motion) into electric energy for self-driving, and work in high humidity or water, providing more potential application scenarios such as heart rate monitoring, organ monitoring and blood vessel wall monitoring. In the biosensor, the bioinformation can also be transformed by a simple Bluetooth system to monitor and collect the data, including moving frequency, the change in angle and physiology information, and thus help to formulate sport plans or adjust sport skills. Figure 1b shows the optical images of the self-powered biosensor and the attached position of the three swimming styles, and the optical micrographs of commercial LEDs connected with the biosensor that is attached to a tester's elbow joint. A simple Bluetooth wireless transmission system using a commercial signal amplification device is used as the launcher and receiver of Bluetooth in Figure 1c. It can be seen that with the increase in the output of piezoelectric voltage of the biosensor, the number of LED lamps that are turned off at the receiving end increases.

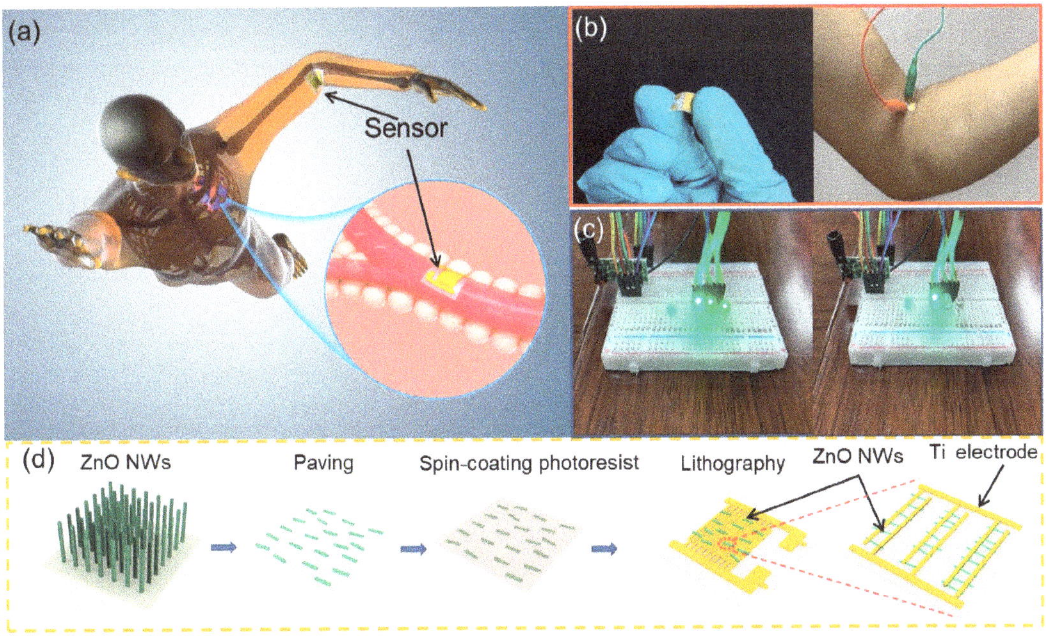

Figure 1. A potential scenario and the process of synthesis of self-powered biosensor in swimming monitoring. (**a**) Simulating the monitoring of athlete's elbow joint angle and heart rate. (**b**) Optical image of biosensor. (**c**) Simple wireless transmitter and information receiver. (**d**) Process of synthesis of self-powered biosensor.

Figure 2 shows the SEM images and XRD pattern of ZnO NWs synthesized from a hydrothermal process and the ZnO-based biosensor, as well as its schematic diagram of the piezoelectric process. It can be seen that ZnO NWs grow in the same direction and show good alignment (Figure 2a). The length of vertical ZnO crystals is about 5–10 μm, which is enough to cover the distance between electrodes (Figure 2b). Figure 2c shows the XRD pattern of ZnO NWs, inserted in the right top corner, and the sharp diffraction peaks indicate good crystalline quality. Figure 2d–i are the SEM images of ZnO nanowires on both ends of a titanium electrode. As shown in Figure 2d, ZnO nanowires are arranged in the same direction on the PET substrate. It provides an opportunity to evaporate Ti electrodes on both ends of ZnO (using photolithography). Figure 2e shows one ZnO NW crossing a pair of electrodes, and Figure 2f is an enlarged view of Figure 2e. We can confirm that the ZnO NWs are well linked with the electrodes to ensure the good transfer of electrons generated by the piezoelectric effect. Figure 2g shows the working mechanism of the ZnO NW. When the nanogenerator is bent under deformation, the two ends of the ZnO NW will provide piezoelectric potential. Figure 2h shows the working mechanism of the ZnO NW under low-humidity conditions. When the ZnO NW is exposed to a humid environment, a large number of oxygen vacancies on the surface of the ZnO NW will adsorb the water molecules in the air [31–37], and the chemical adsorption will produce ionization [38–41]. The H2O molecules dissociate into hydronium ions and hydroxide ions, which enhances the shielding effect, reducing the piezoelectric output. Additionally, as shown in Figure 2i, with the humidity continuously increasing, all the oxygen vacancies on the surface of the ZnO NWs are occupied by water molecules and form a water film. The shielding effect is saturated, so the piezoelectric voltage will remain constant in spite of the change in humidity.

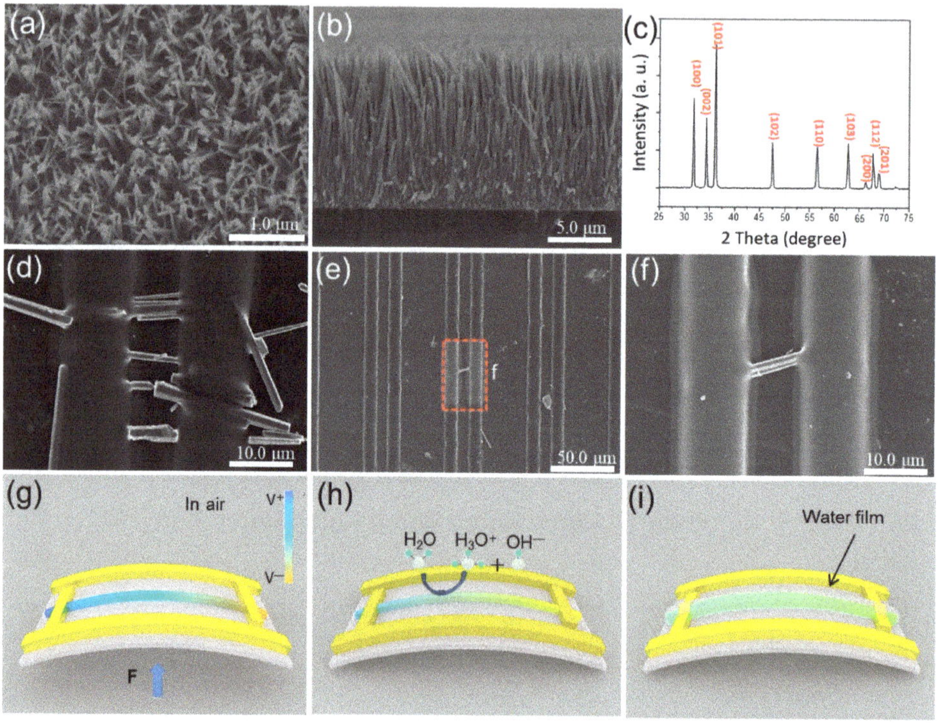

Figure 2. (**a**) Top view SEM image of ZnO. (**b**) Side view SEM image of ZnO. (**c**) XRD image of ZnO. (**d**) SEM image of ZnO NWs crossing a pair of electrodes in the same direction. (**e**) SEM image of a single ZnO NW crossing a pair of electrodes. (**f**) High-magnification morphology of a single ZnO NW crossing a pair of electrodes (Figure 2e). (**g**) Working mechanism of ZnO NW. (**h**) Working mechanism of ZnO NW under low-humidity conditions. (**i**) Working mechanism of ZnO NW under high-humidity conditions.

Figure 3 shows the self-powered biosensor working under different simulated environments and experimental controls. It can be seen that the self-powered biosensor works in different modes of air and liquid, and experimental controls show a different response to the change in humidity of the test environment or the test in water (Figure 3a). The output piezoelectric voltage of the biosensor generated at different motion frequencies is shown in Figure 3b. We can see that the output piezoelectric voltage is 0.718, 0.72, 0.731 and 0.735 V, respectively, when the biosensor is bent at 0.5, 0.75, 1.0 and 1.25 Hz at the same bending angle. The world record of the 50 m men's freestyle in a short pool is 20 " 91.

The number of arm strokes of the world's top male athletes is about 17–20 (from a video of the Olympic Games), so we tested the performance under 5 Hz (in Figure S1). It showed that the sensor can still output a stable piezoelectric signal at a high frequency, which can meet the needs of swimming monitoring. The relationship between output piezoelectric voltage and deformation at different frequencies is shown in Figure 3c. The response of the biosensor can be calculated with the following equation:

$$R\% = \left| \frac{V_0 - V_i}{V_i} \right| \times 100\%, \quad (1)$$

where V_0 is the output piezoelectric voltage under 0.5 Hz, and V_i is the output piezoelectric voltage under other frequencies. When the biosensor is bent at 0.5, 0.75, 1.0 and 1.25 Hz at the same bending angle, the corresponding response of the piezoelectric output is 0, 2, 2.2 and 2.2%. However, the output piezoelectric voltage of the biosensor is hardly changed with the variation in motion frequency, as shown in Figure 3b. From the above result, it can be seen that the output frequency of the piezoelectric voltage increases with the bending frequency, so the performance of the ZnO NW biosensor can be used to monitor the frequency change in the human body (joint). The output piezoelectric voltage of the biosensor at the same frequency and different bending angles is shown in Figure 3d. When the bending angle is set at 38, 28, 20 and 16°, the corresponding output piezoelectric voltage of biosensor is 0.254, 0.163, 0.132 and 0.105 V, respectively. The details of the output piezoelectric voltage of the biosensor as a dependency of the bending angle are plotted in Figure 3e. It can be seen that the larger the bending angle (the greater the deformation of the biosensor) is, the greater the output piezoelectric voltage is. Meanwhile, the response of the biosensor is also proportional to the variation in the bending angle. The V_0 is the output piezoelectric voltage under 38° and V_i is the output piezoelectric voltage under other bending angles. When the bending angle is set at 38, 28, 20 and 16°, the corresponding response is 0, 55.8, 92.4 and 141.9% (Figure 3f). The output piezoelectric voltage of the biosensor under deformation also shows a similar tendency as when it is bent under different angles, so it can also be used to monitor the motion angle of the human body (joint). To explore more potential applications, we tested the output piezoelectric voltage of the ZnO NW biosensor under different humidity conditions, as shown in Figure 3g. The output piezoelectric voltage of the biosensor is steady in regular conditions and a humidity level of more than 45%. This is because a large number of oxygen vacancies on the surface of the ZnO NWs adsorb water molecules [31–34] when the biosensor is exposed to a humid environment. Additionally, chemical adsorption also produces ionization [36–41] which in turn enhances the shielding effect, so the piezoelectric voltage of the ZnO NWs decreases under the same deformation conditions. When the humidity increases to 60%, the piezoelectric voltage remains stable because the oxygen vacancies on the surface of the ZnO NWs are occupied by water molecules, forming a thin water film. Then, the shielding effect does not continue to increase with the increasing humidity [25,42–47]. Furthermore, the piezoelectric voltage is not affected by the change in humidity, so the biosensor can be tested and used to monitor a swimmer in water. In our previous work, we discussed the sensing response of ZnO modified by lactate, and the unmodified ZnO had no sensing performance on sweat [5,44,45]. Sweat appears with swimming and it may be rapidly diluted by water, which may have few effects on our sensor. Therefore, the effects of sweat are not discussed in this paper. From Figure 3h, we can see that the output piezoelectric voltage of the biosensor remains stable after 6 h of continuous operation, indicating its good stability. The above data demonstrate that the designed biosensor has potential applications in sensing motion frequency, angle and humidity, and has a superior waterproof function, contributing toward reliable working life.

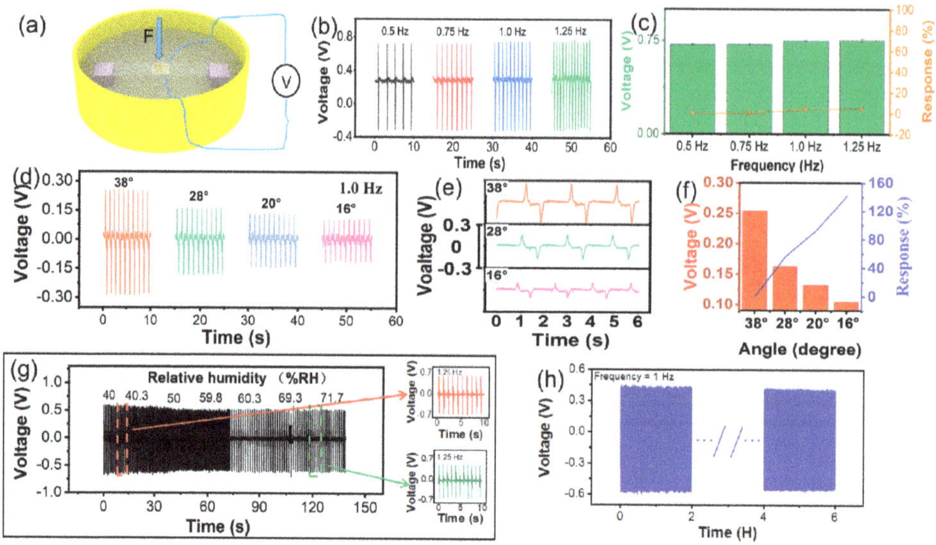

Figure 3. Experimental control of the self-powered biosensor. (**a**) Simulated experimental control of testing environment. (**b**) Output piezoelectric voltage at different motion frequencies. (**c**) Output piezoelectric voltage response at different frequencies. (**d**) Output piezoelectric voltage at the same frequency and different angles. (**e**) Details of output piezoelectric voltage of angle variation. (**f**) Output piezoelectric voltage response of angle variation. (**g**) Output piezoelectric voltage at different humidity levels. (**h**) Biosensor durability.

Figure 4 shows the schematic diagram of the ZnO NW biosensor for simulating an arterial sensing test in vitro and the output piezoelectric voltage, and a potential application scenario for monitoring the heart/internal aortic vessel is proposed. The application scenario of the biosensor is designed so that it can be attached to the blood vessel to monitor the pulse vibration (Figure 4a). As can be seen, the biosensor is attached to the simulated artery, and when the air is pumped in or out, the flexible biosensor deforms according to the simulated artery model shown in Figure 4b. In this way, the output piezoelectric voltage is produced by the biosensor when monitoring different pulse frequencies and the amplitudes of simulated arteries are shown in Figure 4c. When the pulse frequency is set at 30, 36, 48 and 60 times per minute, the output piezoelectric voltage is 0.761, 0.724, 0.557 and 0.583 V, correspondingly. We can clearly observe that the output frequency of the piezoelectric voltage changes with the increase in pulse frequency, and different deformations of the simulated arterial surface are caused by different pulses (pumping out air often leads to large surface deformation of the simulated artery and slow pulse frequency). This can be further verified by the characterization of the output piezoelectric voltage of biosensor. The output response of the piezoelectric voltage is 0, 5, 36.8 and 30.7% when the pulse frequency of the simulated artery is fixed at 30, 36, 48 and 60 times per minute (Figure 4d). Through the application of wireless transmission, the concept of degradable flexible biosensors for pulse or deformation monitoring of the heart and organ surfaces can be applied to more scenarios, such as vascular surgery, early detection of vascular failure [1–3], etc.

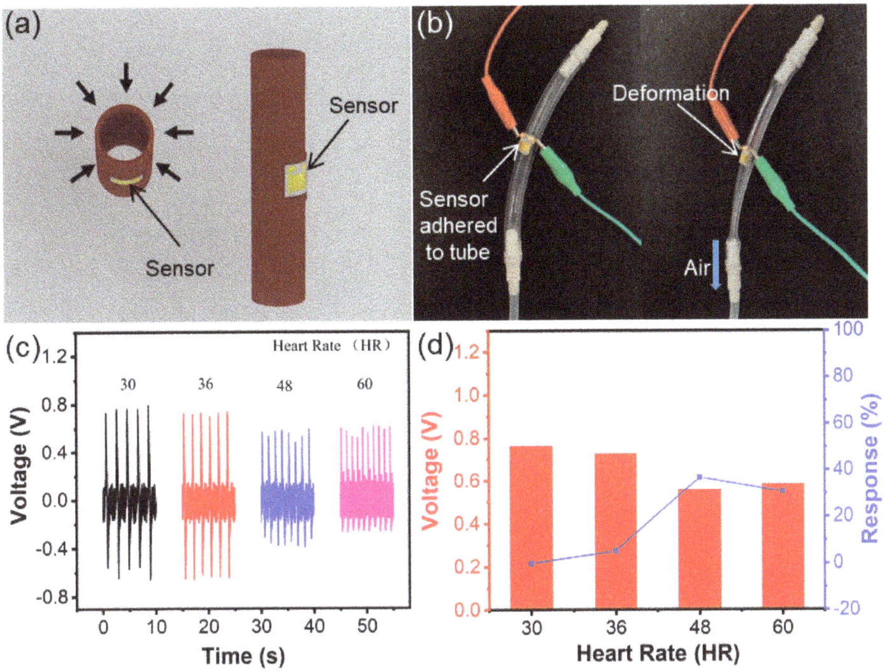

Figure 4. Photo of simulated arterial biosensor and characterization of output piezoelectric voltage. (**a**) Simulation of arterial work and biosensor attachment position. (**b**) Arterial model. (**c**) Output piezoelectric voltage of the arterial model monitored by biosensor. (**d**) Output piezoelectric voltage response.

Figure 5 shows the practical application scenario of a biosensor integrated with a wireless transmitter receiver. The sensor can be easily attached to the inside of the elbow joint between the upper arm and forearm. The rhythmic motions of the arm skills in butterfly stroke are shown in Figure 5a. The output piezoelectric voltage of the biosensor is 1.272, 1.086, 1.072, 1.079, 1.04, 1.067, 1.062, 1.099, 1.086 and 1.084 V. The arm skills of butterfly stroke are divided into four parts: entering, holding, sculling and pushing [9–13]. The output piezoelectric voltage of the biosensor is relatively stable, which indicates that the tester's arm skills are relatively stable in each butterfly stroke part. It is worth noting that the peak's width of the piezoelectric voltage in Figure 5a is slightly wider (within the blue dotted line in Figure 5a). It is assumed that this can be ascribed to the strain applied to the sensor. This part is the technical connection process of the arm from holding to sculling and then to pushing. To verify our claim, we monitored the arm skills of breaststroke, as shown in Figure 5b. The arm skills of breaststroke include five parts: sliding, holding, sculling, hand closing and arm extension. The tester intends to extend the time of hand closing and arm extension in the first three breaststrokes. At this time, we can observe that the angle between the upper arm and forearm is the smallest, while the deformation of the biosensor is the largest, and the output piezoelectric voltage is the highest. After that, the peak width of the output piezoelectric voltage widens (in the red dotted line in Figure 5b) after deliberately extending the hand closing and arm extension. It is believed that the strain applied to the biosensor induces the deformation due to the results of the micro change in the same bending angle of the device. The output piezoelectric voltage of ten breaststroke arm skills is 1.079, 1.042, 0.942, 1.025, 0.95, 1.079, 0.967, 1.064, 0.942 and 0.847 V under stable conditions. For freestyle arm skills, they are generally divided into two main parts: in water and out of water. The action of arms in the water includes entering water, catching water, pulling water and finally pushing water, then immediately becomes out of water action and movement in the air. The output piezoelectric voltage of the freestyle arm skills of the tester is also relatively stable in Figure 5c. By observing the output piezoelectric voltage signal, we can see that the frequency and angle are quite stable, and the performance of motion skills is extremely good. The duration of different swimmers' arm skills is different in each part, and most swimmers are looking for a suitable swimming skill to adjust the frequency and angle of arm skills. Unfortunately, the collection equipment cannot adapt to the wet environment of the swimming pool. In order to prevent the occurrence of unpredictable risks, the above complete swimming skills are not monitored underwater. However, a substitute experiment is conducted to exhibit the potential application in swimming training. In Movie S1, when the sensor is put into the swimming pool water, we can see that the sensor still has piezoelectric output. It shows that the sensor has the potential to be used in underwater swimming skills monitoring. In this way, flexible biosensors can be portable, non-destructive and used in real time to monitor the frequency, angle and other information of swimming skills, so as to help make training plans and improve sport performance. As a result, the data can be analyzed by a simple wireless transmitting and receiving station, as shown in Figure 5d. The output piezoelectric voltage generated by the body motion of the tester is charged to a 4.7 μf capacitor device, and the voltage of 0.72 V (Figure S2) is charged within 80 s. After charging, the wireless information transmission is driven and sent to the receiving station. Movie S2 shows the experimental process. When there is no output piezoelectric voltage, the LED lamps in the receiving station cannot be turned off. When the piezoelectric output increases or the frequency changes, the receiving station turns off different numbers of LED lamps or they flash at the same frequency. Such wireless information transmission functions provide more potential application scenarios for sport big data transmission.

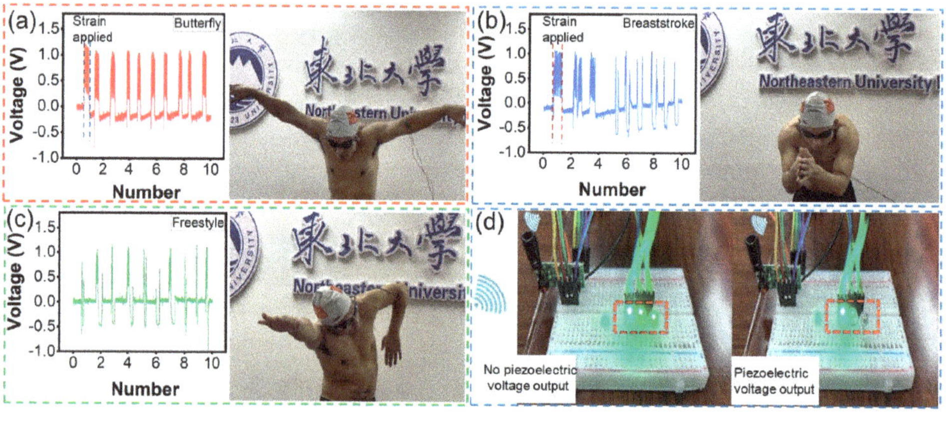

Figure 5. Experimental design of integrated wireless transmitter and receiver for biosensor. (**a**) Output piezoelectric voltage of butterfly stroke. (**b**) Output piezoelectric voltage of breaststroke. (**c**) Output piezoelectric voltage of freestyle stroke. (**d**) Wireless transmission analysis station.

4. Conclusions

In summary, a portable self-powered biosensor based on the electromechanical coupling effect of ZnO NWs has been designed and demonstrated to monitor various swimming styles of swimmers. This work also demonstrates the potential application of ZnO NW biosensors in a simulated scenario of monitoring the aortic pulse and realizing real-time wireless transmission. The biosensor perceives the human body's motion frequency, joint angle and underwater performance through wireless transmission, and uses the information from the receiving station to actively monitor the swimmer's performance. This type of flexible biosensor possesses broad application prospects in human–computer interaction monitoring, infinite sport big data transmission and self-powered portable monitoring systems.

Supplementary Materials: The following are available online at https://www.mdpi.com/article/10.3390/bios11050147/s1. Figure S1: Capacitor charge. Figure S2: Output piezoelectric voltage under 5 Hz. Movie S1: Numbers of LEDs driven by the self-powered sensor under water. Movie S2: LEDs controlled by self-powered sensor.

Author Contributions: Y.M. and B.L. put forward to the concept of the study. The data were collected, sorted out and analyzed by Y.Z., T.Z. and X.L. T.Z. and C.J. were the supervisors. Y.M. carried out the verification, X.L., C.J., Y.L. and M.B. made the visualizations. Y.M., B.L. and T.Z. wrote the manuscript. X.L., Y.L., Y.M. and B.L. finished the writing, reviewing and editing. All authors have read and agreed to the published version of the manuscript.

Funding: This work was supported by the Liaoning Natural Science Foundation Program Guidance Plan: Monitoring and analysis of physiological indexes of biathlon athletes by self-powered biosensor (2019-ZD-0515).

Institutional Review Board Statement: Ethical review and approval were waived for this study, due to the experiments are almost completely safe, and do not cause harm to the subject, and do not involve privacy and moral issues.

Informed Consent Statement: Written informed consent has been obtained from the patient(s) to publish this paper.

Data Availability Statement: The data presented in this study are available in [insert article or supplementary material here].

Conflicts of Interest: The authors declare no conflict of interest. The funders had no role in the design of the study; in the collection, analyses, or interpretation of data; in the writing of the manuscript, or in the decision to publish the results.

References

1. Niu, S.M.; Matsuhisa, N.; Beker, L.; Li, J.; Wang, S.; Wang, J.; Jiang, Y.; Yan, X.; Yun, Y.; Burnetts, W.; et al. A wireless body area sensor network based on stretchable passive tags. *Nat. Electron.* **2019**, *2*, 361–368. [CrossRef]
2. Boutry, C.M.; Kaizawa, Y.; Schroeder, B.C.; Chortos, A.; Legrand, A.; Wang, Z.; Chang, J.; Fox, P.; Bao, Z. A stretchable and biodegradable strain and pressure sensor for orthopaedic application. *Nat. Electron.* **2018**, *1*, 314–321. [CrossRef]
3. Boutry, C.M.; Beker, L.; Kaizawa, Y.; Vassos, C.; Tran, H.; Hinckley, A.C.; Pfattner, R.; Niu, S.M.; Li, J.H.; Claverie, J.; et al. Biodegradable and flexible arterial-pulse sensor for the wireless monitoring of blood flow. *Nat. Biomed. Eng.* **2019**, *3*, 47–57. [CrossRef] [PubMed]
4. Luo, J.; Wang, Z.; Xu, L.; Wang, A.; Han, K.; Jiang, T.; Lai, Q.; Bai, Y.; Tang, W.; Fan, F.; et al. Flexible and durable wood-based triboelectric nanogenerators for self-powered sensing in athletic big data analytics. *Nat. Commun.* **2019**, *10*, 5147. [CrossRef]
5. Mao, Y.; Yue, W.; Zhao, T.; Shen, M.; Liu, B.; Chen, S. A Self-Powered Biosensor for Monitoring Maximal Lactate Steady State in Sport Training. *Biosensors* **2020**, *10*, 75. [CrossRef] [PubMed]
6. Senf, B.; Yeo, W.; Kim, J. Recent Advances in Portable Biosensors for Biomarker Detection in Body Fluids. *Biosensors* **2020**, *10*, 127. [CrossRef]
7. Nugent, F.J.; Comyns, T.M.; Warrington, G.D. Quality Versus Quantity Debate in Swimming: Perceptions and Training Practices of Expert Swimming Coaches. *J. Hum. Kinet.* **2017**, *57*, 147–158. [CrossRef]
8. Fantozzi, S.; Gatta, G.; Mangia, A.L.; Bartolomei, S.; Cortesi, M. Front-Crawl Swimming: Detection of the Stroke Phases through 3d Wrist Trajectory Using Inertial Sensors. *J. Sport Sci. Med.* **2019**, *18*, 438–447.
9. Sanders, R.H.; Gonjo, T.; McCabe, C.B. Reliability of Three-Dimensional Angular Kinematics and Kinetics of Swimming Derived from Digitized Video. *J. Sport Sci. Med.* **2016**, *15*, 158–166.
10. Zacca, R.; Neves, V.; Oliveira, T.D.; Soares, S.; Rama, L.M.P.L.; Castro, F.A.D.; Vilas-Boas, J.P.; Pyne, D.B.; Fernandes, R.J. 5 km front crawl in pool and open water swimming: Breath-by-breath energy expenditure and kinematic analysis. *Eur. J. Appl. Physiol.* **2020**, *120*, 2005–2018. [CrossRef] [PubMed]
11. Burkhardt, D.; Born, D.P.; Singh, N.B.; Oberhofer, K.; Carradori, S.; Sinistaj, S.; Lorenzetti, S. Key performance indicators and leg positioning for the kick-start in competitive swimmers. *Sport Biomech.* **2020**, 1–15. [CrossRef]
12. Gonjo, T.; Fernandes, R.J.; Vilas-Boas, J.P.; Sanders, R. Upper body kinematic differences between maximum front crawl and backstroke swimming. *J. Biomech.* **2020**, *98*, 109452. [CrossRef]
13. Dos Santos, K.B.; Payton, C.; Rodacki, A.L.F. Front crawl arm stroke trajectories of physically impaired swimmers: A preliminary study. *Sci. Sport* **2019**, *34*, 263–266. [CrossRef]

14. Born, D.P.; Stoggl, T.; Petrov, A.; Burkhardt, D.; Luthy, F.; Romann, M. Analysis of Freestyle Swimming Sprint Start Performance After Maximal Strength or Vertical Jump Training in Competitive Female and Male Junior Swimmers. *J. Strength Cond. Res.* **2020**, *34*, 323–331. [CrossRef] [PubMed]
15. Gomes, L.E.; Diogo, V.; Castro, F.A.D.; Vilas-Boas, J.P.; Fernandes, R.J.; Figueiredo, P. Biomechanical analyses of synchronised swimming standard and contra-standard sculling. *Sport Biomech.* **2019**, *18*, 354–365. [CrossRef]
16. Pereira, S.M.; Ruschel, C.; Hubert, M.; Machado, L.; Roesler, H.; Fernandes, R.J.; Vilas-Boas, J.P. Kinematic, kinetic and EMG analysis of four front crawl flip turn techniques. *J. Sport Sci. Med.* **2015**, *33*, 2006–2015. [CrossRef] [PubMed]
17. De Jesus, K.; Figueiredo, P.; Goncalves, P.; Pereira, S.; Vilas-Boas, J.P.; Fernandes, R.J. Biomechanical Analysis of Backstroke Swimming Starts. *J. Sport Sci. Med.* **2011**, *32*, 546–551. [CrossRef] [PubMed]
18. Olstad, B.H.; Zinner, C. Validation of the Polar OH1 and M600 optical heart rate sensors during front crawl swim training. *PLoS ONE* **2020**, *15*, e0231522. [CrossRef] [PubMed]
19. Pollock, S.; Gaoua, N.; Johnston, M.J.; Cooke, K.; Girard, O.; Mileva, K.N. Training Regimes and Recovery Monitoring Practices of Elite British Swimmers. *J. Sport Sci. Med.* **2019**, *18*, 577–585.
20. Song, X.; Liu, X.; Peng, Y.; Xu, Z.; Liu, W.; Pang, K.; Wang, J.; Zhong, L.; Yang, Q.; Meng, J. A graphene-coated silk-spandex fabric strain sensor for human movement monitoring and recognition. *Nanotechnology* **2021**, *32*, 215501. [CrossRef]
21. Luo, J.; Gao, W.; Wang, Z. The Triboelectric Nanogenerator as an Innovative Technology toward Intelligent Sports. *Adv. Mater.* **2021**, *31*, 2004178. [CrossRef]
22. Ong, K.G.; Paulose, M.; Grimes, C.A. A wireless, passive, magnetically-soft harmonic sensor for monitoring sodium hypochlorite concentrations in water. *Sensors* **2003**, *3*, 11–18. [CrossRef]
23. Roy, J.J.; Abraham, T.E.; Abhijith, K.S.; Kumar, P.V.S.; Thakur, M.S. Biosensor for the determination of phenols based on Cross-Linked Enzyme Crystals (CLEC) of laccase. *Biosensors* **2005**, *21*, 206–211. [CrossRef] [PubMed]
24. Liu, B.; Shen, M.; Mao, L.; Mao, Y.; Ma, H. Self-powered Biosensor Big Data Intelligent Information Processing System for Real-time Motion Monitoring. *Z. Anorg. Allg. Chem.* **2020**, *646*, 500–506. [CrossRef]
25. Zhao, T.; Zheng, C.; He, H.; Guan, H.; Zhong, T.; Xing, L.; Xue, X. A self-powered biosensing electronic-skin for real-time sweat Ca2+ detection and wireless data transmission. *Smart Mater. Struct.* **2019**, *28*, 085015. [CrossRef]
26. Tavares, A.; Truta, L.; Moreira, F.; Minas, G.; Sales, M. Photovoltaics, plasmonics, plastic antibodies and electrochromism combined for a novel generation of self-powered and self-signalled electrochemical biomimetic sensors. *Biosens. Bioelectron.* **2019**, *137*, 72–81. [CrossRef]
27. Guan, H.; Zhong, T.; He, H.; Zhao, T.; Xing, L.; Zhang, Y.; Xue, X. A self-powered wearable sweat-evaporation-biosensing analyzer for building sports big data. *Nano Energy* **2019**, *59*, 754–761. [CrossRef]
28. Tarar, A.A.; Mohammad, U.; Srivastava, S.K. Wearable Skin Sensors and Their Challenges: A Review of Transdermal, Optical, and Mechanical Sensors. *Biosensors* **2020**, *10*, 56. [CrossRef]
29. Wu, X.; Jiang, P.; Ding, Y.; Cai, W.; Xie, S.; Wang, Z. Mismatch strain induced formation of ZnO/ZnS heterostructured rings. *Sci. Adv. Mater.* **2007**, *19*, 2319. [CrossRef]
30. Wang, J.; Qu, F.; Wu, X. Synthesis of Ultra-Thin ZnO Nanosheets: Photocatalytic and Superhydrophilic Properties. *Sci. Adv. Mater.* **2013**, *5*, 1052–1059. [CrossRef]
31. Jing, W.; Qu, F.; Xiang, W. Photocatalytic Degradation of Organic Dyes with Hierarchical Ag_2 O/ZnO Heterostructures. *Sci. Adv. Mater.* **2013**, *5*, 1364–1371.
32. Yu, L.; Qu, F.; Wu, X. Facile hydrothermal synthesis of novel ZnO nanocubes. *J. Alloy. Compd.* **2010**, *504*, L1–L4. [CrossRef]
33. Lei, Y.; Qu, F.; Wu, X. Assembling ZnO Nanorods into Microflowers through a Facile Solution Strategy: Morphology Control and Cathodoluminescence Properties. *Nano-Micro Lett.* **2012**, *4*, 45–51. [CrossRef]
34. Yu, L.; Qu, F.; Wu, X. Solution synthesis and optimization of ZnO nanowindmills. *Appl. Surf. Sci.* **2011**, *257*, 7432–7435. [CrossRef]
35. Gong, L.; Wu, X.; Ye, C.; Qu, F.; An, M. Aqueous phase approach to ZnO microspindles at low temperature. *J. Alloy. Compd.* **2010**, *501*, 375–379. [CrossRef]
36. Chakraborty, S.; Settem, M.; Sant, S.B. Evolution of texture and nature of grain growth on annealing nanocrystalline Ni and Ni-18.5%Fe in air. *Mater. Express* **2013**, *3*, 99–108. [CrossRef]
37. Zhang, X.; Wang, H.; Zhang, J.; Li, J.; Liu, B. Enhanced optoelectronic performance of 3C–SiC/ZnO heterostructure photodetector based on Piezo-phototronic effects. *Nano Energy* **2020**, *77*, 105119. [CrossRef]
38. Zhang, X.; Li, J.; Yang, W.; Leng, B.; Liu, B. High-performance flexible UV photodetectors based on AZO/ZnO/PVK/PEDOT:PSS heterostructures integrated on human hair. *ACS Appl. Mater.* **2019**, *11*, 24459–24467. [CrossRef]
39. Zhang, X.; Zhang, J.; Leng, B.; Li, J.; Ma, Z.; Yang, W.; Liu, F.; Liu, B. Enhanced Performances of PVK/ZnO Nanorods/Graphene Heterostructure UV Photodetector via Piezo-Phototronic Interface Engineering. *Adv. Mater. Interfaces* **2019**, *6*, 1970145. [CrossRef]
40. Lin, H.; Liu, Y.; Chen, S.; Xu, Q.; Wang, S.; Hu, T.; Pan, P.; Wang, Y.; Zhang, Y.; Li, N.; et al. Seesaw structured triboelectric nanogenerator with enhanced output performance and its applications in self-powered motion sensing. *Nano Energy.* **2019**, *65*, 103944. [CrossRef]
41. Park, J.Y.; Choi, S.W.; Kim, S.S. A synthesis and sensing application of hollow ZnO nanofibers with uniform wall thicknesses grown using polymer templates. *Nat. Nanotech.* **2010**, *21*, 475601. [CrossRef] [PubMed]
42. Lin, H.; He, M.; Jing, Q.; Yang, W.; Wang, S.; Liu, Y.; Zhang, Y.; Li, J.; Li, N.; Ma, Y.; et al. Angle-shaped triboelectric nanogenerator for harvesting environmental wind energy. *Nano Energy* **2019**, *56*, 269–276. [CrossRef]

43. He, M.; Lin, Y.; Chiu, C.; Yang, W.; Zhang, B.; Yun, D.; Xie, Y.; Lin, Z. A flexible photo-thermoelectric nanogenerator based on MoS2/PU photothermal layer for infrared light harvesting. *Nano Energy* **2018**, *49*, 588–595. [CrossRef]
44. Mao, Y.; Ba, N.; Gao, X.; Wang, Z.; Shen, M.; Liu, B.; Li, B.; Ma, X.; Chen, S. Self-Powered Wearable Sweat-Lactate Analyzer for Scheduling Training of Boat Race. *J. Nanoelectron. Optoelectron.* **2020**, *15*, 212–218. [CrossRef]
45. Mao, Y.; Zhang, W.; Wang, Y.; Guan, R.; Liu, B.; Wang, X.; Sun, Z.; Xing, L.; Chen, S.; Xue, X. Self-Powered Wearable Athletics Monitoring Nanodevice Based on ZnO Nanowire Piezoelectric-Biosensing Unit Arrays. *Sci. Adv. Mater.* **2019**, *11*, 351–359. [CrossRef]
46. Wang, J.X.; Sun, X.; Yang, Y.; Huang, H.; Lee, Y.; Tan, O.; Vayssieres, L. Hydrothermally grown oriented ZnO nanorod arrays for gas sensing applications. *Nat. Nanotech.* **2006**, *17*, 4995–4998. [CrossRef]
47. Lozano, H.; Catalan, G.; Esteve, J.; Domingo, N.; Murillo, G. Non-linear nanoscale piezoresponse of single ZnO nanowires affected by piezotronic effect. *Nat. Nanotech.* **2021**, *32*, 025202. [CrossRef]

biosensors

MDPI

Communication

Numerical Study of Graphene/Au/SiC Waveguide-Based Surface Plasmon Resonance Sensor

Wei Du [1,*], Lucas Miller [1] and Feng Zhao [2,*]

[1] Department of Electrical Engineering and Physics, Wilkes University, Wilkes-Barre, PA 18766, USA; lucas.miller@wilkes.edu

[2] Micro/Nanoelectronics and Energy Laboratory, School of Engineering and Computer Science, Washington State University, Vancouver, WA 98686, USA

* Correspondence: wei.du@wilkes.edu (W.D.); feng.zhao@wsu.edu (F.Z.); Tel.: +1-570-408-4720 (W.D.); +1-360-546-9187 (F.Z.)

Abstract: A new waveguide-based surface plasmon resonance (SPR) sensor was proposed and investigated by numerical simulation. The sensor consists of a graphene cover layer, a gold (Au) thin film, and a silicon carbide (SiC) waveguide layer on a silicon dioxide/silicon (SiO_2/Si) substrate. The large bandgap energy of SiC allows the sensor to operate in the visible and near-infrared wavelength ranges, which effectively reduces the light absorption in water to improve the sensitivity. The sensor was characterized by comparing the shift of the resonance wavelength peak with change of the refractive index (RI), which mimics the change of analyte concentration in the sensing medium. The study showed that in the RI range of 1.33~1.36, the sensitivity was improved when the graphene layers were increased. With 10 graphene layers, a sensitivity of 2810 nm/RIU (refractive index unit) was achieved, corresponding to a 39.1% improvement in sensitivity compared to the Au/SiC sensor without graphene. These results demonstrate that the graphene/Au/SiC waveguide SPR sensor has a promising use in portable biosensors for chemical and biological sensing applications, such as detection of water contaminations (RI = 1.33~1.34), hepatitis B virus (HBV), and glucose (RI = 1.34~1.35), and plasma and white blood cells (RI = 1.35~1.36) for human health and disease diagnosis.

Keywords: waveguide; surface plasmon resonance; graphene; silicon carbide; refractive index; chemical sensor; biosensor

Citation: Du, W.; Miller, L.; Zhao, F. Numerical Study of Graphene/Au/SiC Waveguide-Based Surface Plasmon Resonance Sensor. *Biosensors* **2021**, *11*, 455. https://doi.org/10.3390/bios11110455

Received: 20 October 2021
Accepted: 11 November 2021
Published: 15 November 2021

1. Introduction

Surface plasmons resonance (SPR)-based chemical and biosensors have been widely used for the detection of a variety of chemicals and biomolecules [1–5]. These sensors utilize the surface plasmon polariton (SPP) characteristics to analyze the sensing medium. Change of the analyte concentration on the sensor surface leads to change of local refractive index (RI), and therefore the propagation constant of SPP, which can be measured by optical methods [6]. SPR sensors can be built with several configurations. The most frequently used structures are a prism coupler [7] and a grating coupler [8], in which the resonance angle shifts with the change of RI. However, limitations exist in both sensors, as the prism structure suffers from a relatively large device size, while the grating structure has a small size but complicated fabrication process. Both configurations are not conducive to future photonics integration needs. To address these issues, the optical waveguide-based structures are attracting interest [9–11] since they offer the advantages of good control of light path, easy measurement of input and output light intensity, and a high degree of on-chip integration. These advantages are highly desirable for the next generation of photonic integrated circuits (PICs) [12].

In conventional SPR sensors, a thin metal film is inserted between the light-guiding layer and sensing medium, with the excited surface plasmon wave propagating along the metal and sensing medium interface. Different metal films such as gold (Au), silver (Ag), and aluminum (Al) have been discussed in the literature [13–15]. Among these metals, Au is widely used due to its resistance to chemicals and oxidation. However, the intrinsic high loss of Au film limits the sensitivity. Various methods [3] have been developed to further improve the sensitivity, including the application of metal nanoparticles [16] and nanoslits [17]. Since the precise control of nanostructures is a challenge, these methods complicate the sensor fabrication toward on-chip integration and are not compatible with a silicon (Si) complementary metal–oxide–semiconductor (CMOS) technique. An alternative approach is the application of biomolecular recognition elements (BRE) [3] to functionalize the Au film and enhance the adsorption of analyte on the Au surface.

In this paper, we proposed and numerically simulated a new waveguide-based SPR sensor with a wide bandgap semiconductor silicon carbide (SiC) as the waveguide layer, a Au thin film, and a graphene cover layer as BRE. Due to the wide bandgap energy (2.2 eV of 3C-SiC polytype), the SiC waveguide layer enables the sensor to operate in the visible wavelength range, which avoids the absorption of large amounts of water in the near-infrared range when sensing in a water-based sensing medium [18–20]. The increased adsorption of the analyte on a graphene surface could improve the sensitivity of the sensor [21,22]. The graphene/Au/SiC waveguide SPR sensor structure can be grown and fabricated using standard Si CMOS techniques: SiC can be grown using plasma—enhanced chemical vapor deposition (CVD) [23] on SiO_2/Si substrate, Au can be deposited via evaporation or sputtering with precisely controlled thickness. For graphene, CVD process has been explored extensively to synthesize uniform graphene monolayer and multilayer [24], which can be used to accurately deposit on the SiC surface. Furthermore, the standard photolithography and dry etching processes can be applied to pattern the device.

2. Design and Methods

The cross-sectional schematic of the graphene/Au/SiC waveguide SPR sensor is shown in Figure 1. The width of the sensor was kept at 10 μm, which is attainable via the standard microfabrication process. A SiO_2 layer (RI = 1.45) was inserted between a Si (RI = 3.5) substrate and SiC waveguide layer for optical isolation since the RI of SiC (RI = 2.62) is smaller than Si. The permittivity of Au can be found in [25]. The SiO_2 isolation layer was selected to be 3 μm thick, which is sufficient to prevent optical field leakage onto the Si substrate. Thicknesses of the SiC waveguide layer was kept at 100 nm based on our previous study [26], which showed that the confinement factor of a SiC waveguide sensor increases with the thickness of the SiC layer up to 100 nm. Above this thickness, the coupling effect becomes weak, which reduces the coupling coefficient and confinement factor. Thicknesses of the Au film (from 10 to 100 nm) and graphene layer were investigated in this study. The thickness of the graphene monolayer was 0.34 nm [27] so the total thickness of graphene was $N \times 0.34$ nm, where N varied from 0 (no graphene) to 10 in this study. The sensor was studied by a spectral interrogation method; the resonance wavelength was collected, and its shift with the change in the RI of the sensing medium being compared. This method is different from the angular interrogation method in prism- or grating-based SPR sensors, which use the resonance angle instead of the resonance wavelength.

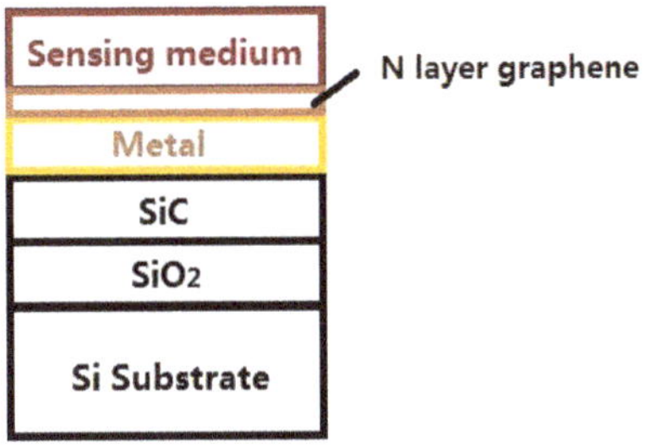

Figure 1. Cross-sectional schematic of graphene/Au/SiC waveguide SPR sensor structure.

The optical properties of a monolayer graphene can be found in [27], which provides the complex RI of graphene in the visible light range:

$$RI_{(graphene)} = 3.0 + i\frac{5.446\ \mu\text{m}^{-1}}{3}\lambda_0 \tag{1}$$

where i is the imaginary unit and λ_0 is the vacuum wavelength. In [27], the optical properties were reported for single and multiple graphene layers and the quantum effects studied. Therefore, application of Equation (1) for the RI of graphene includes quantum effects that could present the multi-layer of graphene. For sensor operation, when the resonance condition is satisfied by a certain RI, the SPP is excited by the incident light, leading to the optical energy distribution in both the waveguide layer and sensing medium. The optical energy being absorbed by the analyte in the sensing medium results in attenuation of the output power. A change of analyte concentration alters the RI near the sensor surface, which consequently changes the propagation constant of SPP and eventually leads to a shift in the resonance wavelength. According to Lambert–Beer's law, in a waveguide structure, the absorbance, A, can be expressed as [28,29]:

$$A = \log\left(\frac{P_0}{P_a}\right) = f\alpha l c \tag{2}$$

where P_0 and P_a are the light intensities without and with energy absorption in the sensing medium, respectively; f is the confinement factor, which is defined as the ratio of the optical power confined in the sensing medium over the total optical power; α is the absorption coefficient; l is the waveguide length; and c is the analyte concentration. The change in c leads to the change in RI. The sensitivity, S, is proportional to the ratio of the change in absorbance, A, over the concentration change in the sensing medium:

$$S = \frac{\Delta A}{\Delta c} = f\alpha l \tag{3}$$

It is clear in Equation (3) that for a given waveguide length, a higher confinement factor value results in an improved sensitivity of the waveguide sensor. In addition, with the graphene layer serving as BRE, the adsorption efficiency is enhanced. This can be defined as the percentage of analyte being effectively adsorbed into the sensor surface, which leads to the change of RI. Therefore, the overall sensitivity, S, is improved by adding graphene layers, as shown in Equation (4):

$$S \propto k \cdot \frac{\Delta A}{\Delta c} = k f \alpha l \tag{4}$$

where k is the enhancement of adsorption efficiency and $k > 1$.

Note that in Equation (4), the values of k and α are generally obtained by experimental measurement. In this study, we applied an effective index method (EIM) [30,31] using COMSOL Multiphysics software to model the graphene/Au/SiC waveguide SPR sensor and calculate the confinement factor *f*. The results were compared with the Au/SiC waveguide SPR sensor without a graphene layer. In the model, a 3-μm thick perfectly matched layer (PML) surrounding the sensor structure was used as the outer boundary condition to truncate the computation region. At the boundary of each layer, the tangential components of the electric and magnetic fields were defined as the continuous inner boundary condition. Since SPP can only be excited by transverse magnetic (TM) polarized light, and the fundamental TM mode (TM_0) in the waveguide has the lowest loss, the TM_0 mode was investigated.

3. Results and Discussion

Figure 2 shows the confinement factor of the TM_0 mode as a function of Au film thickness at its resonance wavelength (675 nm, see inset) in a sensing medium where RI = 1.344. Ten graphene layers were applied to the Au film. The confinement factor increases as the Au film becomes thicker. Considering that thicker Au would lead to higher optical loss, the 50 nm thickness was selected in this sensitivity study of the graphene/Au/SiC waveguide SPR sensor. This thickness allowed for strong coupling between the waveguide and SP modes.

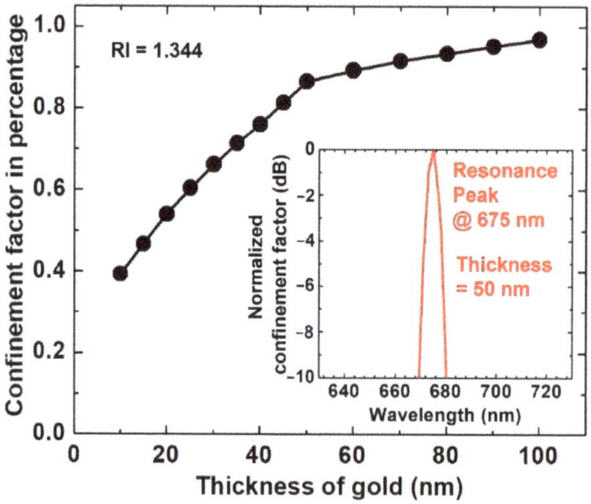

Figure 2. Confinement factor as a function of Au thickness. The number of graphene layers was 10. The RI of the sensing medium was 1.344. Inset: resonant peak at 675 nm with 50 nm thick gold.

The typical resonance wavelength shift for different numbers of graphene layers in a RI = 1.344 sensing medium is shown in Figure 3. It is clear that, as the number of graphene layers increases, the resonance wavelength shifts towards longer wavelengths, from 617 to 675 nm, i.e., a redshift. It is well acknowledged that the resonance wavelength (or frequency) is strongly dependent on the free-electron density of metallic nanostructures [32]. Without the graphene layer, the resonance wavelength is mainly determined by the excited electron density in the Au thin film. When graphene is directly added to the Au film, the electrons excited by SPP can transfer to the graphene, resulting in decreased free-electron density in the Au film. This reduced electron density leads to the redshift of the resonance wavelength. As graphene layers increase, more electrons transfer to the graphene layers and free-electron density further decreases, therefore a more pronounced redshift of the resonance peak is observed. It is worth noting that as the number of graphene layers increases, the linewidth broadens slightly, which may degrade sensing performance. A similar characteristic was also observed in a prism-coupler-based SPR sensor [22]. However, since adding more graphene layers would cause a further shift of the resonance wavelength as shown in Figure 3, this effect is compensated for and the overall sensitivity can still be improved.

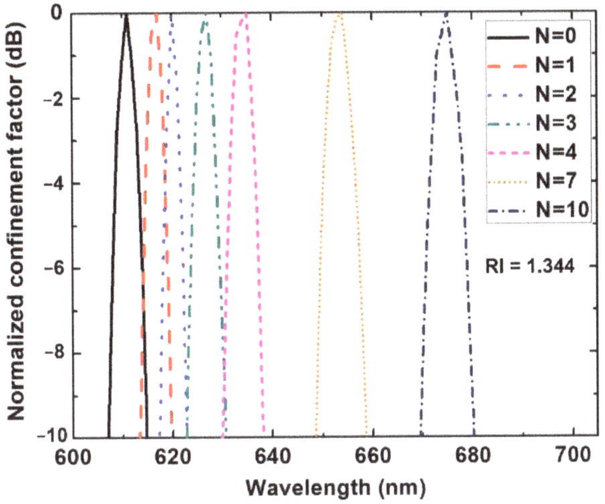

Figure 3. Resonance wavelength for graphene/Au/SiC sensor with different numbers of graphene layers. The gold thickness was 50 nm. The RI of the sensing medium was 1.344.

Modification of the SPP field also improves sensitivity. Figure 4 shows the resonance-wavelength shift of the graphene/Au/SiC waveguide SPR sensor with 10 layers of graphene (blue curves, N = 10) in comparison with the Au/SiC sensor (black curves, N = 0) without graphene; the two RIs mimic the change of analyte concentration. As the RI of the sensing medium increases from 1.33 to 1.36, the resonance wavelength of both sensors shifts to the longer wavelength. The resonance wavelength peak indicates the strongest SPR coupling from waveguide mode to surface plasmon (SP) mode, where the maximum propagation loss of the waveguide occurs. In SP mode, the maximum propagation loss of the waveguide is close to the cutoff wavelength. The increase in RI leads to a shift of the cutoff wavelength towards a longer wavelength and therefore the redshift of the resonance wavelength peak. The graphene/Au/SiC sensor exhibits a redshift of 68.7 nm, corresponding to a sensitivity of 2290 nm/RIU (refractive index unit). While for the Au/SiC sensor, the resonance wavelength shifts 50.8 nm, i.e., a sensitivity of 1693 nm/RIU. An improvement of 35.8% was obtained by adding 10 graphene layers to the Au/SiC waveguide SPR sensor.

The sensitivities in the three RI ranges (1.33~1.34, 1.34~1.35, and 1.35~1.36) are summarized in Figure 5. In each RI range, an increased sensitivity is demonstrated with more graphene layers. For 10 graphene layers, the sensitivities of 1970 nm/RIU, 2090 nm/RIU and 2810 nm/RIU were obtained in each RI range, corresponding to the enhancements of 34.0%, 31.4%, and 39.1%, respectively. There are very useful sensing applications when a graphene/Au/SiC waveguide SPR sensor is used in these RI ranges: detection of contaminations in water [33] in RI = 1.33~1.34, and identification of hepatitis B virus (HBV) [34], glucose [35] in RI = 1.34~1.35, and plasma and white blood cells in RI = 1.35~1.36 [36]. Detection of refractive index change is a useful technique for biosensors and continuously attracting research interest [37–39]. Very small changes in concentration can be detected by utilizing the sensitivity that has been improved by SPR effect.

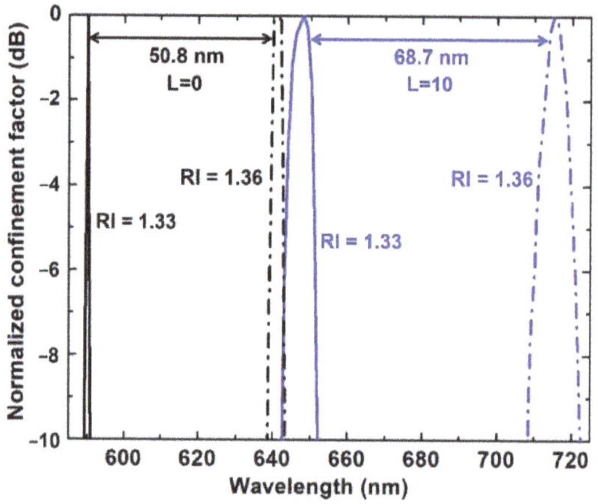

Figure 4. Comparison of resonance wavelength shift for a Au/SiC (black curves, N = 0) and a graphene/Au/SiC (blue curves, N = 10) waveguide-based SPR sensor when the RI of the sensing medium changes from 1.33 (solid curves) to 1.36 (dashed curves).

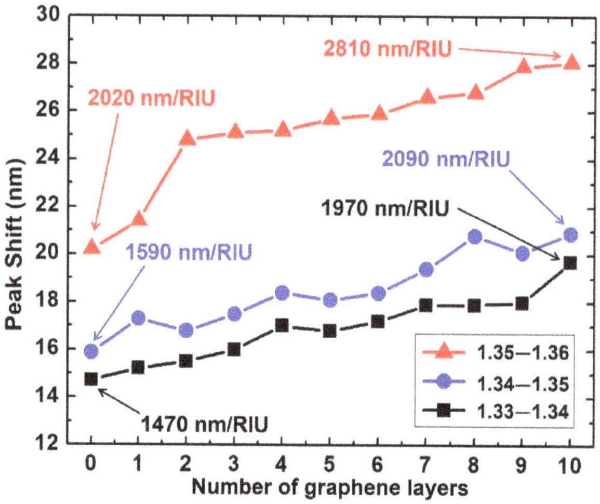

Figure 5. Resonance peak shift with the number of graphene layers. The gold thickness was 50 nm and RI ranges from 1.33 to 1.36.

It is worth noting that according to Equation (4), both the absorption coefficient, α, and the enhanced adsorption efficiency, k, are dependent on analyte materials; therefore, the sensitivity of the waveguide SPR sensor would vary when probing different analytes. Moreover, more sensitivity improvement can be expected since k is always greater than one when adding more graphene layers. However, further coverage of additional graphene layers may not effectively further the transfer of the electrons from the Au film to the graphene. As a result, the resonance peak shift would reach its maximum and no more peak shift could be obtained. On the other hand, the broadened peak linewidth with increased graphene layers also needs to be considered, and the optimal number of graphene layers for maximal sensitivity requires future study.

4. Conclusions

In this work, we proposed and investigated a new graphene/Au/SiC waveguide SPR sensor. The confinement factors of the sensors with 0 to 10 graphene layers were studied by an effective index method, and the sensitivity was studied by a spectral interrogation method by comparing the shift in the resonance wavelength peak. The sensor operates in the visible light range with the wide bandgap SiC as the waveguide layer. When combined with the advantages of good control of light path, easy measurement of input and output light intensity, and high degree of on-chip integration, this sensor is highly desirable for the next generation of PICs. This study shows that when the number of graphene layers is increased, sensitivity increases, and up to 2810 nm/RIU can be achieved in the RI range of 1.33~1.36. The results demonstrate that a graphene/Au/SiC waveguide SPR sensor is promising for important chemical and biological sensing applications.

Author Contributions: Conceptualization, W.D. and F.Z.; Data curation, W.D. and F.Z.; Formal analysis, W.D. and F.Z.; Funding acquisition, W.D.; Investigation, W.D. and L.M.; Methodology, L.M.; Project administration, W.D.; Resources, W.D. and F.Z.; Software, W.D. and L.M.; Supervision, F.Z.; Validation, W.D. and F.Z.; Writing—original draft, W.D.; Writing—review and editing, F.Z. All authors have read and agreed to the published version of the manuscript.

Funding: This research received no external funding.

Institutional Review Board Statement: Not applicable.

Informed Consent Statement: Not applicable.

Data Availability Statement: The data presented in this study are available on request from the corresponding author.

Acknowledgments: W.D. is thankful for the support of Wilkes University Provost's Research and Scholarship Fund.

Conflicts of Interest: The authors declare no conflict of interest.

References

1. Homola, J. Surface Plasmon Resonance Sensors for Detection of Chemical and Biological Species. *Chem. Rev.* **2008**, *108*, 462–493. [CrossRef] [PubMed]
2. Dudak, F.C.; Boyaci, I.H. Rapid and Label-Free Bacteria Detection by Surface Plasmon Resonance (SPR) Biosensors. *J. Biotechnol.* **2009**, *4*, 1003–1011. [CrossRef] [PubMed]
3. Homola, J. Present and Future of Surface Plasmon Resonance Biosensors. *Anal. Bioanal. Chem.* **2003**, *377*, 528–539. [CrossRef]
4. Liedberg, B.; Nylander, C.; Lunström, I. Surface Plasmon Resonance for Gas Detection and Biosensing. *Sens. Actuator* **1983**, *4*, 299–304. [CrossRef]
5. Bai, H.; Wang, R.; Hargis, B.; Lu, H.; Li, Y. A SPR Aptasensor for Detection of Avian Influenza Virus H5N1. *Sensors* **2012**, *12*, 12506–12518. [CrossRef]
6. Raether, H. Surface Plasmons on Smooth Surface. In *Surface Plasmons on Smooth and Rough Surfaces and on Gratings*; Springer: Berlin/Heidelberg, Germany, 1988; p. 19.
7. Kooyman, R.P.H.; Kolkman, H.; van Gent, J.; Greve, J. Surface Plasmon Resonance Immunosensors: Sensitivity Considerations. *Anal. Chim. Acta* **1988**, *213*, 35–45. [CrossRef]
8. Lawrence, C.R.; Geddes, N.J.; Furlong, D.N. Surface Plasmon Resonance Studies of Immunoreactions Utilizing Disposable Diffraction Gratings. *Biosens. Bioelectron.* **1996**, *11*, 389–400. [CrossRef]
9. Debackere, P.; Scheerlinck, S.; Bienstman, P.; Baets, R. Surface Plasmon Interferometer in Silicon-On-Insulator: Novel Concept for an Integrated Biosensor. *Opt. Express* **2006**, *14*, 7063–7072. [CrossRef]
10. Yimit, A.; Rossberg, A.G.; Amemiya, T.; Itoh, K. Thin Film Composite Optical Waveguides for Sensor Applications: A Review. *Talanta* **2005**, *65*, 1102–1109. [CrossRef]
11. Zourob, M.; Lakhtakia, A. Plasmonic-Waveguide Sensors. In *Optical Guided-Wave Chemical and Biosensors*; Springer: Berlin/Heidelberg, Germany, 2010; pp. 133–154.
12. Koch, T.L.; Koren, U. Semiconductor Photonic Integrated Circuits. *IEEE J. Quantum Electron.* **1991**, *27*, 641–653. [CrossRef]
13. Johnsson, B.; Löfås, S.; Lindquist, G. Immobilization of Proteins to a Carboxymethyldextran-Modified Gold Surface for Biospecific Interaction Analysis in Surface Plasmon Resonance Sensors. *Anal. Biochem.* **1991**, *198*, 268–277. [CrossRef]
14. Sherry, L.J.; Chang, S.H.; Schatz, G.C.; Van Duyne, R.P. Localized Surface Plasmon Resonance Spectroscopy of Single Silver Nanocubes. *Nano Lett.* **2005**, *5*, 2034–2038. [CrossRef] [PubMed]
15. Chan, G.H.; Zhao, J.; Schatz, G.C.; Van Duyne, R.P. Localized Surface Plasmon Resonance Spectroscopy of Triangular Aluminum Nanoparticles. *J. Phys. Chem. C* **2008**, *112*, 13958–13963. [CrossRef]
16. Stewart, M.E.; Anderton, C.R.; Thompson, L.B.; Maria, J.; Gray, S.K.; Rogers, J.A.; Nuzzo, R.G. Nanostructured Plasmonic Sensors. *Chem. Rev.* **2008**, *108*, 494–521. [CrossRef]

17. Lee, K.L.; Lee, C.W.; Wang, W.S.; Wei, P.K. Sensitive Biosensor Array Using Surface Plasmon Resonance on Metallic Nanoslits. *J. Biomed. Opt.* **2007**, *12*, 044023. [CrossRef]
18. Du, W.; Zhao, F. Silicon Carbide Based Surface Plasmon Resonance Waveguide Sensor With a Bimetallic Layer for Improved Sensitivity. *Mater. Lett.* **2017**, *186*, 224–226. [CrossRef]
19. Du, W.; Zhao, F. Sensing Performance Study of SiC, A Wide Bandgap Semiconductor Material Platform for Surface Plasmon Resonance Sensor. *J. Sens.* **2015**, *2015*, 341369. [CrossRef]
20. Du, W.; Chen, Z.B.; Zhao, F. Analysis of Single-Mode Optical Rib Waveguide in Silicon Carbide. *Microw. Opt. Technol. Lett.* **2013**, *55*, 2636–2640. [CrossRef]
21. Song, B.; Li, D.; Qi, W.P.; Elstner, M.; Fan, C.H.; Fang, H.P. Graphene on Au(111): A Highly Conductive Material with Excellent Adsorption Properties for High-Resolution Bio/Nanodetection and Identification. *ChemPhysChem* **2010**, *11*, 585–589. [CrossRef]
22. Wu, L.; Chu, H.S.; Koh, W.S.; Li, E.P. Highly Sensitive Graphene Biosensors Based on Surface Plasmon Resonance. *Opt. Expressvol.* **2010**, *18*, 14395–14400. [CrossRef]
23. Chen, Z.; Fares, C.; Elhassani, R.; Ren, F.; Kim, M.; Hsu, S.; Clark, A.E.; Esquivel-Upshaw, J.F. Demonstration of SiO_2/SiC based protective coating for dental ceramic prostheses. *J. Am. Ceram. Soc.* **2019**, *102*, 6591–6599. [CrossRef] [PubMed]
24. Zhang, Y.; Zhang, L.; Zhou, C. Review of Chemical Vapor Deposition of Graphene and Related Applications. *Acc. Chem. Res.* **2013**, *46*, 2329–2339. [CrossRef]
25. Du, W.; Zhao, F. Surface Plasmon Resonance Based Silicon Carbide Optical Waveguide. *Mater. Lett.* **2014**, *115*, 92–95. [CrossRef]
26. Nair, R.R.; Blake, P.; Grigorenko, A.N.; Novoselov, K.S.; Booth, T.J.; Stauber, T.; Peres, N.M.R.; Geim, A.K. Fine Structure Constant Defines Visual Transparency of Graphene. *Science* **2008**, *320*, 1308. [CrossRef]
27. Bruna, M.; Borini, S. Optical Constants of Graphene Layers in the Visible Range. *Appl. Phys. Lett.* **2009**, *94*, 031901. [CrossRef]
28. Raether, H. Collection of the Dielectric Functions of Gold and Silver. In *Surface Plasmons on Smooth and Rough Surfaces and on Gratings*; Springer: Berlin/Heidelberg, Germany, 1988.
29. Pandraud, G.; French, P.J.; Sarro, P.M. Fabrication and Characteristics of a PECVD SiC Evanescent Wave Optical Sensor. *Sens. Actuat. A-Phys.* **2008**, *142*, 61–66. [CrossRef]
30. Tamir, T. Theory of Dielectric Waveguides. In *Integrated Optics*, 1st ed.; Springer: New York, NY, USA, 1975.
31. Batrak, D.V.; Plisyuk, S.A. Applicability of the Effective Index Method for Simulating Ridge Optical Waveguides. *Quantum Electron.* **2006**, *36*, 349–352. [CrossRef]
32. Nan, H.Y.; Chen, Z.Y.; Jiang, J.; Li, J.Q.; Zhao, W.W.; Ni, Z.H.; Gu, X.F.; Xiao, S.Q. The Effect of Graphene on Surface Plasmon Resonance of Metal Nanoparticles. *Phys. Chem. Chem. Phys.* **2018**, *20*, 25078–25084. [CrossRef] [PubMed]
33. Jin, Y.L.; Chen, J.Y.; Xu, L.; Wang, P.N. Refractive Index Measurement for Biomaterial Samples by Total Internal Reflection. *Phys. Med. Biol.* **2006**, *51*, N371–N379. [CrossRef]
34. Chuanga, T.L.; Weib, S.C.; Leec, S.Y.; Lin, C.W. A Polycarbonate Based Surface Plasmon Resonance Sensing Cartridge for High Sensitivity HBV Loop-Mediated Isothermal Amplification. *Biosens. Bioelectron.* **2012**, *32*, 89–95. [CrossRef]
35. Hsieh, H.V.; Pfeiffer, Z.A.; Amiss, T.J.; Sherman, D.B.; Pitner, J.B. Direct Detection of Glucose by Surface Plasmon Resonance with Bacterial Glucose/Galactose-Binding Protein. *Biosens. Bioelectron.* **2004**, *19*, 653–660. [CrossRef]
36. Singh, S.; Kaur, V. Photonic Crystal Fiber Sensor Based on Sensing Ring for Different Blood Components: Design and Analysis. In Proceedings of the Ninth International Conference on Ubiquitous and Future Networks (ICUFN), Milan, Italy, 4–7 July 2017.
37. Zeni, L.; Perri, C.; Cennamo, N.; Arcadio, F.; D'Agostino, G.; Salmona, M.; Beeg, M.; Gobbi, M. A Portable Optical-Fibre-based Surface Plasmon Resonance Biosensor for the Detection of Therapeutic Antibodies in Human Serum. *Sci. Rep.* **2020**, *10*, 11154. [CrossRef] [PubMed]
38. Loyez, M.; Lobry, M.; Hassan, E.M.; DeRosa, M.C.; Caucheteur, C.; Wattiez, R. HER2 Breast Cancer Biomarker Detection Using a Sandwich Optical Fiber Assay. *Talanta* **2021**, *221*, 121452. [CrossRef]
39. Kong, L.X.; Chi, M.J.; Ren, C.; Ni, L.F.; Li, Z.; Zhang, Y.S. Micro-Lab on Tip: High-Performance Dual-Channel Surface Plasmon Resonance Sensor Integrated on Fiber-Optic End Facet. *Sens. Actuators B Chem.* **2022**, *351*, 130978. [CrossRef]

biosensors

MDPI

Communication

The Introduction of a New Diagnostic Tool in Forensic Pathology: LiDAR Sensor for 3D Autopsy Documentation

Aniello Maiese [1], Alice Chiara Manetti [1], Costantino Ciallella [2] and Vittorio Fineschi [2,*]

1 Department of Surgical Pathology, Medical, Molecular and Critical Area, Institute of Legal Medicine, University of Pisa, 56126 Pisa, Italy; aniello.maiese@unipi.it (A.M.); a.manetti3@studenti.unipi.it (A.C.M.)

2 Department of Anatomical, Histological, Forensic and Orthopedic Science, Sapienza University of Rome, 00161 Rome, Italy; costantino.ciallella@uniroma1.it

* Correspondence: vittorio.fineschi@uniroma1.it; Tel.: +39-(06)-49912722

Abstract: Autopsy is a complex and unrepeatable procedure. It is essential to have the possibility of reviewing the autoptic findings, especially when it is done for medico-legal purposes. Traditional photography is not always adequate to record forensic practice since two-dimensional images could lead to distortion and misinterpretation. Three-dimensional (3D) reconstructions of autoptic findings could be a new way to document the autopsy. Besides, nowadays, smartphones and tablets equipped with a LiDAR sensor make it extremely easy to elaborate a 3D model directly in the autopsy room. Herein, a quality and trustworthiness evaluation of 3D models obtained during ten autopsies is made comparing 3D models and conventional autopsy photographic records. Three-dimensional models were realistic and accurate and allowed precise measurements. The review of the autoptic report was facilitated by the 3D model. Conclusions: The LiDAR sensor and 3D models have been demonstrated to be a valid tool to introduce some kind of reproducibility into the autoptic practice.

Keywords: autopsy record; three-dimensional model; LiDAR sensor

Citation: Maiese, A.; Manetti, A.C.; Ciallella, C.; Fineschi, V. The Introduction of a New Diagnostic Tool in Forensic Pathology: LiDAR Sensor for 3D Autopsy Documentation. *Biosensors* **2022**, *12*, 132. https://doi.org/10.3390/bios12020132

Received: 1 January 2022
Accepted: 17 February 2022
Published: 19 February 2022

1. Introduction

Autopsy is a complex and unrepeatable procedure. Therefore, it is essential to document all the procedural steps and findings to achieve legal significance. Traditionally, the forensic pathologist records the autoptic procedure with photographs, and this method is still widely used. However, two-dimensional (2D) images are not always adequate to record forensic practice because they can lead to distortions and misinterpretations, for example, in cases of skin and bone lesions [1]. When discussing a case in court with the purpose of justice, it is fundamental to rely on trustworthy images. In the last years, construct three-dimensional (3D) scanning has been introduced into this field [2,3]. One of the first methods applied was photogrammetry [4,5]. More recently, 3D surface extraction from computer tomography (CT) data and 3D scanning have also been used [6,7]. However, this method has some limits correlated to variability and the need for photographic skills [8]. A light detection and ranging (LiDAR) sensor is a remote sensing device that uses an infrared light pulsed laser to calculate the distance between two points [9]. Those data could then be combined with photographic information and used to construct 3D models of objects and/or surfaces. It is widely used in the engineering and construction field, as well as in many other disciplines [10]. The combination between the LiDAR scanner and the smartphone camera has made it possible to easily obtain 3D images of any objects, with a precise definition of their shape and surface. Before LiDAR, 3D documentation was time consuming and expensive [11]. Besides, usually it requires specific skills, for example, good photographic expertise or specific professional training, particularly in the case of CT 3D reconstruction [11,12]. Moreover, the equipment required for 3D documentation is not present in every facility (e.g., the 3D system "VirtoScan-on-Rails", used by Kottner et al.) [13]. Several studies have demonstrated that 3D models could be a valid tool in forensic practice, in addition to other indispensable analyses (i.e., histology, toxicology, etc.) [14]. Three-dimensional documentation assists in findings visualization and display. Furthermore, it helps in events reconstruction. Additional use of 3D models is for medical education. Tóth et al. demonstrated that 3D reconstructions could be a supplementary tool in medical student training and preparation [15]. In their study, student satisfaction was higher with photogrammetry images than other education methods. Three-dimensional data have also been used to create 3D-printed organs [16,17].

In this work, the LiDAR sensor is presented as a new tool that can help forensic pathologists record their autoptic findings with high-quality 3D images.

2. Materials and Methods

2.1. Subjects

In this study, 3D models of entire corpses, single body-areas, and/or single organs were obtained during ten forensic autopsies using the app TRNIO. Three-dimensional models were then processed by MeshLab. The subjects were six males and four females, the age range was 22–74 y.o. The causes of death were various. Demographic details about the subjects are provided in Table 1.

Table 1. Brief description of the subjects included in this work.

Case Number	Sex	Age (y.o.)
1	M	71
2	M	54
3	F	45
4	M	63
5	F	81
6	M	35
7	F	22
8	F	55
9	M	58
10	M	74

The cases were selected from the autopsy databases of the Institutes of Legal Medicine of the University of Pisa and "Sapienza" University of Rome. All corpses were autopsied between 1 October 2021 and 31 October 2021. Autopsies previously performed were not included because we did not have the LiDAR-equipped device before that time. In all cases, histological analysis of tissues sampled during the autopsy was performed. Toxicological analysis, performed on peripheral blood, was negative for all cases. Table 2 shows the main autoptic (macroscopic and histological) findings of the ten cases included in this study, as well as the causes of death.

Table 2. Autoptic findings and causes of death of the ten cases included in this study.

Case Number	Macroscopic Findings	Microscopic Findings	Cause of Death
1	Entrance gunshot wound in the right side of the trunk, exit gunshot wound in the left side of the trunk	Hemorrhagic infiltration of soft tissues near the gunshot wounds	Gunshot
2	Coronary artery disease (atheromatous plaque)	Myocardial ischemia	Cardiovascular disease

Table 2. *Cont.*

Case Number	Macroscopic Findings	Microscopic Findings	Cause of Death
3	Left ventricular hypertrophy	Diffuse myocardial interstitial fibrosis, myocardial hypertrophy	Cardiovascular disease
4	Diffuse burn lesions in various degrees, soot in the airways	Soot deposition in the medium and small airways' mucosa, intraepidermal and subepidermal separation alongside coagulation necrosis in the skin	Fire burn > 40% body surface
5	Entrance gunshot wound in the oral cavity, several skull fracture	Hemorrhagic infiltration of soft tissues near the gunshot wound	Gunshot
6	Both ventricles dilation	Long and thin myocytes, interstitial fibrosis	Cardiovascular disease
7	Skull base fractures, lower limbs fractures, intracranial hemorrhage, and cerebral lacerations	Subarachnoid hemorrhage, hemorrhagic infiltration of soft tissues	Traffic accident
8	Multiple costal fractures, upper limbs fractures, multiple excoriations, heart lacerations, lungs ecchymoses	Hemorrhagic infiltration of soft tissues	Traffic accident
9	Coronary artery disease (atheromatous plaque)	Myocardial ischemia	Cardiovascular disease
10	Coronary artery disease (atheromatous plaque)	Myocardial ischemia	Cardiovascular disease

2.2. Equipment, Recording Method, and 3D Model Processing

Each autopsy procedural step was documented with a conventional camera and a device equipped with a LiDAR sensor. Therefore, we obtained a complete conventional autopsy photographic record and 3D autopsy record. Any peculiar finding (i.e., external lesions, organ alterations) was specifically documented.

A device equipped with a camera and a LiDAR sensor is required, apart from the conventional autopsy equipment. It is possible to use a tablet (iPad Pro) or a smartphone (iPhone 12 Pro, iPhone 12 Pro Max, iPhone 13 Pro, and iPhone 13 Pro Max); the prices of these devices vary from USD 999 to USD 1299. We used the iPhone 12 Pro, which is produced by Apple. According to the technical specifications provided by the manufacturer, it is sized at "146.7 mm × 71.5 mm", weighs 189 g (6.66 ounces), and has three camera systems: Ultra-Wide ($f/2.4$ aperture and 120° field of view), Wide ($f/1.6$ aperture), and Telephoto ($f/2.0$ aperture) cameras. Additional information could be found at the manufacturer's website [18]. Unfortunately, the manufacturer does not provide further specifications of the LiDAR sensor integrated into the device.

A disposable plastic film cover could be used to protect the device if needed. No specific environmental conditions are required. The device could be used to capture the entire corpse or single organs/body areas. The camera should be pointed to the organ/body perpendicularly and then slowly moved to record all the surfaces of interest, as shown in Figures 1 and 2.

This procedure takes only a few seconds, depending on the dimension of the surface of interest (for example, to record the entire body takes about 60–120 s). For better-quality images, the bearing surface should be flat and smooth. A polished steel table, as classically used for autopsy, is suitable for the purpose.

Two applications could be used to acquire data and then elaborate 3D images: TRNIO or 3D Scanner. Both applications are adequate for the purpose. 3D Scanner is free, TRNIO costs USD 4.99. The 3D reconstruction takes about five to ten minutes to be elaborated by the application.

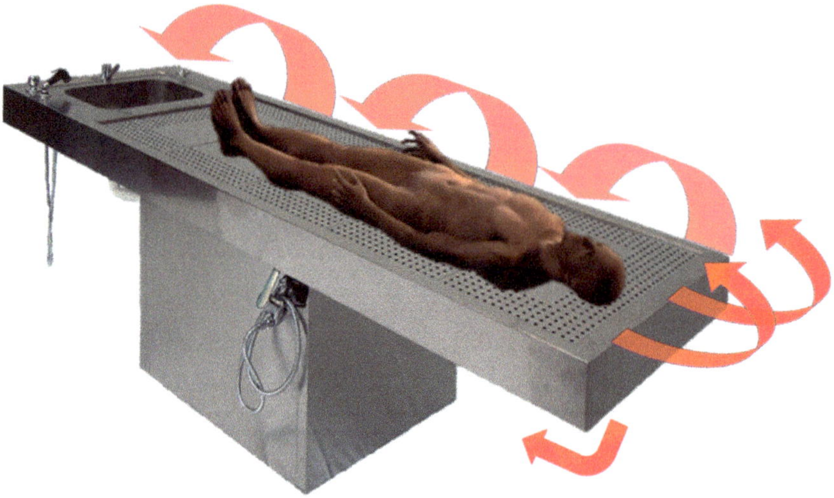

Figure 1. LiDAR 3D reconstruction of a corpse. The corpse was placed on a traditional autoptic steel table. The 3D model was created by capturing the surface data at first horizontally, and then the device was slowly moved to obtain surface data from various degrees. The arrows show how the camera of the device should be pointed, moved, and rotated to allow for capturing all the surfaces. When finished, the corpse should be placed in the prone position and the LiDAR scanning should be repeated.

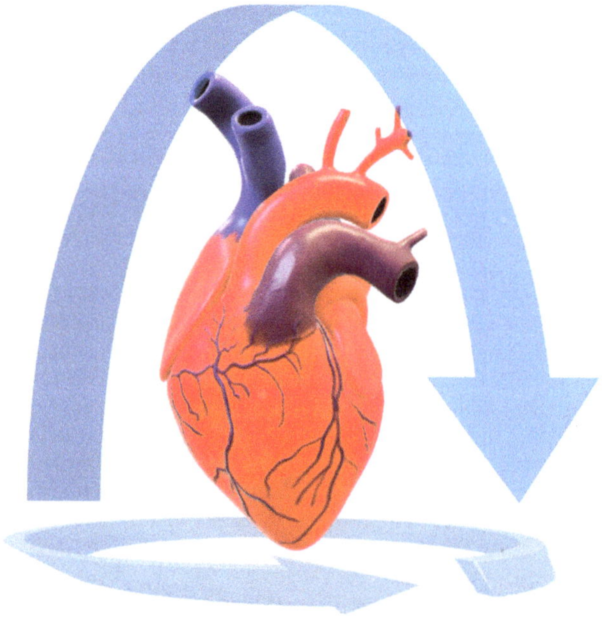

Figure 2. LiDAR 3D reconstruction of a heart. The heart was placed on a white plastic table, lying on its posterior surface. The 3D model was created by capturing the surface data from the anterior surface, then the camera was slowly moved in order to perform a complete rotation around the organ and to capture all the expose surfaces. Then the camera was moved to record the cardiac base. In this way, the heart was completely captured. The procedure should be repeated with the heart lying on its anterior surface.

It is possible to process the 3D models by MeshLab, an open-source tool for the visualization and processing of 3D models. MeshLab also provides a specific tool to measure any length of interest directly on the 3D model. The operator must select two points on the surface of interest (for example, two different lesions or the extremities of the same lesion), then the application provides the length between them in a few seconds. Besides, MeshLab could be used to process raw 3D digitization data for preparing models for 3D printing. MeshLab is freely available for all the major platforms (Windows, MacOS, Linux) [19].

2.3. *Quality and Trustworthiness Evaluation*

To evaluate the trustworthiness of 3D models, a comparison with conventional photography was then done, comparing:

- Conventional autopsy photographic records vs. 3D reconstruction: qualitative evaluation by consensus.
- Body/lesion measurement attained during the autoptic examination vs. body/lesion measurement attained from the 3D model. When a discrepancy was noticed, remeasurements were obtained.
- Lesion description and autopsy revaluation from conventional autopsy photograph records vs. from 3D image review: qualitative evaluation was performed by two forensic pathologists who did not attend the autopsy and did not have knowledge about the cases.

2.4. *3D Printing*

MeshLab was also used to process a heart 3D model for 3D printing. The model was then 3D printed.

3. Results

In all the cases, 3D models met our quality expectations. Three-dimensional images, compared to conventional autopsy photographic records, were realistic and accurate, the color rendering was truthful. Three-dimensional reconstruction was a valid method in recording autoptic findings. In Figure 3 and Video S1 (in Supplementary Materials), an example of 3D reconstruction is provided.

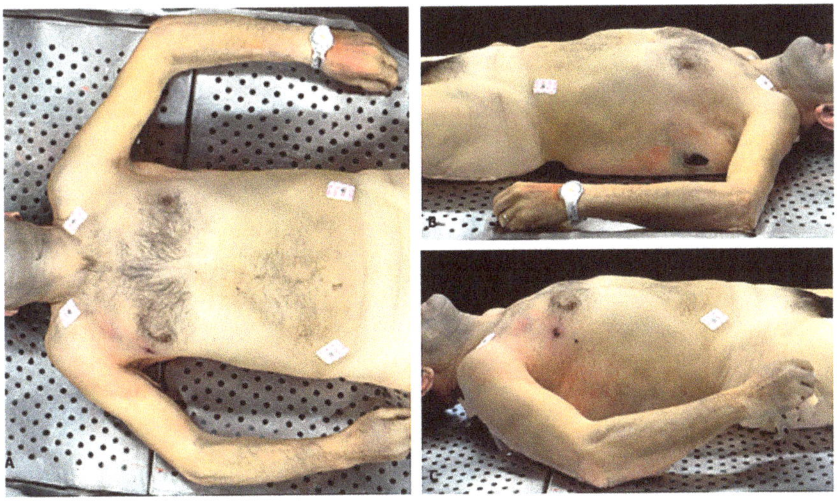

Figure 3. 3D reconstruction of a corpse's trunk and upper limbs (case 1). (**A**) gunshot wound is evident on both sides of the trunk (entrance on the right, exit on the left). (**B**) The reconstruction is realistic, accurate, and detailed. (**C**) Details that could allow personal recognition have been censored.

The measurement of lesions or body parameters (i.e., body length) assessed on 3D models were trustworthy, even more so than the measurement obtained during the autopsy. In fact, in two cases we noticed a discrepancy between the "hand" measurement and the digital measurement, but when we re-measured the body/lesion of interest, we found out the reason was an operator inaccuracy, instead of LiDAR imprecision. Figure 4 shows an example of the comparison between traditional measurement and 3D model measurement.

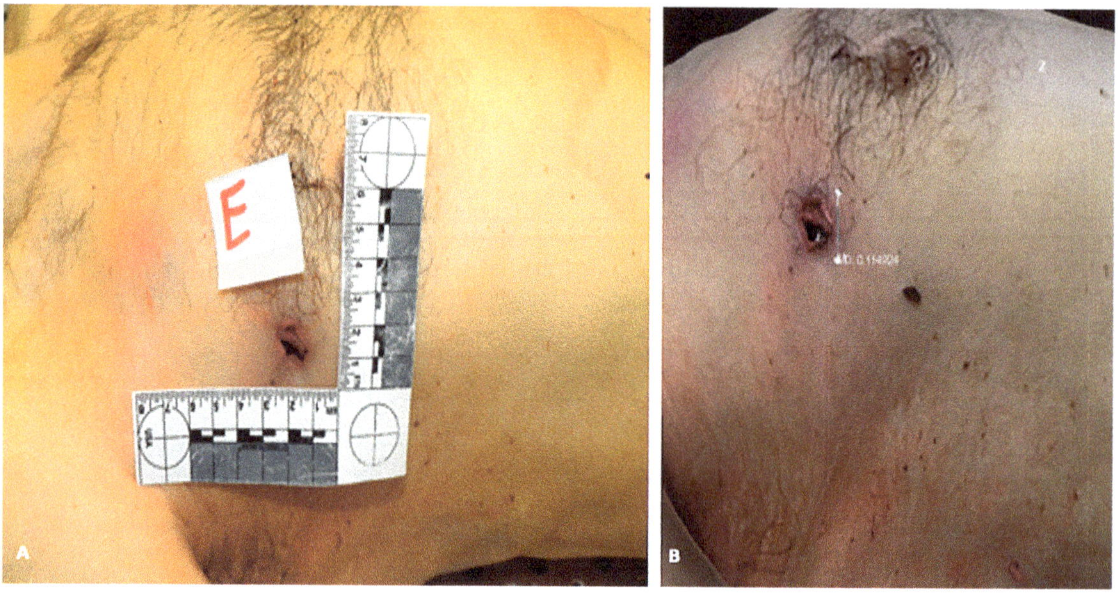

Figure 4. Comparison between 2D picture and 3D reconstruction of a corpse's trunk (case 1). (**A**) shows the 2D picture with a ruler next to the gunshot wound (unit of measurement: centimeter). (**B**) shows the measurement of the gunshot wound diameter obtained from the 3D model (unit of measurement: decimeter). In this case, the initial "hand" measurement of the diameter of the lesion was 1.3 cm. We immediately checked it on the 3D model, which provided 1.14 cm, as shown in Figure 1B. We then re-measured the lesion and confirmed the true measure was the one provided by the 3D model.

Besides, when reviewing the autoptic procedure, the 3D model allows for more precise measurements than traditional images, because there is no 2D-induced distortion. We asked two forensic pathologists, who did not attend the autopsy and did not have knowledge about the cases, to re-evaluate both the conventional autopsy photograph record and the LiDAR reconstructions, in order to assess if 3D models could be used to audit forensic practice. The experts conveyed that external examination of the body and lesion measurements were accurate when performed on 3D reconstruction. In cases 2, 9, and 10 (see Table 2), the cause of death was fatal myocardial ischemia due to acute coronary artery disease. In these cases, the 3D reconstructions allowed the reviewer to measure the diameter of the coronary artery and to evaluate the percentage of lumen obstruction. In case 3, left ventricular hypertrophy was seen at the macroscopic examination of the heart. The reviewer easily suspected this cardiac alteration by reviewing the 3D reconstruction of the heart slides (Figure 5).

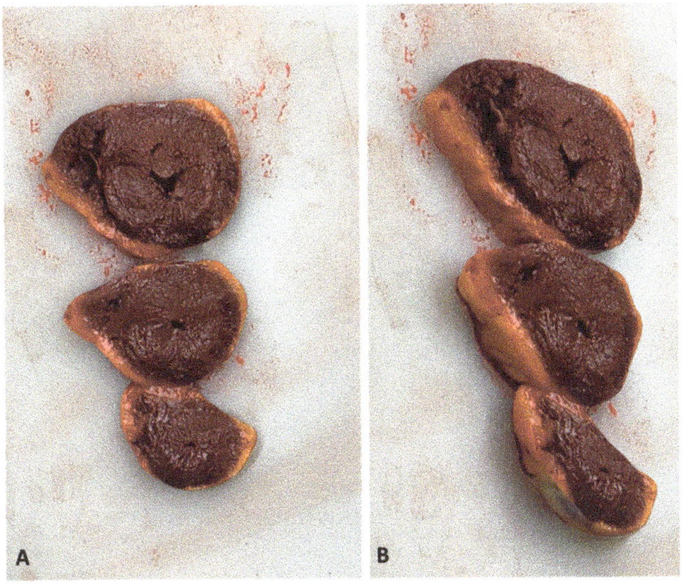

Figure 5. Three-dimensional reconstruction of the heart slides performed at the macroscopic examination of the heart (case 3). (**A**) shows a perpendicular view of the 3D model. (**B**) shows a lateral view. The myocardial wall is precisely measurable in the 3D model, sustaining the hypothesis of myocardial hypertrophy. In this case, the histologic examination confirmed the diagnosis.

Furthermore, 3D images allowed us to evaluate the degree of depth of some lesions. This was obviously not possible with traditional pictures. In cases of complex traumatic lesion patterns, the audit of the autoptic process was facilitated by LiDAR reconstruction, because 3D images better showed the anatomical relationships between body structures (for example, the description of skull base fractures in case 7 and multiple costal fractures in case 8). Figure 6 shows the 3D reconstruction of a >40% burned body (case 4).

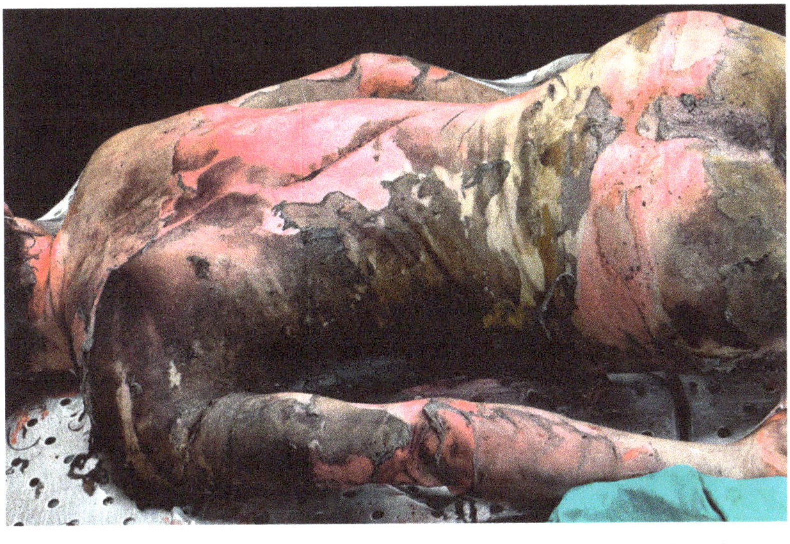

Figure 6. Three-dimesnional reconstruction of a corpse burned >40% of the body surface (case 4).

As a supplementary activity, we also 3D printed the model of a heart. The reproduction was very accurate, as can be seen in Figure 7. Video S2 shows the heart 3D model.

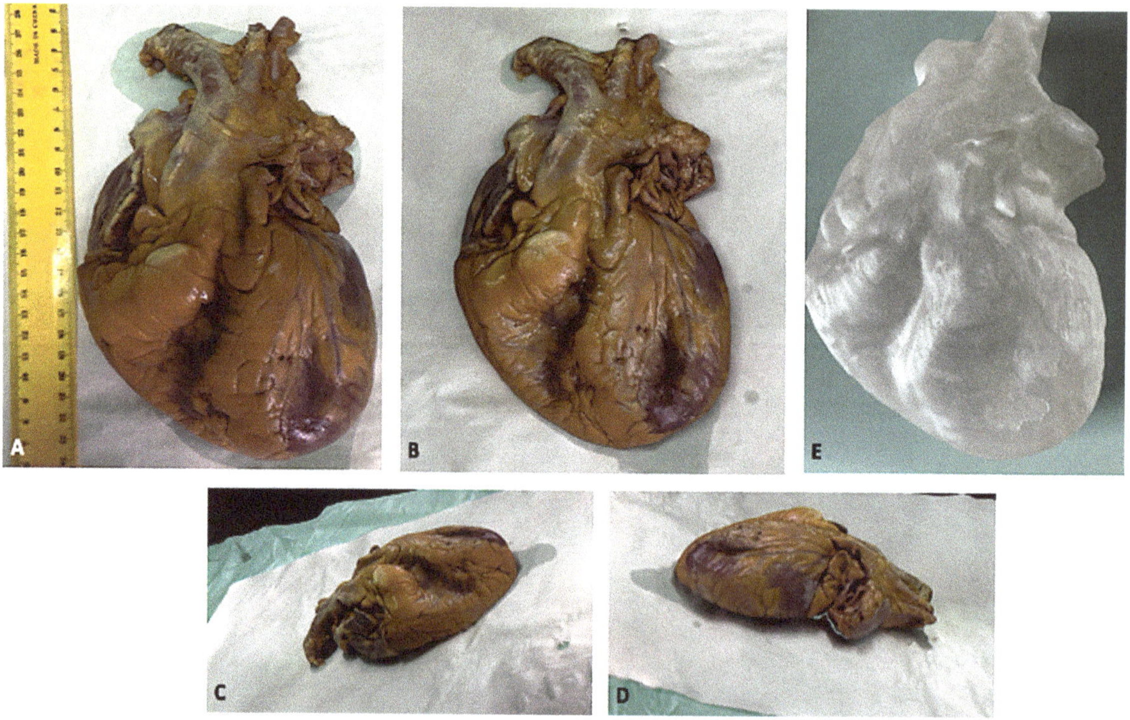

Figure 7. 3D model of a formalin-fixed heart. (**A**) shows the traditional picture. (**B–D**) show the 3D reconstruction. (**E**) shows the 3D-printed heart.

4. Discussion

In our study, 3D models applied to the autoptic examination met the expectations and demonstrated trustworthiness in terms of quality and measurement accuracy. This technique preserves information in all three dimensions and so it is very useful in cases of traumatic lesions. Furthermore, measurements performed on the 3D reconstruction allowed us to avoid operator-related errors, not only associated with measurement imprecision but also in case the operator missed measuring or describing some finding during the autoptic examination.

Autopsy intrinsically destructs the object of its analysis, the corpse. Besides, putrefactive processes irreversibly altered the cadaver, and so, after a certain amount of time, exhuming and re-examining the body could be pointless. Photography allows one to maintain archival data and to audit the forensic practice. However, the quality and reliability of the photographic record and the autopsy report are not always guaranteed [20]. Technical requirements and good photographic skills are indispensable to perform a good photographic report, minimizing distortions and misinterpretations [21,22].

The introduction of radiological examinations into the forensic practice provided another way to record the pathological findings [23–26]. Nevertheless, post-mortem imaging entails considerable expenditure, both for the corpse transportation to the radiology facility and for the exam itself, and to perform those examinations is also time consuming. In the last years, 3D reconstruction has supplemented medico-legal activities, first of all in crime scene reconstruction [27–29]. Forensic pathologists also benefit from 3D surface documentation, but usually complex, expensive, and/or unwieldy instrumentations are required [1,30,31]. The introduction of photogrammetry has made 3D documentation easier than in the past since the required equipment consists basically of a camera and a computer [2,3,32–35]. However, this method has some limits. At first, the variability correlated to the type of camera [5]. Formerly, photographic skills are still necessary because the computer application needs good traditional photographs to create the 3D model. Besides, it requires a two-steps procedure: taking pictures during the autopsy and then, in a second moment, computer elaboration. It means that it is not possible to directly evaluate the 3D reconstruction quality in the autopsy room, so you cannot re-take a picture if you later discover it is not adequate.

Recently, LiDAR technology has met the mobile and tablet industry and nowadays smartphones/tablets with a LiDAR sensor next to the traditional camera have been placed on the market. This makes it extremely manageable to obtain 3D models of surfaces: you just need to point the camera at the object of interest (the body, the organ, the lesion) and slightly move, in order to create a complete reconstruction. No peculiar abilities or skills are required, and an everyday device is used for the purpose. TRNIO and 3D Scanner take from five to ten minutes to create the 3D model, so it is possible to verify the reconstruction directly in the autopsy room and to re-take it if necessary. In addition, this method is quite cheap if compared with other diagnostics examinations. The mobiles and tablets with a LiDAR sensor integrated cost about USD 1000, while other imaging machines cost thousands of dollars.

It is foreseeable that 3D models and 3D printing presentations in court would make medico-legal dissertations more effective and understandable. Besides, 3D printing could be useful in crime scene and traumatic dynamic reconstruction.

The introduction of this technology into the autoptic practice would also provide a new tool to review the autoptic findings. Unfortunately, the autopsy is not always followed by a good-quality report [36,37]. Sometimes, it could be necessary to audit the autopsy report, for example, when the process proceeds among the levels of justice. Three-dimensional models would guarantee a new form of reproducibility to the autopsy practice.

5. Conclusions

The autopsy is an unrepeatable procedure, but the autopsy report and the autopsy photographic record do not always meet the demanded standard of quality. In the last years, photogrammetry (3D images elaborated by photographs of the autoptic procedure) has been introduced into forensic practice. However, this technology still presents some limits.

The recent arrival on the scene of smartphones and tablets equipped with LiDAR sensors, in addition to the traditional camera, allows us to use this new technology in the autopsy room. Creating a 3D model of corpses, organs, and lesions has been made extremely easy and quick. In this study, 3D images obtained during autopsies were accurate and precise and have been demonstrated to be a valid tool in auditing and reviewing autoptic procedures.

Furthermore, displaying 3D models and 3D printings in court as evidence would probably improve the effectiveness and understandability of medico-legal dissertation. In conclusion, LiDAR technology could be a valid instrument that helps to introduce some kind of reproducibility into the autoptic practice.

Supplementary Materials: The following supporting information can be downloaded at: https://www.mdpi.com/article/10.3390/bios12020132/s1, Video S1. 3D reconstruction of a corpse's trunk and upper limbs (case 1). Details that could allow personal recognition have been censored. Video S2. 3D model of a formalin-fixed heart.

Author Contributions: Conceptualization, A.M.; methodology, V.F.; formal analysis, A.C.M.; investigation, A.M.; writing—original draft preparation, A.M. and A.C.M.; writing—review and editing, A.M. and C.C.; supervision, V.F. All authors have read and agreed to the published version of the manuscript.

Funding: This research received no external funding.

Institutional Review Board Statement: Not applicable.

Informed Consent Statement: Not applicable.

Conflicts of Interest: The authors declare no conflict of interest.

References

1. Thali, M.J.; Braun, M.; Dirnhofer, R. Optical 3D surface digitizing in forensic medicine: 3D documentation of skin and bone injuries. *Forensic Sci. Int.* **2003**, *137*, 203–208. [CrossRef] [PubMed]
2. Gitto, L.; Donato, L.; Di Luca, A.; Bryant, S.M.; Serinelli, S. The Application of Photogrammetry in the Autopsy Room: A Basic, Practical Workflow. *J. Forensic Sci.* **2020**, *65*, 2146–2154. [CrossRef]
3. Schweitzer, W.; Röhrich, E.; Schaepman, M.; Thali, M.J.; Ebert, L. Aspects of 3D surface scanner performance for post-mortem skin documentation in forensic medicine using rigid benchmark objects. *J. Forensic Radiol. Imaging* **2013**, *1*, 167–175. [CrossRef]
4. Thali, M.J.; Braun, M.; Brueschweiler, W.; Dirnhofer, R. 'Morphological imprint': Determination of the injury-causing weapon from the wound morphology using forensic 3D/CAD-supported photogrammetry. *Forensic Sci. Int.* **2003**, *132*, 177–181. [CrossRef]
5. Villa, C. Forensic 3D documentation of skin injuries. *Int. J. Leg. Med.* **2016**, *131*, 751–759. [CrossRef] [PubMed]
6. Sansoni, G.; Cattaneo, C.; Trebeschi, M.; Gibelli, D.; Porta, D.; Picozzi, M. Feasibility of contactless 3d optical measureme for the analysis of bone and soft tissue lesions: New technologies and perspectives in forensic sciences. *J. Forensic Sci.* **2009**, *54*, 540–545. [CrossRef]
7. Grassberger, M.; Gehl, A.; Püschel, K.; Turk, E. 3D reconstruction of emergency cranial computed tomography scans as a tool in clinical forensic radiology after survived blunt head trauma—Report of two cases. *Forensic Sci. Int.* **2011**, *207*, e19–e23. [CrossRef]
8. American Geosciences Institute. Available online: https://www.americangeosciences.org/critical-issues/faq/what-lidar-and-what-it-used (accessed on 11 February 2021).
9. Cabaleiro, M.; Riveiro, B.; Arias, P.; Caamaño, J.; Vilán, J. Automatic 3D modelling of metal frame connections from LiDAR data for structural engineering purposes. *ISPRS J. Photogramm. Remote Sens.* **2014**, *96*, 47–56. [CrossRef]
10. Bolliger, S.A.; Thali, M.J. Imaging and virtual autopsy: Looking back and forward. *Philos. Trans. R. Soc. B Biol. Sci.* **2015**, *370*, 20140253. [CrossRef]
11. Shintaku, H.; Yamaguchi, M.; Toru, S.; Kitagawa, M.; Hirokawa, K.; Yokota, T.; Uchihara, T. Three-dimensional surface models of autopsied human brains constructed from multiple photographs by photogrammetry. *PLoS ONE* **2019**, *14*, e0219619. [CrossRef]
12. Grabherr, S.; Baumann, P.; Minoiu, C.; Fahrni, S.; Mangin, P. Post-mortem imaging in forensic investigations: Current utility, limitations, and ongoing developments. *Res. Rep. Forensic Med Sci.* **2016**, *6*, 25–37. [CrossRef]
13. Kottner, S.; Schaerli, S.; Fürst, M.; Ptacek, W.; Thali, M.; Gascho, D. VirtoScan-on-Rails—An automated 3D imaging system for fast post-mortem whole-body surface documentation at autopsy tables. *J. Forensic Med. Pathol.* **2019**, *15*, 198–212. [CrossRef] [PubMed]
14. Kottner, S.; Schulz, M.M.; Berger, F.; Thali, M.; Gascho, D. Beyond the visible spectrum—Applying 3D multispectral full-body imaging to the VirtoScan system. *Forensic Sci. Med. Pathol.* **2021**, *17*, 565–576. [CrossRef] [PubMed]
15. Tóth, D.; Petrus, K.; Heckmann, V.; Simon, G.; Poór, V.S. Application of photogrammetry in forensic pathology education of medical students in response to COVID-19. *J. Forensic Sci.* **2021**, *66*, 1533–1537. [CrossRef]
16. Yoo, S.-S. 3D-printed biological organs: Medical potential and patenting opportunity. *Expert Opin. Ther. Patents* **2015**, *25*, 507–511. [CrossRef]
17. Schubert, C.; Van Langeveld, M.C.; A Donoso, L. Innovations in 3D printing: A 3D overview from optics to organs. *Br. J. Ophthalmol.* **2014**, *98*, 159–161. [CrossRef]
18. iPhone 12 Pro Technical Specifications. Available online: https://support.apple.com/kb/SP831?locale=it_IT&viewlocale=en_US (accessed on 10 February 2022).
19. Cignoni, P.; Callieri, M.; Corsini, M.; Dellepiane, M.; Ganovelli, F.; Ranzuglia, G. MeshLab: An open-source mesh processing tool. In Proceedings of the 6th Eurographics Italian Chapter Conference, Salerno, Italy, 2–4 July 2008.
20. Roberts, I.S.; Benamore, R.E.; Benbow, E.W.; Lee, S.H.; Harris, J.N.; Jackson, A.; Mallett, S.; Patankar, T.; Peebles, C.; Roobottom, C.; et al. Post-mortem imaging as an alternative to autopsy in the diagnosis of adult deaths: A validation study. *Lancet* **2012**, *379*, 136–142. [CrossRef]
21. Henham, A.P.; Lee, K.A.P. Photography in forensic medicine. *J. Audiov. Media Med.* **1994**, *17*, 15–20. [CrossRef]
22. Gouse, S.; Karnam, S.; Girish, H.; Murgod, S. Forensic photography: Prospect through the lens. *J. Forensic Dent. Sci.* **2018**, *10*, 2–4. [CrossRef]
23. Urschler, M.; Bornik, A.; Scheurer, E.; Yen, K.; Bischof, H.; Schmalstieg, D. Forensic-Case Analysis: From 3D Imaging to Interactive Visualization. *IEEE Comput. Graph. Appl.* **2012**, *32*, 79–87. [CrossRef]
24. Maiese, A.; Gitto, L.; dell'Aquila, M.; Bolino, G. When the hidden features become evident: The usefulness of PMCT in a strangulation-related death. *Leg. Med. (Tokyo)* **2014**, *16*, 364–366. [CrossRef] [PubMed]
25. Thali, M.; Dirnhofer, R.; Vock, P. *The Virtopsy Approach: 3D Optical and Radiological Scanning and Reconstruction in Forensic Med-icine*, 1st ed.; CRC: New York, NY, USA, 2009; pp. 3–10.

26. Bertozzi, G.; Cafarelli, F.P.; Ferrara, M.; Di Fazio, N.; Guglielmi, G.; Cipolloni, L.; Manetti, F.; La Russa, R.; Fineschi, V. Sudden Cardiac Death and Ex-Situ Post-Mortem Cardiac Magnetic Resonance Imaging: A Morphological Study Based on Diagnostic Correlation Methodology. *Diagnostics* **2022**, *12*, 218. [CrossRef] [PubMed]
27. Buck, U.; Naether, S.; Räss, B.; Jackowski, C.; Thali, M.J. Accident or homicide—Virtual crime scene reconstruction using 3D methods. *Forensic Sci. Int.* **2013**, *225*, 75–84. [CrossRef] [PubMed]
28. Wang, J.; Li, Z.; Hu, W.; Shao, Y.; Wang, L.; Wu, R.; Ma, K.; Zou, D.; Chen, Y. Virtual reality and integrated crime scene scanning for immersive and heterogeneous crime scene reconstruction. *Forensic Sci. Int.* **2019**, *303*, 109943. [CrossRef] [PubMed]
29. Ma, M.; Zheng, H.; Lallie, H. Virtual Reality and 3D Animation in Forensic Visualization. *J. Forensic Sci.* **2010**, *55*, 1227–1231. [CrossRef] [PubMed]
30. Leipner, A.; Baumeister, R.; Thali, M.J.; Braun, M.; Dobler, E.; Ebert, L.C. Multi-camera system for 3D forensic documentation. *Forensic Sci. Int.* **2016**, *261*, 123–128. [CrossRef]
31. Sieberth, T.; Ebert, L.C.; Gentile, S.; Fliss, B. Clinical forensic height measurements on injured people using a multi camera device for 3D documentation. *Forensic Sci. Med. Pathol.* **2020**, *16*, 586–594. [CrossRef]
32. Brüschweiler, W.; Braun, M.; Dirnhofer, R.; Thali, M. Analysis of patterned injuries and injury-causing instruments with forensic 3D/CAD supported photogrammetry (FPHG): An instruction manual for the documentation process. *Forensic Sci. Int.* **2003**, *132*, 130–138. [CrossRef]
33. Urbanová, P.; Hejna, P.; Jurda, M. Testing photogrammetry-based techniques for three-dimensional surface documentation in forensic pathology. *Forensic Sci. Int.* **2015**, *250*, 77–86. [CrossRef]
34. Flies, M.J.; Larsen, P.K.; Lynnerup, N.; Villa, C. Forensic 3D documentation of skin injuries using photogrammetry: Photographs vs. video and manual vs. automatic measurements. *Int. J. Leg. Med.* **2018**, *133*, 963–971. [CrossRef]
35. Slot, L.; Larsen, P.K.; Lynnerup, N. Photogrammetric Documentation of Regions of Interest at Autopsy-A Pilot Study. *J. Forensic Sci.* **2013**, *59*, 226–230. [CrossRef] [PubMed]
36. The Coroner's Autopsy: Do We Deserve better? A Report of the National Confidential Enquiry into Patient Outcome and Death, 2006. Available online: https://www.ncepod.org.uk/2006Report/Downloads/Coronial%20Autopsy%20Report%202006.pdf (accessed on 11 February 2021).
37. Arunkumar, P.; Maiese, A.; Bolino, G.; Gitto, L. Determined to Die! Ability to Act Following Multiple Self-inflicted Gunshot Wounds to the Head. The Cook County Office of Medical Examiner Experience (2005–2012) and Review of Literature. *J. Forensic Sci.* **2015**, *60*, 1373–1379. [CrossRef] [PubMed]

biosensors

MDPI

Article

A Wearable and Real-Time Pulse Wave Monitoring System Based on a Flexible Compound Sensor

Xiaoxiao Kang [1,2,3], Jun Zhang [1,2,3], Zheming Shao [1,2,3], Guotai Wang [1,2,3], Xingguang Geng [1,3], Yitao Zhang [1,3] and Haiying Zhang [1,2,3,*]

1 Institute of Microelectronics of Chinese Academy of Sciences, Beijing 100029, China; kangxiaoxiao@ime.ac.cn (X.K.); zhangjun@ime.ac.cn (J.Z.); shaozheming@ime.ac.cn (Z.S.); wangguotai@ime.ac.cn (G.W.); gengxingguang@ime.ac.cn (X.G.); zhangyitao@ime.ac.cn (Y.Z.)
2 University of Chinese Academy of Sciences, Beijing 100049, China
3 Beijing Key Laboratory for Next Generation RF Communication Chip Technology, Beijing 100029, China
* Correspondence: zhanghaiying@ime.ac.cn

Abstract: Continuous monitoring of pulse waves plays a significant role in reflecting physical conditions and disease diagnosis. However, the current collection equipment cannot simultaneously achieve wearable and continuous monitoring under varying pressure and provide personalized pulse wave monitoring targeted different human bodies. To solve the above problems, this paper proposed a novel wearable and real-time pulse wave monitoring system based on a novel flexible compound sensor. Firstly, a custom-packaged pressure sensor, a signal stabilization structure, and a micro pressurization system make up the flexible compound sensor to complete the stable acquisition of pulse wave signals under continuously varying pressure. Secondly, a real-time algorithm completes the analysis of the trend of the pulse wave peak, which can quickly and accurately locate the best pulse wave for different individuals. Finally, the experimental results show that the wearable system can both realize continuous monitoring and reflecting trend differences and quickly locate the best pulse wave for different individuals with the 95% accuracy. The weight of the whole system is only 52.775 g, the working current is 46 mA, and the power consumption is 160 mW. Its small size and low power consumption meet wearable and portable scenarios, which has significant research value and commercialization prospects.

Keywords: wearable; flexible compound sensor; wrist pulse signal; real-time monitoring; the varying trend of pulse wave peak; best pulse wave positioning

Citation: Kang, X.; Zhang, J.; Shao, Z.; Wang, G.; Geng, X.; Zhang, Y.; Zhang, H. A Wearable and Real-Time Pulse Wave Monitoring System Based on a Flexible Compound Sensor. *Biosensors* **2022**, *12*, 133. https://doi.org/10.3390/bios12020133

Received: 7 January 2022
Accepted: 18 February 2022
Published: 20 February 2022

Publisher's Note: MDPI stays neutral with regard to jurisdictional claims in published maps and institutional affiliations.

1. Introduction

Pulse wave diagnosis has a glorious history both in China and India. Studies have shown that pulse waves are the intuitive reflection of the state of the internal heart and blood vessels [1–5]. It has been proven in modern medicine to be able to predict and reflect a variety of diseases, such as cardiovascular disease [6] and diabetes [7]. The intensity of the radial artery pulse wave is considered an indicator for the diagnosis of many diseases. Moreover, its characteristics of non-invasiveness, non-radiation, and relatively simple processes have been widely accepted and concerned [8].

Wearable and continuous monitoring of physiological signals such as pulse wave has gradually become a research hotspot [9–12]. Some studies have used wearable sensors to monitor arterial waveforms such as photoplethysmography (PPG) signals, combined with novel machine learning algorithms, to establish new ways to advance the progress of physiological health monitoring, and made remarkable progress [9,11]. Pulse wave diagnosis can obtain the varying trend of pulse wave peak by applying different levels of static pressure to the radial artery, which can reflect the current physical state of the observer [10,12]. Since each person has different static pressure ranges, it is necessary to measure the pressure of the radial artery to obtain an individualized varying trend of pulse wave peaks. Traditional pulse wave diagnosis mainly relies on the experience of Traditional Chinese Medicine (TCM), and the diagnostic criteria vary from person to person. Objective and quantitative diagnostic equipment has been a research hotspot for decades [13].

There are some problems with the pulse wave sensor. The main categories of pulse wave pressure sensors include photoelectric sensors [14–17], piezoresistive sensors [18,19], ultrasonic sensors [20], and pressure sensors [21]. Photoelectric sensors, such as PPG sensors, which have made some notable progress [14,16,17], are susceptible to light interference from external sources, and cannot measure the trend of pulse wave pressure under continuously varying pressure. The sensitivity of the piezoresistive sensor [18] is inversely proportional to the pressure range, so when the applied pressure is much larger than the pulse wave, it is difficult to detect the weak pulse wave signal and obtain high-quality data. The pressure sensor converts the mechanical pressure into an electrical signal, which imitates the doctor's tactile sense of pulse in practice, which is considered to be a better choice. The flexible pressure sensor based on Polyvinylidene fluoride (PVDF) piezoelectric sensor can be used for wearable pulse measurement, such as [22], it is still unable to obtain the pulse wave and applied pressure information under continuously varying pressure during the test.

There are also some defects in the existing pulse wave acquisition equipment. In our previous work [1,2], we proposed a new type of pulse wave acquisition device that can automatically pressurize the radial artery in sections, but the device is large in size, poor in portability, and high in power consumption, which cannot meet the needs of continuous pulse wave collection and real-time monitoring. This problem also exists in other jobs [22]. There are also some wearable pulse wave acquisition devices that have been verified in principle, but there are still problems such as the inability to perform real-time calculations or to apply continuously changing pressure [23–25]. Building a wearable pulse wave monitoring system to obtain simultaneously pulse wave and pressure information under continuously varying pressure is one of the urgent problems to be solved.

To solve the above problems, this paper proposed a wearable and real-time monitoring system based on a flexible compound sensor, which can simultaneously obtain pulse wave and pressure information under continuously varying pressure. Firstly, the flexible compound sensor includes a custom-packaged pulse pressure sensor, a signal stabilization structure, and a micro pressurization system. While applying continuously changing static pressure to the radial artery, it achieves stable acquisition of pulse wave signals. Then, a conditioning circuit was designed for pulse signal processing and an algorithm was developed to obtain the varying trend of the pulse wave peak under varying pressure in real-time, so as to calculate the characteristic parameters of the pulse wave. Finally, experiments are carried out to verify the accuracy, repeatability, and effectiveness of the flexible compound sensor. The results show that the compound sensor has good accuracy and repeatability, and the system can not only obtain the pulse wave under continuously varying pressure, but also analyze the varying trend of the pulse wave peak with pressure in real-time, which can be used by different people and quickly locate the strongest point of pulse wave.

2. Materials and Methods

2.1. System Overview

The wearable and real-time pulse wave monitoring system proposed in this paper includes a flexible compound sensor that is worn on the human wrist to complete the pulse wave signal acquisition, a circuit structure to accomplish the signal processing and transmission, and a real-time algorithm to realize the calculation of the pulse wave under different static pressures. Specifically, the flexible compound sensor consists of three parts: a pulse wave pressure sensor to collect pulse wave signals, a signal stabilization structure customized to ensure signal quality, and a micro pressurization system to apply continuous varying pressure to the radial artery. The schematic diagram of the monitoring system is shown in Figure 1a and the photograph of the monitoring system is shown in Figure 1b.

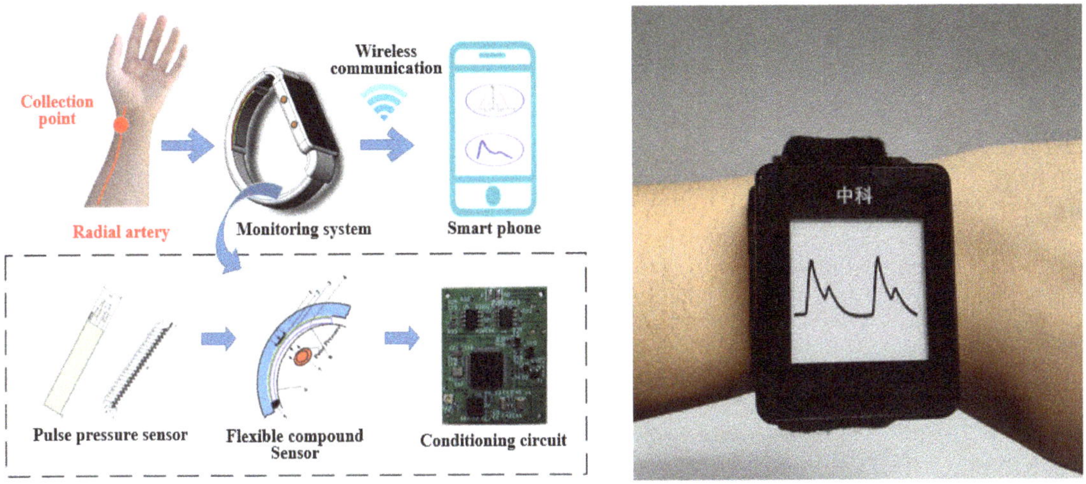

(**a**) (**b**)

Figure 1. The proposed pulse wave monitoring system. (**a**) Schematic diagram of the monitoring system, based on a flexible compound sensor; (**b**) Photograph of the monitoring system.

Firstly, the pulse wave signal is collected by the flexible compound sensor under the continuously varying pressure, and then transmitted to the circuit, conveyed to the microprocessor for real-time algorithm processing to obtain information such as the varying trend of pulse wave peak. Simultaneously, it was formed feedback based on the calculation results to control the micro pressurization system. The original data and algorithm results can be displayed on the low-power ink screen that comes with the system. Furthermore, they can be transmitted to a PC or smartphone via wireless communication for real-time monitoring. The weight of the whole system is only 52.775 g, the maximum working current is approximately 46 mA, and the power consumption of the whole machine is approximately 160 mW, which meets the requirements of wearable and portable scenarios.

2.2. Flexible Compound Sensor

The flexible compound sensor is the key to the design of the entire wearable system that is designed to support the stable and effective collection of pulse waves under continuously varying pressure. In order to closely fit the human wrist to collect pulse waves, the flexible compound sensor consists of a pulse pressure sensor, a signal stabilization structure, and a customized micro pressurization system. A schematic diagram of the flexible compound sensor is shown in the Figure 2a. The solid line shows the specific component, and the broken line indicates the name of the specific component.

2.2.1. Pulse Pressure Sensor

To obtain an effective pulse wave signal, we designed the pulse pressure sensor based on the PVDF piezoelectric sensor, which has high sensitivity and meets the frequency characteristics of the pulse signal. Its dynamic range completely covers the pulse beating range and can effectively cover the pulse wave collection site on the wrist. The characteristic table of the sensor is shown in Table 1.

To collect the pulse wave stably and effectively, considering the sensing, protection, and external connection, we customized the pulse pressure sensor into a five-layer structure. The schematic diagram of the package structure is shown in Figure 2b. From top to bottom, they are the top protective layer, the positive conductive layer, and the PVDF piezoelectric thin film sensor (28 μm), the negative conductive layer, and the bottom protective layer. The top and bottom protective layers are made of polyester film. On the one hand, it protects the

PVDF film material and conductive layer inside the sensor from being damaged by moisture and mechanical friction. On the other hand, it can also provide mechanical strength for the pins. The positive and negative conductive layers are printed with silver ink on both sides of the film as electrodes on both sides of the film. When the PVDF piezoelectric sensor is deformed by force, polarized charges are generated on both sides of the film, and the positive charge side passes through the positive conductive layer. It is transferred to the positive pin, and the negative charge side is transferred to the negative pin through the negative conductive layer. The photograph of the pulse pressure sensor is shown in Figure 2c. The sensitive area of the sensor is determined by the PVDF piezoelectric sensor, which is 40 × 10 mm and can effectively cover the pulse wave collection site on the wrist. The distance between the boundary of the shape and the boundary of the sensitive surface is 0.5 mm. The connector uses a pin with a length of 10 mm to conduct the charge out.

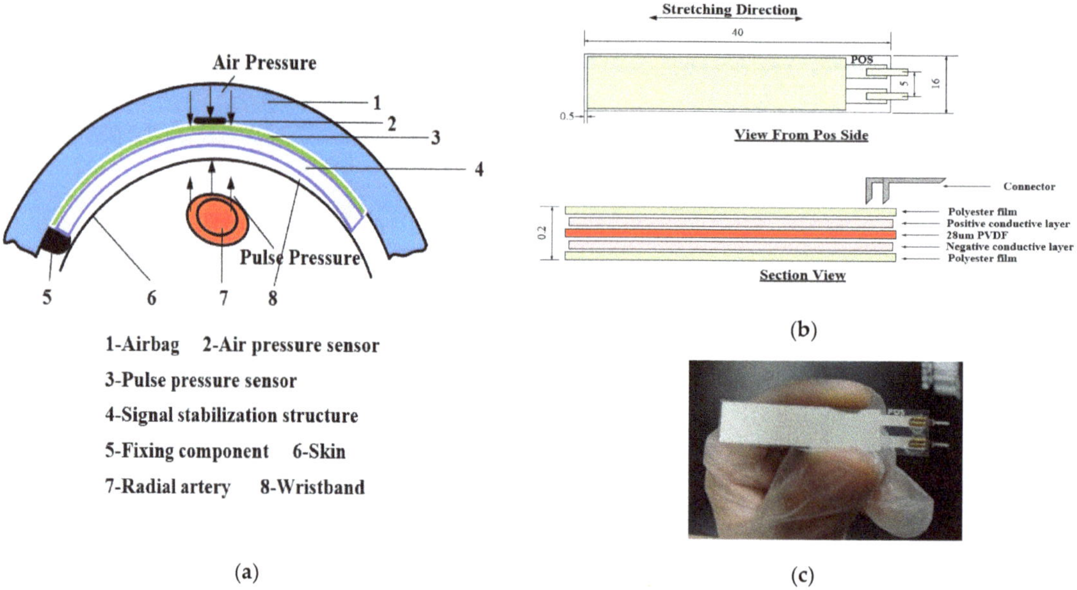

Figure 2. Flexible compound sensor: (**a**) Schematic diagram of the flexible compound sensor; (**b**) Schematic diagram of the package structure of the pulse pressure sensor; (**c**) Photograph of the pulse pressure sensor.

Table 1. Parameters of PVDF piezoelectric sensor.

Variables	Parameters
Density	1.78×10^3 kg/m^3
Active area	40 mm × 10 mm
Thickness	28 μm
Capacitance	1.6 nF
Young's Modulus	2×10^9 N/m^2
Mylar	5 mil
Sensitivity	14.4 V/N

Considering the design of the package, we try to fix the shape of the film itself and consider trying our best to reduce the interference caused by the space electromagnetic and the stability of the connector. Firstly, to prevent the fluctuation of the shape of the film itself from generating noise, we use packaging and pulse signal stabilization structure to limit the freedom of the film shape in the application. Secondly, the sensor lead is connected with a twisted pair when it is connected to the pin, which can not only transmit the signal of the PVDF piezoelectric sensor but also shield the external electromagnetic interference. Finally, to ensure the stability of the connector, in our research, the sensor is connected by a pin and the lead is connected by solder.

2.2.2. Pulse Signal Stabilization Structure

To enhance the sensor sensitivity and effectively collect pulse waves, based on the above package structure, we have customized a signal stabilization structure using soft rubber (length: 50 mm, width: 10 mm, thickness: 3 mm, Shore hardness: A30, 3D printing), which is applied between the skin and the sensor. The schematic diagram of the signal stabilization structure is shown in Figure 3a. Soft rubber has good toughness and elasticity, high heat resistance, tear resistance, and soft texture, which can fit the wrist closely and increase the friction between the skin and the sensor so that the stability of the pulse signal is at the sensor position. The photograph of the signal stabilization structure is shown in Figure 3b. The zigzag shape design of the module can effectively transmit the deformation of the PVDF film. The schematic diagram of stress analysis of the signal stabilization structure is shown in 3c. The stress analysis of the signal stabilization structure shows that when the pulse wave pressure acts on the lower surface, it can be regarded as a rigid body in a steady state. After being transmitted to the upper surface, the pressure at the contact points on the upper surface can be increased to make the signal more stable and sensitive to capture by the PVDF sensor structure.

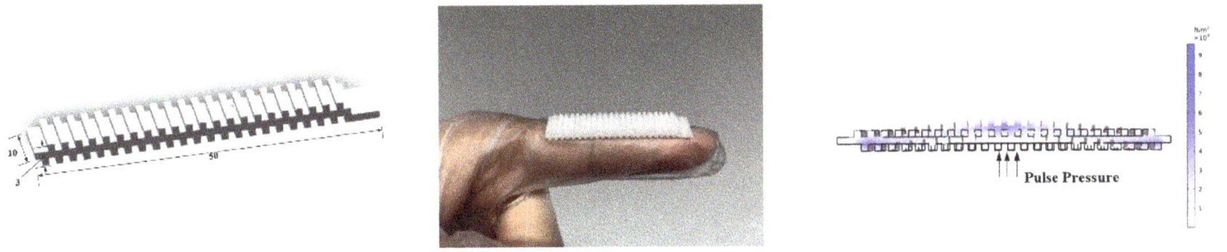

(a) (b) (c)

Figure 3. Signal stabilization structure: (**a**) Schematic diagram of the signal stabilization structure; (**b**) Photograph of the signal stabilization structure; (**c**) Schematic diagram of stress analysis of the signal stabilization structure.

2.2.3. Micro Pressurization System

To obtain the varying trend of the pulse wave peak of the pulse wave under continuously varying pressure, we designed a micro pressurization system to apply continuously varying pressure on the radial artery. The pressure range is from 0 mmHg to 180 mmHg, which is in line with the small size and low power consumption design to meet wearable and portable scenarios. The micro pressurization system mainly includes an integrated pump, air pressure sensor (MPS20N0040D-S), and inflatable wrist strap. To meet the needs of wearable and portable design, we customized an integrated air pump (thickness is only 6 mm and weight is only 2.48 g) that combines an air pump and a solenoid valve. The integrated pump is controlled by the microcontroller unit (MCU) to inflate the customized micro wristband, maintain the pressure, and deflate the pressure. The air pressure sensor has good repeatability and long-term stability, which is used to measure the air pressure in the micro pressurization system and feedback the current air pressure value to the MCU for further control.

To keep the air pressure stable, we propose an integrated air pump control method based on the Proportion Integration Differentiation (PID) algorithm. Flow chart of air pressure stabilization control is shown in Figure 4. The difference between the expected air pressure value and the actual air pressure value is used as the algorithm input. Through proportional and differential adjustment, the output feedback error drive voltage is superimposed on the original drive voltage. The MCU controls the driving voltage by changing the duty cycle of the Pulse Width Modulation (PWM) wave to change the pressing speed. To stabilize the air pressure, adjust the air pressure so that it stabilizes at the optimal air pressure value and fluctuates no more than 3%. According to the personalized inflation speed, the integrated air pump can be controlled by MCU to perform stable inflation and deflation; also, the air pump achieved to inflate to any pressure value and maintain it continually.

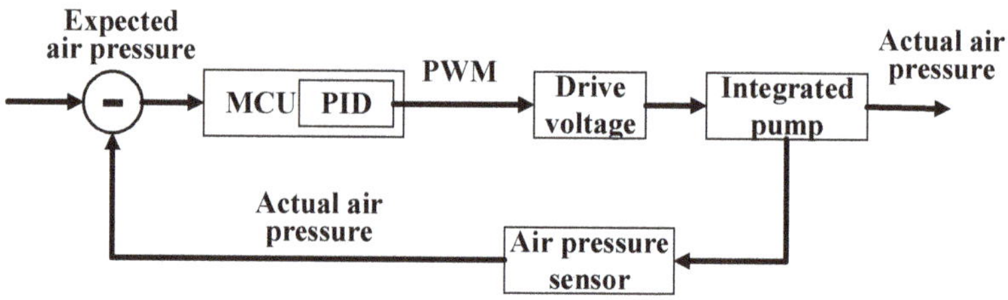

Figure 4. Flow chart of air pressure stabilization control.

When the pulse wave is collected, the flexible compound sensor is pressed above the radial artery of the wrist, and the micro pressurization system applies a continuously changing static pressure to the radial artery. The force generated by the pulse is transmitted through the skin and the pulse signal stable structure. The sensitive area of the sensor captures the deformation, the sensor generates a polarized charge based on the piezoelectric effect, and then the charge is transferred to the pin, through the pre-amplifier circuit, to complete the collection of the pulse wave electrical signal.

2.3. *Signal Processing*

2.3.1. Circuit Architecture

To meet the needs of a wearable and mobile monitoring system, the circuit architecture adopts low power consumption and miniaturization design, which mainly includes signal processing circuit, analog-digital converter (ADC) circuit, control circuit, and power supply module. Schematic diagram of circuit architecture is shown in Figure 5. The voltage supply is powered by a 4.2 V rechargeable lithium battery with a rated capacity of 270 mAh. The wrist skin is connected to the system ground through a wire, and the reference ground electrode is introduced on the skin to reduce the interference of space charge on the PVDF signal acquisition, which can effectively eliminate the 50 Hz power frequency signal and greatly simplifies the circuit.

In the signal acquisition process, firstly, the pulse pressure sensor transfers the polarized charge to the pre-charge amplifier circuit through the pins and leads. The high-impedance input can well capture the weak charge generated by the PVDF film. Then a preamplification circuit is a voltage amplifier with a voltage gain of 11 times. After that the signal is conveyed to the MCU to calculate the varying trend of the pulse wave peak in real-time and transmitted to the smartphone or PC via wireless communication. The signal sampling frequency is 250 Hz.

2.3.2. Real-Time Calculation Algorithm

To ensure the real-time performance of the calculation, we calculate the varying trend of pulse wave peak on the MCU. The calculation result can be output and displayed on the screen of the system in real-time, or transmitted to the PC or smartphone via wireless communication. Before this, the collected signal will be filtered to remove noise. We use a median filter to remove abnormal points in the sampling process, and an average filter and a low-pass filter with a cutoff frequency of 15 Hz to filter out the interference of baseline drift. The filtered pulse wave signal and air pressure signal is shown in Figure 6b.

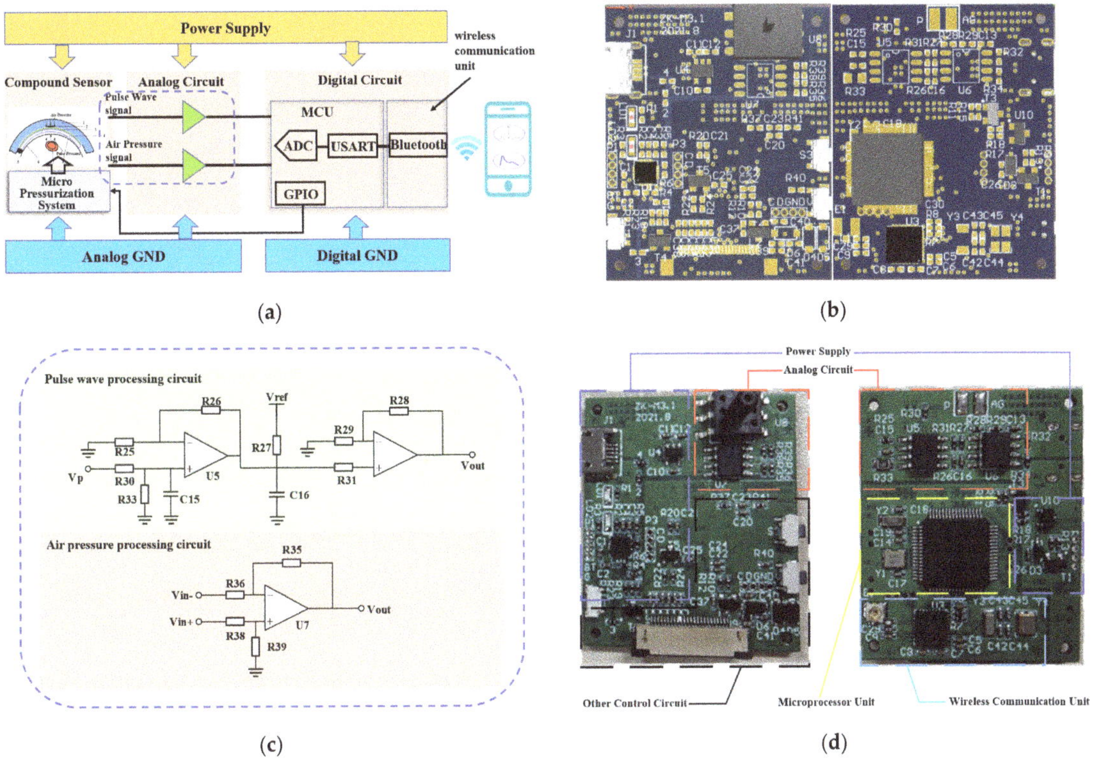

Figure 5. Schematic diagram of the circuit system: (**a**) Circuit system function diagram; (**b**) Detailed design in the blue dash frame in (**a**); (**c**) Printed circuit board layout view; (**d**) Photograph of the circuit system.

To calculate the pulse wave parameters and the varying trend of pulse wave peaks in real-time, we proposed a calculation method based on a sliding window. The schematic diagram of the real-time algorithm is shown in Figure 6a. The schematic diagram of sliding window is shown in Figure 6c. The size of sliding window is 1024 sampling points, and the sliding step size is set to 250 sampling points. For the pulse wave signal in the window, shown in Figure 6d, firstly, locate the pulse wave starting point for real-time period division, shown in Figure 6e. Secondly, according to the position of the characteristic point, calculate the pulse wave peak, pulse rate, and other parameters. The pulse wave in the signal sequence is monitored to obtain the static pressure corresponding to the pulse wave with the strongest amplitude, to realize the accurate positioning and continuous monitoring of the best pulse wave of different individuals.

The dynamic pulse pressure curve generated by a sensor takes the peak value under static pressure as the horizontal axis, and the air pressure value of the pulse wave peak value as the vertical axis of the varying trend of pulse wave peak. It depicts the varying trend of the wrist pulse wave peak under continuously varying pressure, hereinafter referred to as the pressure-height (P-H) curve, shown in Figure 6f, which fully describes the depth information of the radial artery.

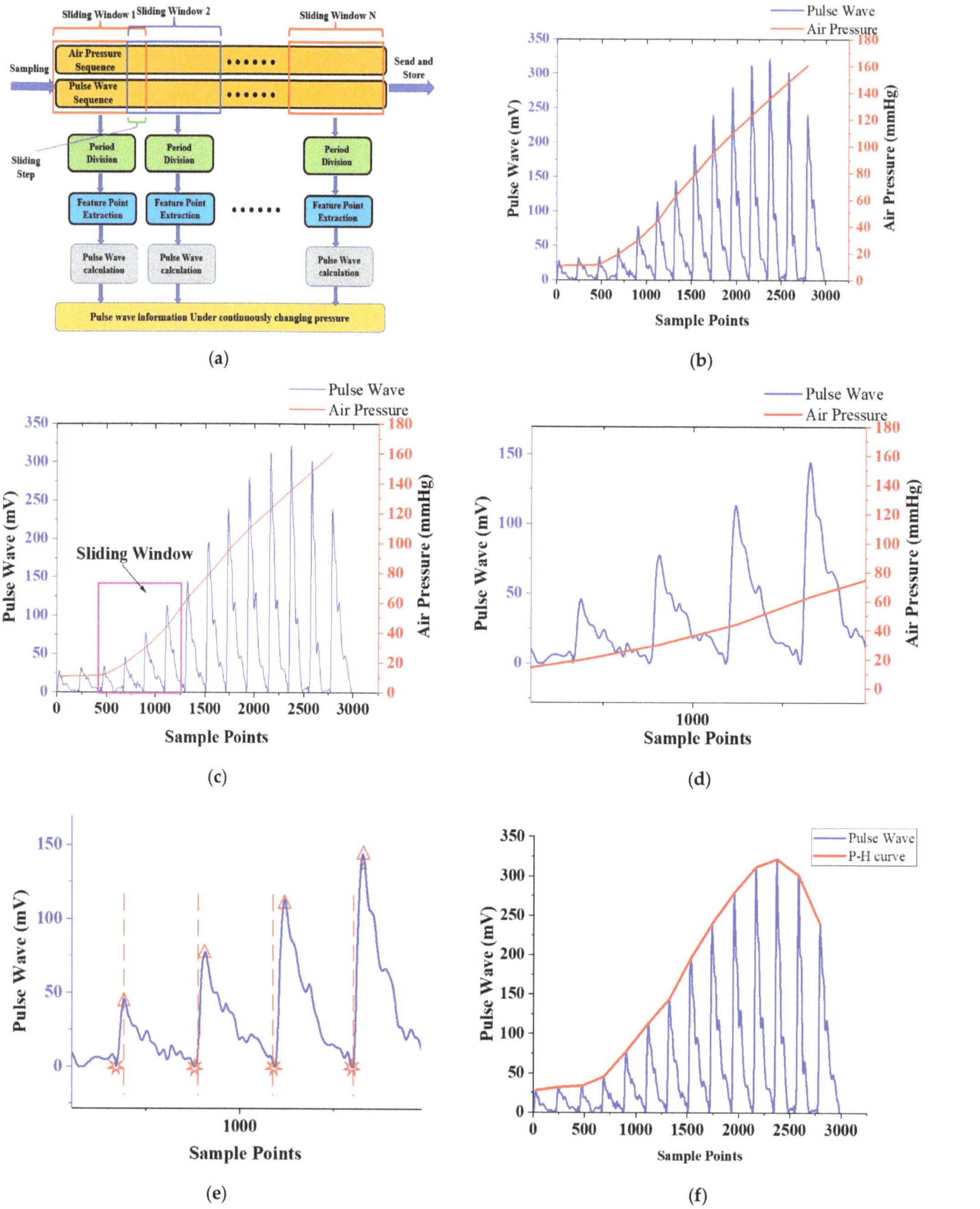

Figure 6. Real-time calculation algorithm: (**a**) Schematic diagram of the real-time algorithm diagram; (**b**) Filtered pulse wave signal and air pressure signal; (**c**) Schematic diagram of sliding window; (**d**) The signal in the sliding window in Figure 5c; (**e**) Location of the starting point of the pulse wave and period division; (**f**) Pulse wave and P-H curve.

3. Experimental Results and Discussion

3.1. Test Device for Performance Test of the Flexible Compound Sensor

To verify the reliability, consistency, and effectiveness of the flexible compound sensor, we employed a standard pulsation signal source, the MM-4 pulse simulator, shown in Figure 7a. The equipment based on bionic simulation and waveform synthesis methods, develops bionic hands and radial artery blood vessels with polymer material formulas, and uses stepping speed-regulating motors and special oil pumps to simulate the dilation and contraction of the human heart. It can output a variety of standard finger-sensing real pulse wave signals at the radial artery of the bionic hand. We can set the shape of the pulse wave independently. Figure 7 shows the pulse shapes called Ping, Xian, Hua, Ji, and Chi generated by the pulse simulator, which are considered as the five common pulse sharps in TCM.

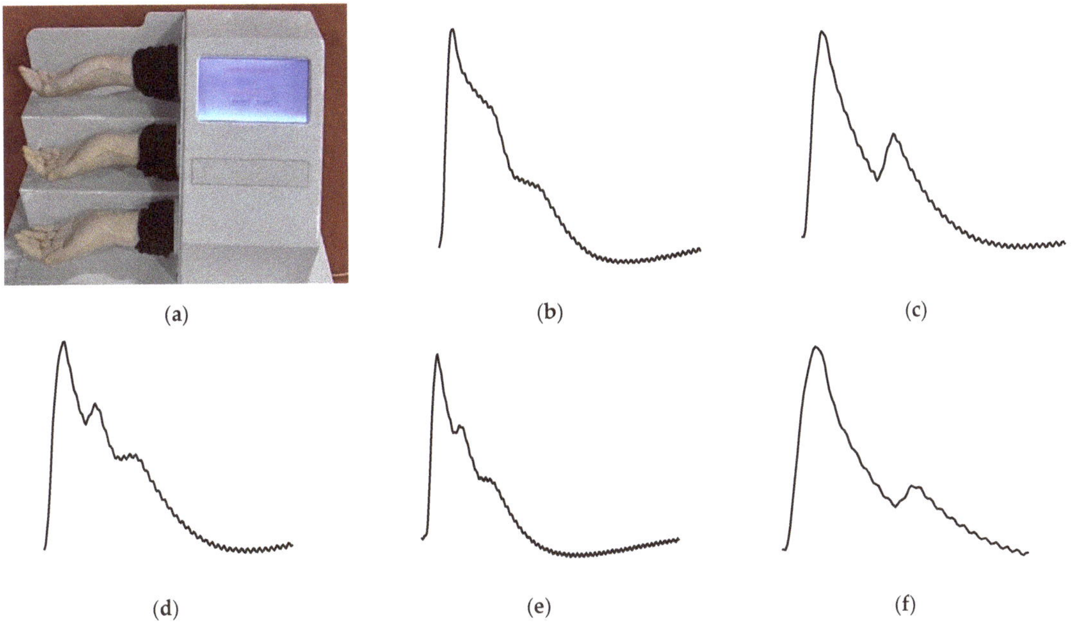

Figure 7. Test device for the flexible compound sensor. (**a**) Photograph of the test device; (**b–f**) the pulse generated by the test device called, respectively, Ping, Xian, Hua, Ji, and Chi.

3.2. Verification of Airtightness

The micro pressurization system provides a continuously changing static pressure for the flexible compound sensor, which is an important part of the entire system. Initially, the airtightness test of the micro pressurization system in the flexible compound sensor is carried out. Firstly, wear the sensor on the simulated wrist of the simulator, then control the micro pressurization system to inflate to 150 mmHg, turn off the integrated air pump, and keep it for a while. Finally, record the air pressure value in the micro pressurization system measured by the air pressure sensor to verify the micro pressurization system airtightness. Repeat the above experiment five times. As shown in Figure 8, within the 40 s after the integrated air pump is turned off, the air pressure can remain above 96.5% of the closed air pressure, which means that the airtightness of the system is excellent.

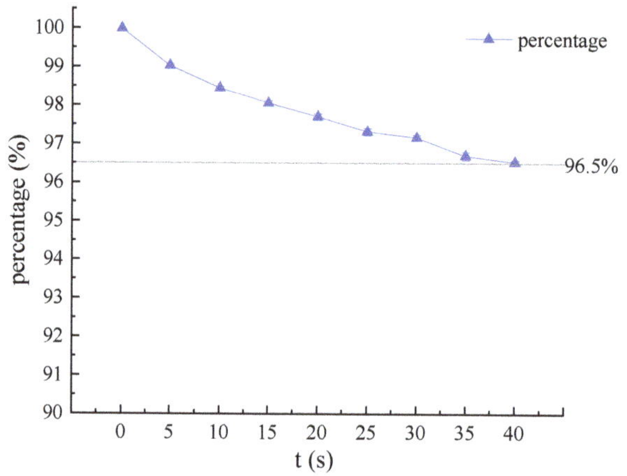

Figure 8. Air tightness of the flexible compound sensor under 150 mmHg airbag pressure for 40 s.

3.3. Consistency of Different Positioning of the Sensor

To verify the consistency of different positionings of the sensor, we choose three positions A, B, and C on the sensor, whose positions are shown in Figure 9. Among them point B is the center position of the sensitive area of the sensor. After the assembly is completed, press the three points A, B, and C of the sensor on the test device, respectively, to collect pulse wave information at the three positions. The above experiment was repeated three times, and the average amplitudes of the pulse wave at the three positions were shown in the Figure 9.

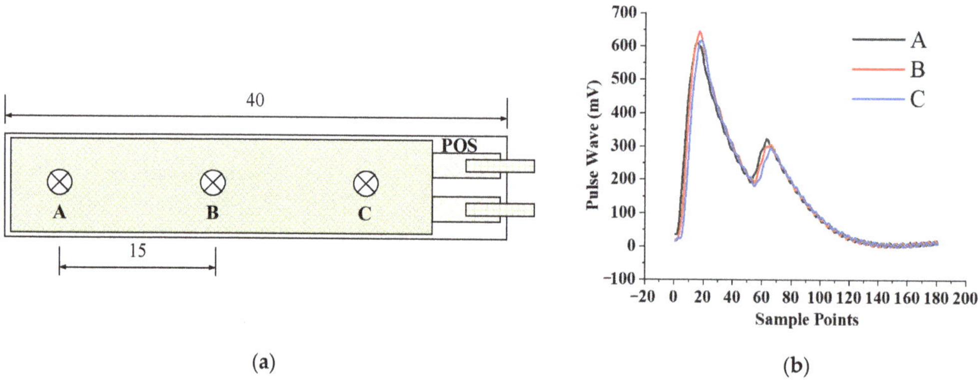

Figure 9. Consistency test of different positioning of the sensor: (**a**) The positions of the three points A, B, and C; (**b**) Pulse wave measured at three points A, B, C.

The experimental results show that the pulse wave amplitude collected at point B is the largest, the pulse wave amplitude collected at point A is 4.76% smaller than that of point B, and the amplitude of pulse wave collected at point C is 4.19% smaller than that of point B, which are all less than 5%. Therefore, different positioning of the sensor has little influence on measuring results. In the following experiments, unless otherwise specified, we collect pulse waves at the position point B of the sensor, which can not only obtain the maximum signal amplitude, but also help to cover a sufficient range to ensure that the pulse wave can be monitored.

3.4. Repeatability of Flexible Compound Sensor

To verify the repeatability of the applied variable pressure of the micro pressurization system, we performed a pressure test on the flexible compound sensor. The sensor is worn on the simulated wrist of the simulator. Control the micro pressurization system to inflate to 150 mmHg and record the change in the value of the air pressure sensor during the entire pressurization process. Repeat the above experiment five times.

To evaluate the repeatability of the flexible compound sensor, which also reveals the reliability and stability of the sensor, the equation for calculating the repeatability of the sensor is shown as follows:

$$s_i^2 = \frac{1}{m-1}\sum_{j=1}^{m}\left(y_{ij} - \overline{y}_i\right)^2 \quad (1)$$

$$s = \sqrt{\frac{1}{2n}\sum_{i=1}^{n} s_i^2} \quad (2)$$

where y is the measured value, s_i is the variance of the measurement point i, m represents the number of repetitions of test experiment, in this experiment, the value is five, n is the number of measurement points.

When the micro pressurization system applies continuous pressure to the sensor, the pulse pressure signal and the applied static pressure signal are recorded and used to evaluate the repeatability of the composite pressure sensor. The curve drawn by repeating the above process is shown in Figure 10. The standard deviation of each measurement point is calculated according to Equations (1) and (2). It can be seen from the Figure 10 that the air pressure value and the pulse pressure value under continuously varying pressure show a great linear correlation and stable standard deviation. To check the standard deviation more specifically, we sample the standard deviation every 1 s, and the relative standard deviation values of approximately 18 s are shown in Table 2.

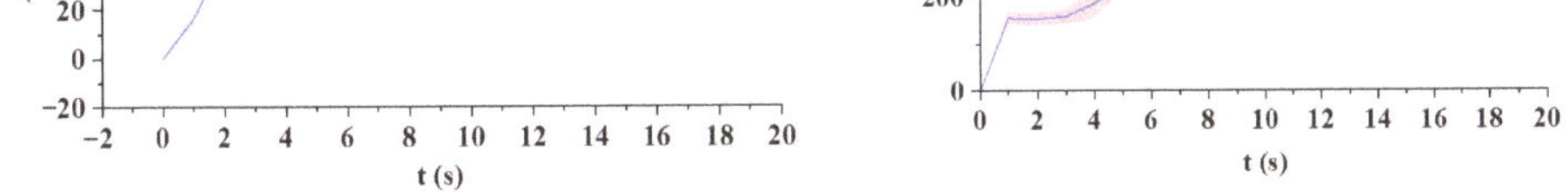

(**a**) (**b**)

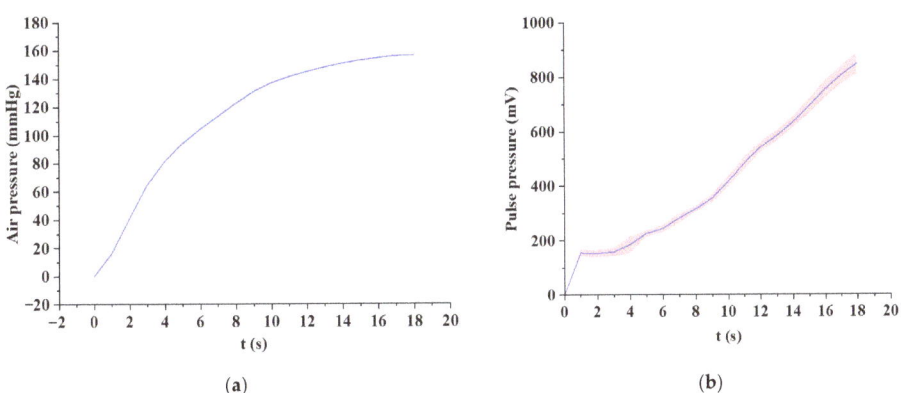

Figure 10. Repeatability test of the flexible compound sensor. Mean and standard deviation of air pressure (**a**) and pulse pressures (**b**) under 0–150 mmHg.

Table 2. Relative standard deviations (RSD) of air pressure and pulse pressures.

Time (s)	1	2	3	4	5	6	7	8	9	10	11	12	13	14	15	16	17	18
RSD of Pulse Pressure	8.7%	9.0%	10.7%	16.7%	5.4%	5.9%	6.4%	3.4%	4.5%	5.0%	5.0%	3.6%	3.5%	3.4%	4.0%	4.2%	5.3%	5.9%
RSD of Air Pressure	33.2%	13.2%	7.8%	5.6%	4.5%	4.1%	3.8%	3.5%	3.5%	2.4%	2.1%	1.9%	1.7%	1.5%	1.1%	0.8%	0.7%	0.8%

As shown in Table 2, the relative standard deviation of pulse pressure and the relative standard deviation of air pressure in the low-pressure stage (1 s to 4 s) is greater than in the medium pressure and high-pressure stages, and the relative standard deviation values are also unstable. This phenomenon is caused by the fact that the wristband is less inflated in the initial stage and the sensor is not completely in close contact with the test equipment. With the gradual increase of airbag pressure, the relative standard deviations of static pressure and dynamic pressure in the middle-pressure section and the high-pressure section gradually decrease and become stable. The relative standard deviation of static pressure is reduced from 5.6% to 1.5% in high-pressure sections, showing good stability. The relative standard deviation of pulse pressure produced large fluctuations during the entire compression process and the value was much larger than the relative standard deviation of static pressure. However, the relative standard deviation of the pulse pressure was always kept in a low range (from 16.7% Reduced to 3.4%), which will not have a major impact on data analysis. Therefore, during the entire pressurization process, the relative standard deviation of the pulse pressure and the air pressure is kept at a low value, which proves that the pulse pressure sensor and the barometric pressure sensor work stably during the entire process.

3.5. Verification of Pulse Pressure and Air Pressure Collection

To evaluate the effectiveness of the flexible compound sensor, we compared the sensor we proposed with the sensor on the ZM-300 [1], which meets TCM's technical standards for pulse wave detection, and is generally considered to be a standard pulse wave detection system. A verification experiment is designed, as shown in Figure 11. The pulse simulator is used to generate the five most common specific waveforms in TCM to simulate the pulse wave of the human body, and then let our proposed sensor and the ZM-300 sensor measure. The default unit of the output value of the ZM-300 sensor is g/cm^2, which is converted to kPa to keep the unit consistent with the output value of our sensor. Then, the ratio of the amplitude of the waveform captured by the two sensors is calculated. We have measured five kinds of pulse, namely Ping, Xian, Hua, Ji, and Chi. For each group of pulse waveforms, and we tested them ten times.

The amplitude of the pulse simulator is much larger than the usual pulse wave amplitude, ensuring that the pulse wave can always be recorded without loss. The test results of these five pulse waveforms are shown in Figure 11. From the perspective of waveform similarity, five kind of pulse waveforms were collected with high similarity by our system and ZM-300, respectively. As shown in Table 3, The Pearson correlations between the five kind of pulse waves are 0.99, 0.97, 0.97, 0.98 and 0.99 separately, which means that the pulse wave waveform acquired by our system is very similar to the ZM-300. From the perspective of amplitude, the amplitude ratios of these five kinds of pulse are 1.06, 1.04, 0.97, 1.08 and 0.98 separately, and the average amplitude ratio is 1.03, which shows that the linearity of our flexible compound sensor is only slightly different from that of the ZM-300. The standard deviation of the amplitude ratio of these five types of pulse is 4.00%, which proved that the consistency of the sensor is outstanding. However, our system can automatically collect. Compared with the ZM-300 manual collection, the time required for collection from 5 min is greatly shortened to 30 s.

Table 3. Pearson correlation between the five kind of pulse waves collected by our system and ZM-300.

Pulse Type	Ping	Xian	Hua	Chi	Ji
Pearson correlation	0.99	0.97	0.97	0.98	0.99

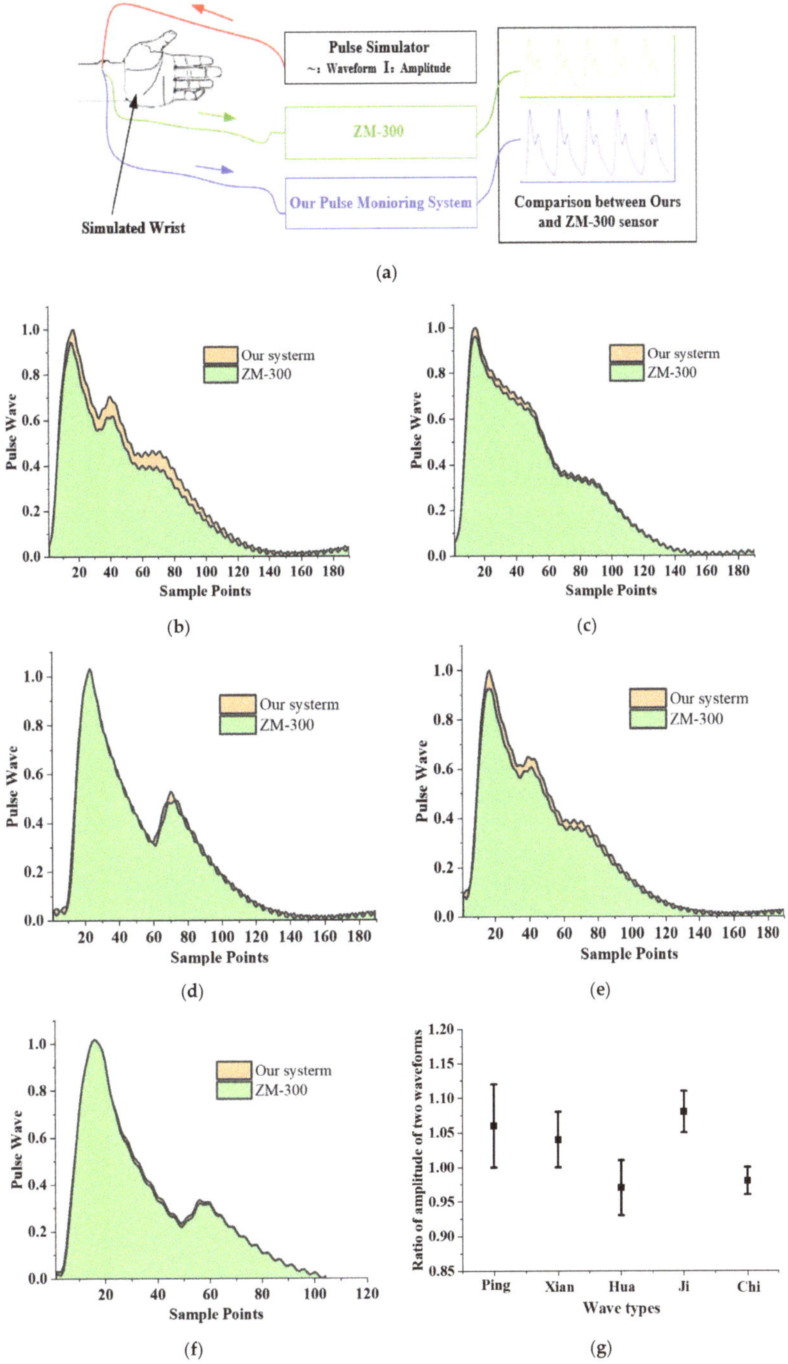

Figure 11. Verification experiment of dynamic characteristics between our sensor and ZM-300 sensor: (**a**) Schematic diagram of the experiment; (**b**–**f**) Result of waveform comparison of five kinds of pulse, Ping, Xian, Hua, Chi, and Ji; (**g**) Result of amplitude comparison of five kinds of pulse, Ping, Xian, Hua, Chi, and Ji.

3.6. Verification of Best Pulse Wave Positioning

To test the performance of best pulse wave positioning of the pulse wave monitoring system we proposed, firstly, the system is worn on the simulated wrist of the simulator. Control the micro pressurization system to inflate, and record the variation in the value of the pulse wave and air pressure during the entire pressurization process. After real-time processing by the algorithm, the experimental result is shown in Figure 12. The system can locate the best pulse wave and corresponding air pressure.

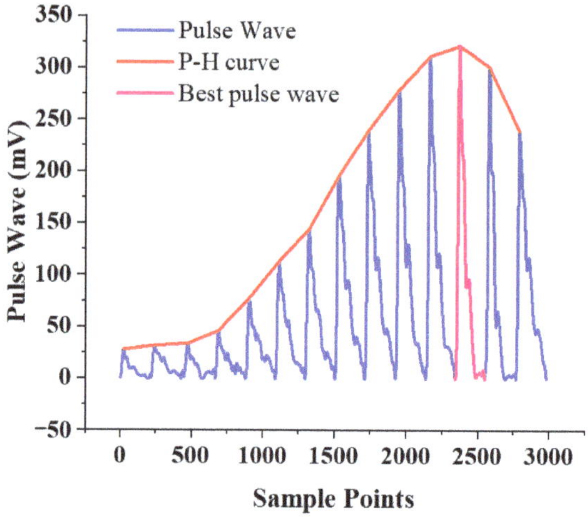

Figure 12. Experimental result of best pulse wave positioning.

To verify that the system has the same performance for different individuals, 20 volunteers in our institute are recruited for measurement. Each volunteer was asked to sit still for five minutes before the test. Table 4 shows the basic information of the volunteers and the experimental result of best pulse wave positioning. There were 19 of 20 people who could correctly locate the best pulse wave, while one person failed to locate it because the volunteer had vigorous movement during the collection process, which is also our next step: to develop algorithms to eliminate interference from motion artifacts. In summary, the accuracy was 95% in 20 people whose differences are obvious, meaning that the proposed system shows good performance for best pulse wave positioning.

Table 4. Basic information of 20 volunteers and the experimental result of best pulse wave positioning.

Variables	Parameters	Experimental Result		
		YES	NO	Accuracy
Gender				
Male	10			
Female	10			
Age (year)	29 ± 5.0 (22–46)	19	1	95%
Height (cm)	174.6 ± 7.4 (153–190)			
Weight (Kg)	72.5 ± 18.3 (41–115)			
BMI	22.04 ± 3.4 (16.1–38.9)			

3.7. Pulse Wave Continuous Monitoring

To verify the features for continuous pulse wave monitoring, the pulse wave monitoring system we proposed was worn on a volunteer's wrist and automatically measured every hour. The main peak of best pulse of the measurement and the corresponding air pressure were calculated in real-time. The experimental result of continuous monitoring from 8 a.m. to 12 p.m. is shown in Figure 13.

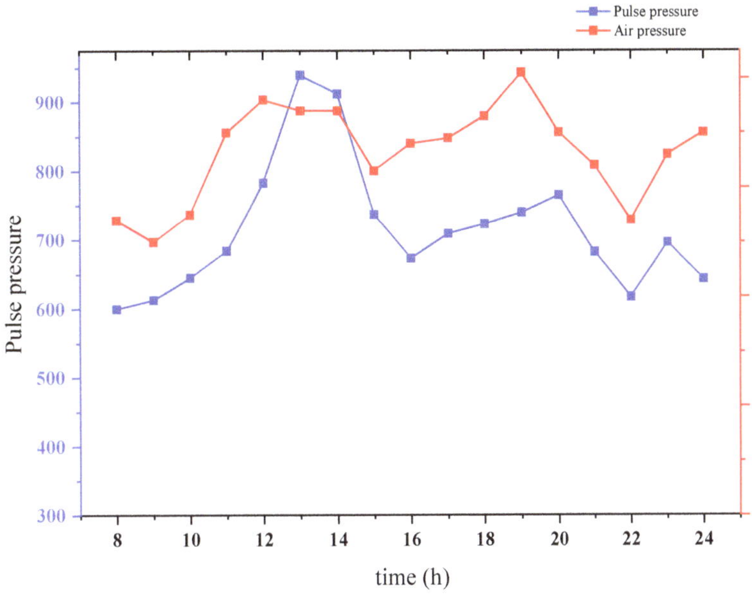

Figure 13. Experimental result of continuous monitoring from 8 a.m. to 12 p.m.

According to the experimental results, we can see the varying trend of the main peak of this volunteer's best pulse wave during the day, which is consistent with the description in TCM. It means that the proposed pulse wave monitoring system based on the flexible compound sensor could indicate the capability of continuous monitoring and reflecting trend differences.

4. Conclusions

This study proposed a novel wearable and real-time pulse wave monitoring system based on a flexible compound sensor, which achieved stable acquisition of pulse wave signals under continuously varying pressure. The weight of the whole system is only 52.775 g, the maximum working current is less than 46 mA, and the power consumption of the whole system is less than 160 mW, which meets the requirements of wearable and portable scenarios. Simultaneously, the real-time algorithm we proposed can complete the analysis of the pulse wave and the trend of the best pulse wave peak under continuously varying pressure, which can quickly locate the strongest pulse wave for different individuals. Within 40 s the air tightness can remain above 96.5%. The experiments to verify the reliability, consistency, and effectiveness show that the wearable pulse wave monitoring system can not only realize best pulse wave positioning and pulse wave monitoring under continuously varying pressure, but also indicate the capability of continuous monitoring and reflecting trend differences.

The proposed system and other pulse measurement devices presented in recent studies are summarized in Table 5. Chen [1] and Liu [2] are the previous works used to develop effective pulse wave acquisition devices. Jessica [25] proposed a wearable pulse-taking device. J.C. [24] proposed a wearable pulse acquiring system using airbags. Hsieh [26] proposed a portable pulse tactile recorder system to collect pulse palpation forces and vibrations. Chen J. [27] proposed flexible piezoresistive sensors for pulse monitoring and Li [28] used flexible pressure-sensors to realize the acquisition of arterial pulse signals in the time domain.

Table 5. Comparisons with other pulse measurement systems.

System	Jessica et al. [25]	Liu et al. [2]	J.C. et al. [24]	Chen C. et al. [1]	Hsieh et al. [26]	Chen J. et al. [27]	Li et al. [28]	Proposed
Wearable	YES	NO	YES	NO	YES	YES	YES	YES
Real-time	NO	NO	NO	NO	NO	NO	NO	YES
Weight	Not mentioned	1164.4 g	~800 g	Not mentioned	10 g	Not mentioned	Not mentioned	52.8 g
Portable	NO	NO	NO	NO	YES	YES	NO	YES
Flexible	NO	YES	NO	YES	NO	YES	YES	YES
Pulse-taking pressure acquiring	NO	YES	YES	YES	NO	NO	YES	YES
Measure under continuously changing pressure	NO	NO	YES	NO	NO	NO	NO	YES
Pressurization method	Manually	Pump and air bag	Pump and air bag	Pump and air bag	Manually	Manually	Manually	Integrated air pump (weight: 2.48 g) and air bag
Year of publication	2017	2018	2019	2020	2021	2021	2021	2022

In conclusion, the system is feasible for stable acquisition of pulse wave signals under continuously varying pressure, and the analysis of the varying trend of the best pulse wave peak, which is beneficial to pulse diagnosis. Moreover, its small size and low power consumption meet the needs of wearable and portable scenarios, which will play an important role in health monitoring and disease warning. Combining the above advantages, the system has significant research value and commercialization prospects.

In the future, we will improve the function of the system and develop algorithms to eliminate interference from motion artifacts to meet the requirements of exercise monitoring. In addition, we will study the subject in long-term use for users. Furthermore, we will carry out more experiments to make the system more accurate and standardized. This is of important significance to pulse diagnosis and health monitoring.

5. Patents

The works presented in this paper are subject to pending China and international patents filed by Institute of Microelectronics of Chinese Academy of Sciences (IMECAS) in China (202110808586.4, 202111553703.3).

Author Contributions: Conceptualization, X.K., J.Z., Z.S., Y.Z. and H.Z.; methodology, X.K. and J.Z.; software, X.K., G.W. and Z.S.; validation, X.K., J.Z. and Y.Z.; formal analysis, X.K. and X.G.; investigation, X.K.; resources, J.Z., Y.Z. and H.Z.; data curation, X.K., Y.Z. and X.G.; writing—original draft preparation, X.K.; writing—review and editing, X.K., J.Z., Z.S., Y.Z. and H.Z.; project administration, J.Z., Y.Z. and H.Z. All authors have read and agreed to the published version of the manuscript.

Funding: This research was supported by the Key Research Program of the Chinese Academy of Sciences, Grant NO.ZDRW-ZS-2021-1.

Institutional Review Board Statement: Ethical review and approval were waived for this study, due to the experiments are almost completely safe, and do not cause harm to the subject, and do not involve privacy and moral issues.

Informed Consent Statement: Informed consent was obtained from all subjects involved in the study. Written informed consent has been obtained from the patients to publish this paper.

Data Availability Statement: The raw/processed data required to reproduce these findings cannot be shared at this time as the data also form part of an ongoing study.

Acknowledgments: All authors of this manuscript have directly participated in the planning, execution, and/or analysis of this study. The contents of this manuscript have not been copyrighted or published previously. All authors have no objection to the ranking order.

Conflicts of Interest: The authors declare no conflict of interest.

References

1. Chen, C.; Li, Z.; Zhang, Y.; Zhang, S.; Hou, J.; Zhang, H. A 3D Wrist Pulse Signal Acquisition System for Width Information of Pulse Wave. *Sensors* **2020**, *20*, 11. [CrossRef] [PubMed]
2. Liu, S.; Zhang, S.; Zhang, Y.; Geng, X.; Zhang, J.; Zhang, H. A novel flexible pressure sensor array for depth information of radial artery. *Sens. Actuators A Phys.* **2018**, *272*, 92–101. [CrossRef]
3. Zhang, Z.; Zhang, Y.; Yao, L.; Song, H.; Kos, A. A Sensor-Based Wrist Pulse Signal Processing and Lung Cancer Recognition. *J. Biomed. Inform.* **2018**, *79*, 107–116. [CrossRef] [PubMed]
4. He, D.; Wang, L.; Fan, X.; Yao, Y.; Geng, N.; Sun, Y.; Xu, L.; Qian, W. A New Mathematical Model of Wrist Pulse Waveforms Characterizes Patients with Cardiovascular Disease—A Pilot Study. *Med. Eng. Phys.* **2017**, *48*, 142–149. [CrossRef] [PubMed]
5. Moura, N.; Ferreira, A. Pulse Waveform Analysis of Chinese Pulse Images and Its Association with Disability in Hypertension. *J. Acupunct. Meridian Stud.* **2016**, *9*, 93–98. [CrossRef] [PubMed]
6. Lee, Q.Y.; Chan, G.S.H.; Redmond, S.J.; Middleton, P.M.; Steel, E.; Malouf, P.; Critoph, C.; Flynn, G.; O'Lone, E.; Lovell, N.H. Classification of low systemic vascular resistance using photoplethysmogram and routine cardiovascular measurements. In Proceedings of the 2010 Annual International Conference of the IEEE Engineering in Medicine and Biology, Buenos Aires, Argentina, 31 August–4 September 2010; Volume 2010, pp. 1930–1933.
7. Wang, D.; Zhang, D.; Lu, G. A Novel Multichannel Wrist Pulse System with Different Sensor Arrays. *IEEE Trans. Instrum. Meas.* **2015**, *64*, 2020–2034. [CrossRef]
8. Malinauskas, K.; Palevicius, P.; Ragulskis, M.; Ostaševičius, V.; Dauksevicius, R. Validation of Noninvasive MOEMS-Assisted Measurement System Based on CCD Sensor for Radial Pulse Analysis. *Sensors* **2013**, *13*, 5368–5380. [CrossRef] [PubMed]
9. Convertino, V.A.; Schauer, S.G.; Weitzel, E.K.; Cardin, S.; Stackle, M.E.; Talley, M.J.; Sawka, M.N.; Inan, O.T. Wearable Sensors Incorporating Compensatory Reserve Measurement for Advancing Physiological Monitoring in Critically Injured Trauma Patients. *Sensors* **2020**, *20*, 6413. [CrossRef] [PubMed]
10. Chung, C.Y.; Cheng, Y.W.; Luo, C.H. Neural network study for standardizing pulse-taking depth by the width of artery. *Comput. Biol. Med.* **2015**, *57*, 26–31. [CrossRef]
11. Convertino, V.A.; Sawka, M.N. Wearable compensatory reserve measurement for hypovolemia sensing. *Appl. Physiol.* **2018**, *124*, 442–451. [CrossRef] [PubMed]
12. Yoo, S.K.; Shin, K.Y.; Lee, T.B.; Jin, S.O. New pulse wave measurement method using different hold-down wrist pressures according to individual patient characteristics. *SpringerPlus* **2013**, *2*, 1–8. [CrossRef] [PubMed]
13. Chen, Y.-Y.; Chang, R.-S.; Jwo, K.-W.; Hsu, C.-C.; Tsao, C.-P. A Non-Contact Pulse Automatic Positioning Measurement System for Traditional Chinese Medicine. *Sensors* **2015**, *15*, 9899–9914. [CrossRef] [PubMed]
14. Chan, M.; Ganti, V.G.; Heller, J.A.; Abdallah, C.A.; Etemadi, M.; Inan, O.T. Enabling Continuous Wearable Reflectance Pulse Oximetry at the Sternum. *Biosensors* **2021**, *11*, 521. [CrossRef]
15. Martín-Escudero, P.; Cabanas, A.M.; Fuentes-Ferrer, M.; Galindo-Canales, M. Oxygen Saturation Behavior by Pulse Oximetry in Female Athletes: Breaking Myths. *Biosensors* **2021**, *11*, 391. [CrossRef]
16. Nam, D.-H.; Lee, W.-B.; Hong, Y.-S.; Lee, S.-S. Measurement of Spatial Pulse Wave Velocity by Using a Clip-Type Pulsimeter Equipped with a Hall Sensor and Photoplethysmography. *Sensors* **2013**, *13*, 4714–4723. [CrossRef]
17. Warren, K.M.; Harvey, J.R.; Chon, K.H.; Mendelson, Y. Improving pulse rate measurements during random motion using a wearable multichannel reflectance photoplethysmograph. *Sensors* **2016**, *16*, 342. [CrossRef] [PubMed]
18. Chen, Y.; Lu, B.; Chen, Y.; Feng, X. Biocompatible and Ultra-Flexible Inorganic Strain Sensors Attached to Skin for Long-Term Vital Signs Monitoring. *IEEE Electron Device Lett.* **2016**, *37*, 496–499. [CrossRef]
19. Wang, Z.; Wang, S.; Zeng, J.; Ren, X.; Chee, A.J.Y.; Yiu, B.Y.S.; Chung, W.C.; Yang, Y.; Yu, A.C.H.; Roberts, R.C.; et al. High Sensitivity, Wearable, Piezoresistive Pressure Sensors Based on Irregular Microhump Structures and its Applications in Body Motion Sensing. *Small* **2016**, *12*, 3827–3836. [CrossRef] [PubMed]
20. Huang, C.; Ren, T.-L.; Luo, J. Effects of parameters on the accuracy and precision of ultrasound-based local pulse wave velocity measurement: A simulation study. *IEEE Trans. Ultrason. Ferroelectr. Freq. Control* **2014**, *61*, 2001–2018. [CrossRef] [PubMed]
21. Murphy, J.C.; Morrison, K.; Mclaughlin, J.; Manoharan, G.; Adgey, A.J. An innovative piezoelectric-based method for measuring pulse wave velocity in patients with hypertension. *J. Clin. Hypertens.* **2011**, *13*, 497–505. [CrossRef] [PubMed]
22. Kan-heng, Z.; Peng, Q.; Chun-ming, X.; Yi-qin, W. Research on a Novel Three-Channel Self-Pressurized Wrist Pulse Acquisition System. In *Biomedical Engineering Systems and Technologies*; Springer: Berlin/Heidelberg, Germany, 2015; pp. 49–59.
23. Fu, Y.; Zhao, S.; Zhu, R. A Wearable Multifunctional Pulse Monitor Using Thermosensation-Based Flexible Sensors. *IEEE Trans. Biomed. Eng.* **2018**, *66*, 1412–1421. [CrossRef] [PubMed]

24. Jin, C.; Xia, C.; Zhang, S.; Wang, L.; Wang, Y.; Yan, H. A Wearable Combined Wrist Pulse Measurement System Using Airbags for Pressurization. *Sensors* **2019**, *19*, 386. [CrossRef] [PubMed]
25. Kabigting, J.E.T.; Chen, A.D.; Chang, E.J.; Lee, W.; Roberts, R.C. Mems pressure sensor array wearable for traditional Chinese medicine pulse-taking. In Proceedings of the IEEE 14th International Conference on Wearable and Implantable Body Sensor Networks (BSN), Eindhoven, The Netherlands, 9–12 May 2017.
26. Hsieh, T.-C.; Wu, C.-M.; Tsai, C.-C.; Lo, W.-C.; Wang, Y.-M.; Smith, S. Portable Interactive Pulse Tactile Recorder and Player System. *Sensors* **2021**, *21*, 4339. [CrossRef] [PubMed]
27. Chen, J.; Zhang, J.; Hu, J.; Luo, N.; Sun, F.; Venkatesan, H.; Zhao, N.; Zhang, Y. Ultrafast-Response/Recovery Flexible Piezoresistive Sensors with DNA-Like Double Helix Yarns for Epidermal Pulse Monitoring. *Adv. Mater.* **2022**, *34*, 2104313. [CrossRef] [PubMed]
28. Chen, J.; Sun, K.; Zheng, R.; Sun, Y.; Yang, H.; Zhong, Y.; Li, X. Three-Dimensional Arterial Pulse Signal Acquisition in Time Domain Using Flexible Pressure-Sensor Dense Arrays. *Micromachines* **2021**, *12*, 569. [CrossRef] [PubMed]

biosensors

MDPI

Article

Highly Sensitive Immunoresistive Sensor for Point-Of-Care Screening for COVID-19

Tianyi Li [1], Scott D. Soelberg [2], Zachary Taylor [1], Vigneshwar Sakthivelpathi [1], Clement E. Furlong [2], Jong-Hoon Kim [3], Sang-gyeun Ahn [4], Peter D. Han [5,6], Lea M. Starita [5,6], Jia Zhu [7] and Jae-Hyun Chung [1,*]

1 Department of Mechanical Engineering, University of Washington, Seattle, WA 98195, USA; lit24@uw.edu (T.L.); zntaylor@uw.edu (Z.T.); viggysak@uw.edu (V.S.)
2 Departments of Medicine, Division of Medical Genetics and Genome Sciences, University of Washington, Seattle, WA 98195, USA; scottjs@uw.edu (S.D.S.); clem@uw.edu (C.E.F.)
3 School of Engineering and Computer Science, Washington State University, Vancouver, WA 98686, USA; jh.kim@wsu.edu
4 Industrial Design, University of Washington, Seattle, WA 98195, USA; ahnsang@uw.edu
5 Department of Genome Sciences, University of Washington, Seattle, WA 98195, USA; petedhan@uw.edu (P.D.H.); lstarita@uw.edu (L.M.S.)
6 Brotman Baty Institute for Precision Medicine, Seattle, WA 98195, USA
7 Department of Laboratory Medicine and Pathology, University of Washington, and Vaccine and Infectious Disease Division, Fred Hutchinson Cancer Research Center, Seattle, WA 98195, USA; jiazhu@uw.edu
* Correspondence: jae71@uw.edu; Tel.: +1-206-543-4355

Abstract: Current point-of-care (POC) screening of Coronavirus disease 2019 (COVID-19) requires further improvements to achieve highly sensitive, rapid, and inexpensive detection. Here we describe an immunoresistive sensor on a polyethylene terephthalate (PET) film for simple, inexpensive, and highly sensitive COVID-19 screening. The sensor is composed of single-walled carbon nanotubes (SWCNTs) functionalized with monoclonal antibodies that bind to the spike protein of SARS-CoV-2. Silver electrodes are silkscreen-printed on SWCNTs to reduce contact resistance. We determine the SARS-CoV-2 status via the resistance ratio of control- and SARS-CoV-2 sensor electrodes. A combined measurement of two adjacent sensors enhances the sensitivity and specificity of the detection protocol. The lower limit of detection (LLD) of the SWCNT assay is 350 genome equivalents/mL. The developed SWCNT sensor shows 100% sensitivity and 90% specificity in clinical sample testing. Further, our device adds benefits of a small form factor, simple operation, low power requirement, and low assay cost. This highly sensitive film sensor will facilitate rapid COVID-19 screening and expedite the development of POC screening platforms.

Keywords: single-walled carbon nanotubes; immunoresistive sensor; resistance ratio; COVID-19; point-of-care diagnosis

Citation: Li, T.; Soelberg, S.D.; Taylor, Z.; Sakthivelpathi, V.; Furlong, C.E.; Kim, J.-H.; Ahn, S.-g.; Han, P.D.; Starita, L.M.; Zhu, J.; et al. Highly Sensitive Immunoresistive Sensor for Point-of-Care Screening for COVID-19. *Biosensors* **2022**, *12*, 149. https://doi.org/10.3390/bios12030149

Received: 19 January 2022
Accepted: 24 February 2022
Published: 28 February 2022

1. Introduction

The emerging SARS-CoV-2 virus, including its reemerging coronavirus variants, continues to pose a serious threat to global public health and economy. As of 3 January 2022, the World Health Organization (WHO) reported worldwide 281,808,270 confirmed cases, including a total of 5,411,759 deaths due to SARS-CoV-2 infection caused Coronavirus Disease 2019 (COVID-19) [1]. The novel coronavirus has impacted industry, economy, and many facets of our daily life. Currently, COVID-19 continues to spread rapidly in communities around the world.

The diagnosis of COVID 19 is based on respiratory system assessment, nucleic acid-based method, and immunoassays. Respiratory system assessment, such as chest CT and wearable breath monitoring, lacks specificity [2,3]. Alternatively, respiratory rate, oxygen saturation, and heart rate are used for symptom management [4]. For an accurate diagnosis, nucleic acid amplification tests (NAATs) such as quantitative reverse transcription-polymerase chain reaction (qRT-PCR) assay [5,6] are considered the gold standard for COVID-19 screening [7]. These methods are currently used for screening patients for COVID-19 infection. However, these commercial assays require 4~6 h of assay time, as well as expensive, bulky equipment and skilled technicians [8]. More recently, a loop-mediated isothermal amplification (LAMP) assay has been developed to accelerate the screening. By combining a shorter screening time with a more convenient detection tool such as colorimetry, a POC NAAT detection assay could be developed. For example, a colorimetric reverse-transcriptional LAMP assay was developed for the detection of SARS-CoV-2 [9].

Many rapid tests have been developed to detect whole virus, viral RNA, immunoglobulin from infection, and antigens without nucleic acid amplification [10]. For example, the volatile organic compounds (VOCs) of exhaled gas could be detected for screening [11]. Among these, many commercially available rapid tests detect antigens. For example, lateral flow immunoassays (LFIA) rely on fluorescent, colorimetric, or electrochemical detection methods to detect the presence of SARS-CoV-2 viral proteins. Such antigen tests are being used as pre-screening or home screening tools under the Emergency Use Authorization (EUA) [12]. These devices are simple, fast, and low cost but are limited to sensitivity. The BinaxNOW™ COVID-19 Antigen Self Test was reported to have a lower limit of detection (LLD) of 10^4 copies/mL, which is 100-fold less sensitive than qRT-PCR tests [13]. Other Ag-based commercial POC antigen tests have a limit of detection (LOD) greater than 10^6 copies/mL [14]. These reported levels are not sensitive enough to detect the target virus in nasal swab samples at an early stage of infection where the viral load can be lower than 100 copies/mL, according to a clinical study [15]. Immunoglobulin tests detecting Immunoglobulin G (IgG) or Immunoglobulin M (IgM) lack specificity, do not respond to early-stage infection, and may produce false positives for the vaccinated population [16–18]. Other detection methods are more promising in accuracy and screening time. Some of them are antibody-coated field-effect transistors [19,20], paper-based electrochemical sensors [21], nanoparticles (NP) based electrochemical sensors [22], optical sensors [23], surface plasmon resonance (SPR) [24], and surface-enhanced Raman spectroscopy (SERS) [25].

Single-walled carbon nanotubes (SWCNTs) are one of the potential candidates for simple and inexpensive detection with high sensitivity and specificity. Resistive SWCNT sensors can detect target binding by electrostatic interaction or work function modification [26–29]. Viral particles and bacteria can be detected by monitoring this resistance change. Using similar technology, the LLD of the swine influenza virus (H1N1) was 177 TCID50 (50% tissue culture infective dose)/mL [30]. SWCNTs functionalized with heparin detected dengue virus at concentrations as low as 840 TCID50/mL [31]. For detecting H1N1, the LLD was 1 plaque-forming unit (PFU)/mL [32]. In our previous report, *Mycobacterium tuberculosis* (MTB) was detected at 100 CFU/mL in sputum samples using SWCNT sensors combined with magnetic particles [33]. However, this assay did not demonstrate sufficient sensitivity for detecting early-stage SARS-CoV-2 patients. Also, because the sensor substrate was made on silicon chips, the fabrication and integration costs were too high for an inexpensive screening assay.

In this paper, we constructed a resistive SWCNT biosensor on a polyethylene terephthalate (PET) film for low-cost COVID-19 screening. An array of silver electrodes were silkscreen-printed on SWCNTs for large-scale production. The sensitivity and specificity were characterized for SARS-CoV-2 in phosphate-buffered saline (PBS) and nasal swabs. The relative resistance ratio of both control and sensor was measured upon binding of the spike protein of SARS-CoV-2. The SWCNT sensor also detected the virus in positive nasal swabs previously screened with qRT-PCR. The presented biosensor will facilitate the development of a POC COVID-19 rapid screening platform that has high sensitivity, low assay cost, and low power requirements.

2. Materials and Methods

2.1. Sensor Configuration and Operation

The SWCNT immunosensor was designed to handle a minimally processed nasal swab sample suspended in 1 mL of PBS, yielding a 'Yes or No' answer. The prototype device (Figure 1a) was composed of two linear motors for vertical sensor movement (dipping, withdrawal, and rinsing) and horizontal sample cup movement (solution change and mixing). Resistance was measured for both sensor and control electrodes. A heater was embedded under a sample cup to maintain a temperature of 36 °C to speed up the antibody-antigen binding and maintain a consistent temperature through the assay steps and between samples.

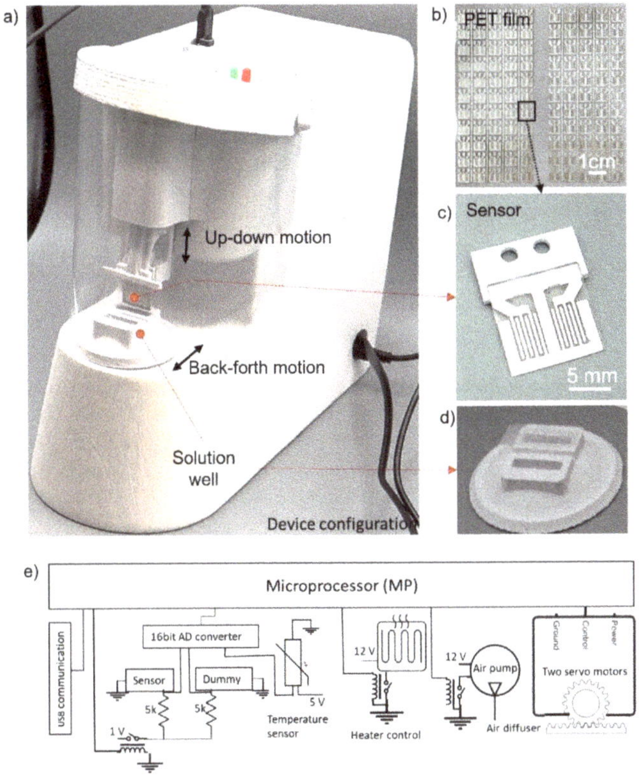

Figure 1. (**a**) Analyzer for rapid COVID-19 screening. (**b**) Sensors are made on a PET film coated with single-walled carbon nanotubes immobilized with antibodies. (**c**) A sensor consists of a SARS-CoV-2 sensor and a control sensor. (**d**) Sample cup containing 1×PBS with 1mL-target analyte and 1.1 mL-DI water. (**e**) Configuration of the electric circuit. USB communication unit, resistance measurement units, temperature sensing unit, heating and control unit, air blow with a diffuser, and two servo motors for vertical and horizontal movements.

The SWCNT sensor was fabricated by spin-coating SWCNTs onto a PET film and silkscreening silver electrodes over the SWCNT surface (Figure 1b). A SWCNT sensor was composed of a sensing electrode and a control electrode (Figure 1c). The SWCNTs on the sensing electrode were covalently conjugated with monoclonal antibodies specific to the spike protein of SARS-CoV-2. The SWCNTs on the control electrode element were conjugated with bovine serum albumin (BSA). The interdigitated electrodes offered a large surface area for high sensitivity.

The sample cup had two liquid compartments: one held 1×PBS from a nasal swab sample, and the other held deionized (DI) water for the washing steps (Figure 1d). For immunocomplex formation, a buffered solution (PBS) was needed. Since the electrostatic interaction of SWCNTs with antigen was a key mechanism for detection, the masking effect by ions in the PBS needed to be reduced by rinsing the sensor with DI water. The vertical motion of the sensor played two roles in detection. One was to eliminate nonspecific binding, and the other was to rinse and dry the sensor completely. By carefully controlling the sensor withdrawal step, the capillary and viscous forces removed the nonspecifically bound molecules.

The sensor surface was mostly dried by using a low withdrawal speed (1 mm/s). The remaining water drop at the edge of the sensor surface was removed by an air diffuser designed to blow air uniformly over the sensor surface. An air pump (flow rate: 4 L/min) was connected to the air diffuser, which was powered on only at the withdrawal step. The air pump operated at a low flow rate so that aerosols could not be generated but the sensor surface could completely dry. The resistance measurement confirmed the complete dryness of the sensor surface. A sensor with residual water yielded low and unpredictable resistance readings, while a dry sensor showed stable values. If a sensor remains wet, the silver electrode on the sensor surface could be quickly oxidized due to the potential.

Figure 1e shows the configuration of the control and electrical units, including a microcontroller (Atmega 328p). The resistance measurement units were installed to measure the resistance change of the sensor elements. A joule heating element with a temperature sensor was installed to maintain the temperature between 35 and 37 °C. An air pump was controlled with a relay switch. Two servo motors were combined with a rack and pinion gear to provide accurate linear movements.

The major innovation of the SWCNT sensor was to use the ratio of the resistance change of a sensing electrode in comparison to that of a control electrode. In our previous work [33], the sensing mechanism was characterized. Despite the high sensitivity, the previous sensor was susceptible to temperature change and aging. In this SWCNT sensor, such effects could be calibrated by comparing the resistance change of sensing and control electrodes. Based on the comparison, we could identify the subtle resistance change from the target binding by negating environmental changes.

The use of PET films as sensor substrates significantly reduces the material and manufacturing costs in comparison to silicon chips. However, the rough surface on a PET film made the contact resistance higher. According to our study previously performed using an atomic force microscope, the roughness of the surface ranges from 15 to 80 nm. By patterning silver electrodes on the SWCNT surface, the contact resistance could be stably controlled [33].

For the screening protocol, a swab was used to collect a sample from inside the nostrils (Figure 2). The sample swab was then immersed and stirred in 1.2 mL-1×PBS. A sample cup containing 1.1 mL-DI water was installed in the analyzer. One mL of the 1×PBS solution containing the swab sample was then transferred to the sample cup. After sensor installation, the 15 min-screening protocol was initiated. Once the measurement was completed, the data were analyzed and transferred to a laptop computer.

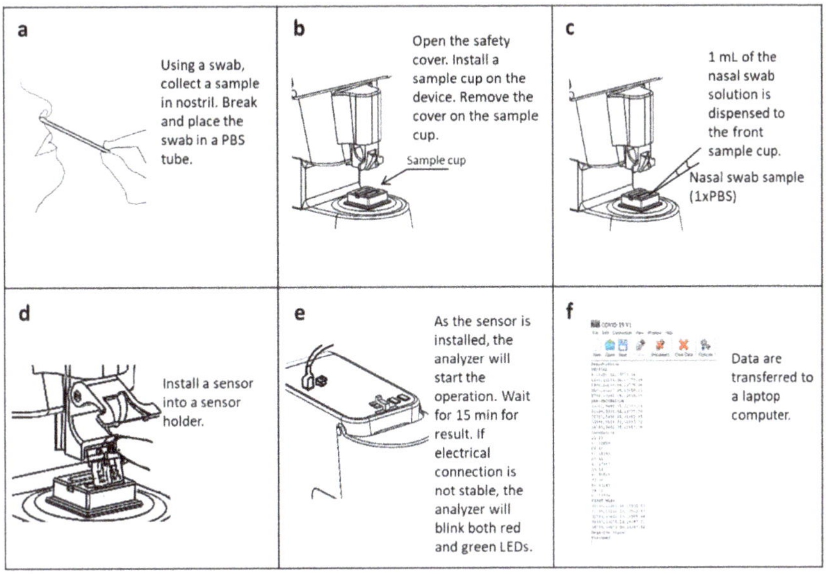

Figure 2. Screening protocol (**a**) Nasal swab sample is collected from nostril. The nasal swab is immersed and eluted in 1×PBS. (**b**) Install a sample cup where 1.1 mL DI water is contained. (**c**) A nasal swab sample of 1 mL is transferred to a sample cup. (**d**) Install a sensor with inspection of electrical connection. (**e**) Press a reset switch to begin detection protocol. (**f**) Data are collected after 15 min.

For the screening protocol, the resistances of the sensing and control electrodes were measured five times during the course of one assay. The resistance measurement steps are described with the detection protocol in Table 1. At the initial stage, the resistances of the sensing and control electrodes were measured (R_{0_s} and R_{0_c}). Subsequently, the sensor was immersed into the DI water for 10 seconds, withdrawn, and dried with an air pump for 40 s. The resistances were measured after air dry with an average of five readings (R_{1_s} and R_{1_c}). The resistance values from DI water showed the initial status of SWCNT sensors. If the ratio ($P_1 = P_{1\_s} / P_{1\_c}$) was in the range of 0.9~1.1, the measurement went to the next step. If the ratio was not in the range, the screening was halted due to poor sensor functionality. Once the quality control step passed, the sensor was then dipped into the sample cup containing the nasal swab sample in 1 mL of 1×PBS. The sensor was agitated in this sample at a speed of 1mm/second back and forth for 10 min with the liquid temperature at 36 °C. After a 10 min incubation, the sensor was rinsed in the DI water well at a stirring speed of 2 mm/s for 10 s. The sensor was subsequently air-dried, and the resistance values of R_{2_s} and R_{2_c} were measured. The same dipping rinse steps were repeated without stirring twice, during which a set of (R_{3_s}, R_{3_c}) and (R_{4_s}, R_{4_c}) was measured.

Table 1. Screening protocol, resistance measurement, parameters, and screening time.

Resistance Measurement Step	Resistance Values and Ratios	Parameters	Time (minutes) Total Time = 15 min
Before testing	$P_{0\_s} = R_{0\_s} / R_{0\_s}$; $P_{0\_c} = R_{0\_c} / R_{0\_c}$	$P_0 = P_{0\_s} / P_{0\_c} = 1$	0.5
Prewash in DI water	$P_{1\_s} = R_{1\_s} / R_{0\_s}$; $P_{1\_c} = R_{1\_c} / R_{0\_c}$	$P_1 = P_{1\_s} / P_{1\_c}$	1
Incubation	Not Measured	None	10
Wash 1	$P_{2\_s} = R_{2\_s} / R_{0\_s}$; $P_{2\_c} = R_{2\_c} / R_{0\_c}$	$P_2 = P_{2\_s} / P_{2\_c}$	1
Wash 2	$P_{3\_s} = R_{3\_s} / R_{0\_s}$; $P_{3\_c} = R_{3\_c} / R_{0\_c}$	$P_3 = P_{3\_s} / P_{3\_c}$	1
Wash 3	$P_{4\_s} = R_{4\_s} / R_{0\_s}$; $P_{4\_c} = R_{4\_c} / R_{0\_c}$	$P_4 = P_{4\_s} / P_{4\_c}$	1

Regarding the quality control step, the initial resistance measurement was used to find the functionalization quality of a sensor in comparison to control. It was found that the errors were caused by the activation and deactivation step of the carboxyl group on the SWCNT surface. The errors could occur due to small differences in the manual fabrication steps, including pipetting and incubation steps. In our test, the fabrication yield was ~70%. In the future, quality control needs to be improved to increase the fabrication yield.

2.2. Sensor Fabrication

An SWCNT sensor was prepared by screen-printing silver electrodes on an SWCNT-coated polyethylene terephthalate (PET) substrate (Figure 3a). Polyethyleneimine solution (0.1% PEI in DI water) was prepared by diluting a stock solution (50%, Millipore-Sigma, St. Louis, MI, USA). The diluted PEI solution was spin-coated on a 100 μm-thick PET film (3M Highland 903) at 3000 rpm for 3 min. SWCNTs were spread on the PET surface (200 × 200 mm^2). Using a radius of 100 mm, the relative centrifugal field (RCF) was 1006*g*. The spin-coater we used was VTC-50A (MTI Corporation, Richmond, CA, USA). The PEI-coated film was cured at 100 °C for 10 min. Carboxylic acid-functionalized SWCNTs (SWCNT-COOH, Millipore-Sigma) were dispersed in double-distilled water (ddH$_2$O, Millipore-Sigma) at 0.3 mg/mL. Using a horn-type sonicator, SWCNTs were dispersed for 20 min. The SWCNT suspension was spin-coated on a PEI-coated PET film at 3000 rpm for 3 min, followed by curing at 100 °C for 10 min. Silver ink was used to silkscreen electrodes onto the SWCNT-coated sensor surface. The silver we used was AG-510 conductive ink (Kayaku Advanced Materials, Westborough, MA, USA). The screen printer was the LS-34 (New Long, Japan). And the screen-printing mask was fabricated by Sefar Inc. (Depew, NY, USA). After patterning, the silver ink was cured at 120 °C for 15 min. The sensor was composed of two resistive sensing sections; the left section detected the SARS-CoV-2 virus, and the right section served as a control electrode. Both sections contain two interdigitated electrodes whose fingers were separated by 0.3 mm (Figure 3a).

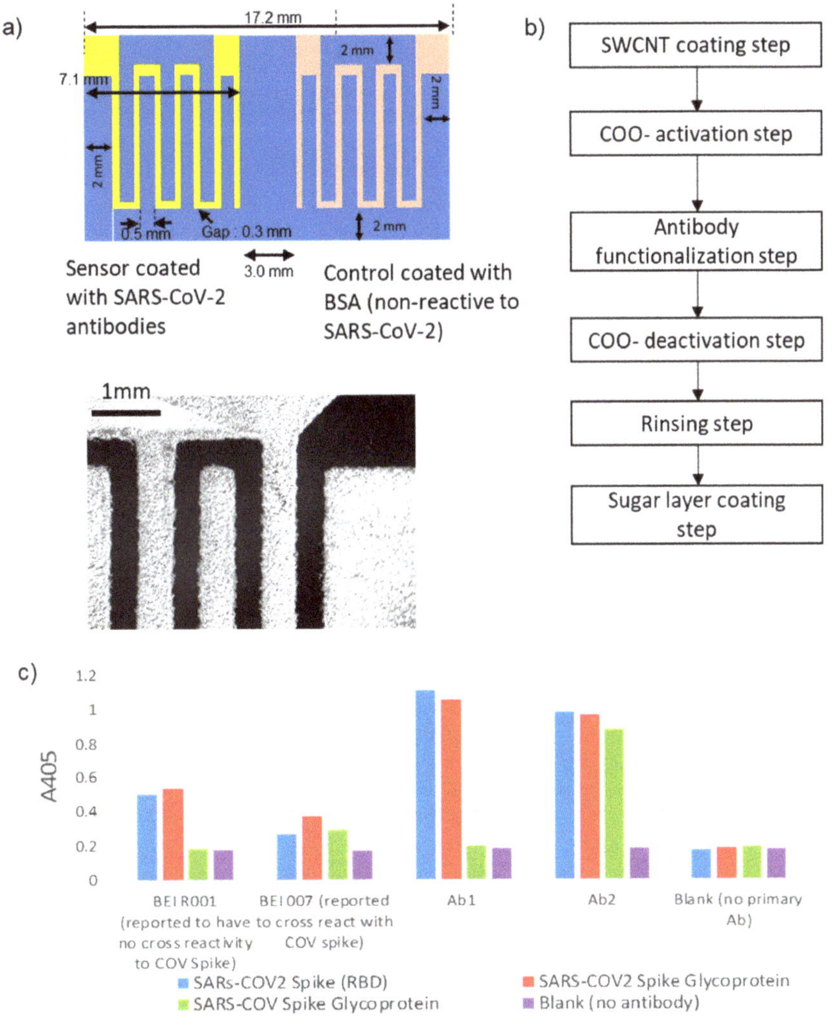

Figure 3. (**a**) Sensor configuration. Sensor electrodes are coated with SARS-CoV-2 antibodies. Control electrodes are with BSA. (**b**) Antibody functionalization step on SWCNTs. (**c**) Specificity test results to SARS-CoV and SARS-CoV-2 of antibodies using ELISA.

To covalently immobilize antibodies onto the SWCNT-COOH, a protocol was modified from the reference [34] to activate carboxyls on the SWCNT for covalently bonding to amino groups on antibodies (Figure 3b). A solution of 38.5 mg/mL EDC (Thermo #22980) and 11 mg/mL S-NHS (Thermo #PG8-2071) in DI water was prepared. 60 µL of this solution was pipetted onto each side of the sensor and incubated for 15 min at room temperature. Sensors were then washed with DI water from a wash bottle and dried with a stream of air from a compressor. A 20 µg/mL solution of either virus-specific antibody or BSA was then added (left side = 80 µL Ab, right side = 80 µL BSA) and incubated at room temperature for 2 h. Sensors were then rinsed with DI water and dried with a stream of air from a compressor. To quench any remaining amine-reactive groups, the pH was raised to 8.0 to speed hydrolysis. This was done by adding 300 µL PBS (pH 8) to cover both sides of each sensor and incubating overnight at room temperature. Sensors were then rinsed with DI water and dried with a stream of air from a compressor. A layer of a trehalose and dextran mixture was added to protect the antibody surface during storage. Each sensor was dipped in a trehalose/dextran solution [2.5% trehalose, 2.5% dextran (average MW 500,000)] [35] to cover the lower 2/3 of the sensing area. Sensors were then cured for 2 H in a 37 °C incubator. In the following tests, all the sensors were stored at room temperature and used within one week.

2.3. Antibody Characterization

We compared four commercial antibodies for binding to spike protein of both SARS-CoV and SARS-CoV-2. Antibody cross-reactivity was measured to SARS-CoV-2 whole spike protein (BEI NR-52308), SARS-CoV-2 receptor-binding domain (RBD) section of spike protein (Sino Biological 40592-V05H), and SARS coronavirus whole spike (S) Protein (BEI NR-722).

For this experiment, two antibodies were previously tested for cross-reactivity with both SARS-CoV and SARS-CoV-2 spike protein (both whole and RBD). Sino Biological 40150-R007 has been previously shown to be specific to the SARS-CoV-2 spike S1 domain and spike receptor-binding domain (RBD) and has also shown to be cross-reactive with the SARS-CoV Spike S1 domain and RBD. Sino Biological 40150-R001 was specific to the SARS-CoV-2 spike protein RBD as shown previously in ELISA, with cross-reactivity to the SARS-CoV-2 spike S1 protein. However, cross-reactivity was not observed in ELISA with S1 glycoproteins from SARS-CoV.

Protein binding plates (Immulon 2HB, ThermoFisher Scientific 3455) were coated with 100 μL of a 2 μg/mL antigen (spike protein) solution for 24 H at room temperature. Following antigen binding, plates were washed w/DPBS from a wash bottle and then blocked with a 1 mg/mL BSA solution in DPBS (200 μL) and incubated for 30 min at 37 °C. After washing excess BSA from the plate with DPBS from a wash bottle, a solution of the primary antibody (100 μL of 1 μg/mL in DPBS) was added and incubated for 30 min at 37 °C. The plate was then washed with DPBS, and a 100 μL of anti-rabbit conjugated HRP (Invitrogen 31460) at a 1:2000 dilution was added and incubated at 37 °C. After 30 min, the excess secondary antibody was removed by washing with DPBS, then 100 μL ABTS substrate (ThermoFisher 37615) was added and incubated for 10 min at room temperature. The plate was then read for absorbance on a microplate reader at A405nm.

The ELISA results showed the specific binding of BEI R001 and Ab1 to SARS-CoV-2 whole spike and RBD, while Ab2 shows additional cross-reactivity to SARS-CoV whole spike protein (Figure 3c).

2.4. Sensor Characterization

The sensor resistance change was characterized for sensors with and without antibodies. According to our observations, the functionalization step to activate and deactivate carboxyl groups on the SWCNT surface dominated the sensor resistance change. After the carboxyl groups were activated, the sensor resistance change was not consistent. By comparing the resistance change of sensors with and without antibodies, deactivation steps could be modified to result in a predictable change of SWCNT resistances. The resistance values for each step were measured as shown in Table 1. By considering the resistance change of the sensor without antibodies as a control, the functionalization protocol for the sensors with antibodies was optimized. The resistance change was compared for each step. For the comparison tests, 1mL of 1×PBS was used as the target solution with 1.1 mL of DI water. In addition, an initial test was conducted to study the resistance ratio change for 1×PBS, and 1×PBS spiked with SARS-CoV-2 (1000 genome equivalents/mL).

2.5. Sensitivity Tests

To test the sensitivity, various concentrations of inactivated SARS-CoV-2 [BEI #NR-52287 (Irradiated, Novel Coronavirus, 2019-nCoV/USA-WA1/2020)] were suspended in PBS buffer. The SARS-CoV-2 source consisted of the cell lysate and supernatant from Cercopithecus aethiops kidney epithelial cells infected with SARS-CoV-2. The virus was gamma-irradiated for inactivation. The initial concentration from BEI resources was 1.7×10^9 genome equivalents/mL. The initial stock solution was serially diluted to 10 particles/mL by serial 10 fold dilutions. A 1 mL solution of the prepared virus sample was loaded into a sample cup. After the initial resistance measurement, an SWCNT sensor was dipped in DI water, followed by air-drying and the 2nd resistance measurement. The SWCNT sensor was then immersed in 1 mL of a virus solution for 10 min with an agitation (3 mm/s), followed by an air-dry and the first washing. Two more dipping, air drying, and washing steps were repeated to measure all resistance changes. Based on the initial resistance value, all the normalized resistance values were calculated for data processing. For the control experiments, $1\times$PBS buffer without target virus was used.

2.6. Test Using Nasal Swab Samples

To evaluate the lower limit of detection for SARS-CoV-2, nasal swab samples were collected from deidentified healthy volunteers. After the complete drying of swabs for a few hours in air, the swab samples were immersed in 1 mL PBS for 1 min with gentle stirring. Subsequently, 500 µL of the target analyte (SARS-CoV-2) in PBS was mixed with 500 µL of the eluted swab solution. The 1 mL solution was used to test the LLD. The spiked concentrations of SARS-CoV-2 ranged from 10^2 to 10^5 genome equivalents/mL in steps of 10-fold dilutions. The resistance values were measured and processed as previously described.

Additional sensitivity tests were conducted for the SARS-CoV-2 concentrations of 100, 250, 500, and 1000 genome equivalents/mL in order to estimate LOD. Based on the results, a linear analysis was conducted to estimate the accurate detection limit.

2.7. Cross-Reactivity Test

For cross-reactivity study, the response for SARS-CoV-2 (10^3 genome equivalents/mL) was compared with Staphylococcus Epidermidis (S. Epi at 10^3 CFU/mL), Mycobacterium Tuberculosis (MTB at 10^3 CFU/mL), and Staphylococcus Aureus (SA) at 10^3 CFU/mL, respiratory syncytial virus (RSV, 10^6 genome equivalents/mL) and influenza A (H1N1, 10^6 genome equivalents/mL). The nontargeted samples were suspended in $1\times$PBS, which was mixed with nasal swab samples. Each sample was repeated three times (N = 3).

2.8. Test Using Clinical Samples

To validate the assay performance, 12 positive and 10 negative patient samples were tested from previously determined RT-qPCR assayed samples. The samples were collected by anterior nares swabs for the Husky Coronavirus Testing research study (IRB) that provided testing to faculty, staff, and students at the University of Washington in Seattle, WA, USA (PMID: 34805425). Dry samples were transported and eluted in 1 mL Tris-EDTA (PMID: 34286830) and stored at −80 °C. Among the samples, 12 positive and 10 negative samples were randomly chosen and deidentified for sensor testing. The positive samples included alpha and delta variants of SARS-CoV-2. The sample collection and testing procedure were approved by the institutional review board (IRB) at the University of Washington (Husky Testing number: STUDY00011148).

Since the collected sample volume after RT-qPCR assays was only 100 µL, the sample was diluted to 1 mL using $1\times$PBS. The 1mL samples were tested by the prepared SWCNT sensors in a non-blinded fashion. RT-qPCR Ct values were determined after thawing and dilution to serve as a direct comparator to the SWCNT.

The clinical testing lab was approved for SARS-CoV-2 screening assay based on RT-qPCR [36]. The Northwest Genomics Center (NWGC) SwabDirect SARS-CoV-2 detection assay was validated for the workflow of COVID-19 screening. The sensitivity, specificity, accuracy, and precision of an extraction-free protocol were validated through the evaluation of the contrived positive specimens along with known positive and negative clinical specimens.

3. Results and Discussion

3.1. Sensor Characterization

When the sensor was fabricated without antibodies, the average resistance values were 9.88 ± 1.51 kΩ (N = 12). When the antibodies were immobilized on the sensor surface, the average resistance values increased to 24.5 ± 2.69 kΩ. The normalized difference between the sensor and control resistances was 0.037 ± 0.010 for the sensors immobilized without antibodies (N = 6). The normalized difference between the sensor and control resistances was −0.057 ± 0.061 for the sensors with immobilized antibodies (N = 6). Before antibody immobilization, the normalized resistance difference between sensing and control electrodes was positive. After antibody immobilization, the normalized resistance difference changed to a negative value due to the difference between SARS-CoV-2 antibodies and BSA on the electrodes.

To study the resistance change for the sensors with and without antibodies, both sensors were tested by the analyzer using the screening protocol (Figure 4). For this experiment, 1×PBS was used without any target analytes. As described in Table 1, the initial resistance values (R_0) were collected from the sensor (R_{0_s}) and control (R_{0_c}) electrodes. The initial resistance values served as a baseline for the following measurements. Figure 4a,b show P_{i_s} and P_{i_c} value changes and their ratio change P_i (i = 0, 1, 2, 3, and 4) for the sensors without antibodies. The normalized resistances of P_{i_s} and P_{i_c} were close to 1 at the prewash step in DI water, followed by an increase at the first rinsing step. The increase of the normalized resistance values was caused by the ion adsorption on the surface when the sensor was immersed in 1×PBS. The normalized resistance values decreased at the second and third rinsing steps as the ions were depleted in DI water.

Figure 4c,d present the P_{i_s} and P_{i_c}, and P_i value changes with antibodies, respectively. With immobilization of antibodies, the prewash values of P_{1_s} and P_{1_c} reduced to 0.67, but the overall trend was similar to the sensors without antibodies. The P_i value showing the relative change ratio between the sensing and control electrodes showed an increased response at the first wash. The P_3 and P_4 values corresponding to the second and third rinsing showed a trend converging to 1. According to the initial characterization, the trend for the P_i values with and without antibodies approached 1 with multiple rinsing steps.

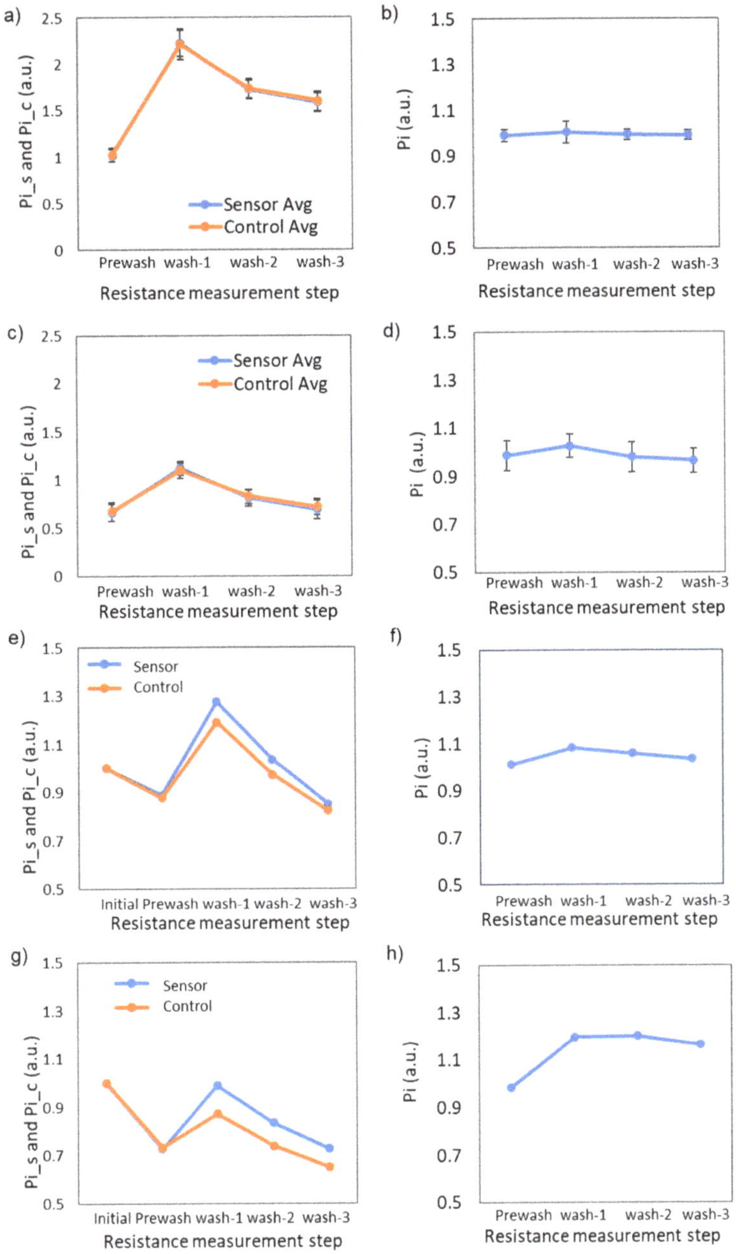

Figure 4. (**a**) P_{i_s} and P_{i_c} changes for the sensors without antibodies (N = 6). (**b**) P_i changes for the sensors without antibodies (N = 6). (**c**) P_{i_s} and P_{i_c} changes for the sensors with antibodies (N = 6). (**d**) P_i changes for the sensors with antibodies (N = 6). (**e**) P_{i_s} and P_{i_c} changes for the antibody-immobilized sensors for a negative nasal swab sample. (**f**) P_i changes for the antibody-immobilized sensors for a negative nasal swab sample. (**g**) P_{i_s} and P_{i_c} changes for the antibody-immobilized sensors for a negative nasal swab sample spiked with SARS-CoV-2 (10^3 genome equivalents/mL). (**h**) P_i changes for the antibody-immobilized sensors for a negative nasal swab sample spiked with SARS-CoV-2 (10^3 genome equivalents/mL).

Table 2 shows one example of the measured resistance values for sensing and control electrodes. The resistance values were converted to the resistance ratio in Figure 4c. If the sensor resistance was greater than 40 kOhm, the sensor was not used due to an unpredictable sensitivity. If the resistance was lower than 10 kOhm, the SWCNTs were too abundant to achieve adequate sensitivity.

Table 2. Resistance values for negative control shown in Figure 4c.

	Sensor (kΩ)	Control (kΩ)
Initial resistance	23.368	24.048
pre-wash	13.140	13.115
wash 1	24.239	23.551
wash 2	16.822	17.075
wash 3	13.518	14.379

An example of the resistance change ratios for the negative control in a nasal swab sample is shown in Figure 4e,f. The P_{i_s} and P_{i_c} values for sensing and control electrodes appeared to diverge more than pure PBS solution (Figure 4e), but the P_i values between sensor and control remained close to 1 (Figure 4f). Figure 4h are examples of the resistance changes for the positive control of 10^3 genome equivalents/mL in nasal swab samples. When the target viruses were captured on the sensor surface, the P_{i_s} and P_{i_c} became larger at the rinsing steps (Figure 4g). The P_i values clearly showed the difference between sensing and control electrodes in Figure 4h. In comparison to the negative control signal in Figure 4f, the positive control signal in Figure 4h showed the normalized value >1 due to the resistance change difference for sensing and control electrodes.

3.2. *Signal Processing and Sensitivity Tests*

Before the dose-response tests in nasal swab samples, the P_i value changes were monitored for negative and positive nasal swab samples to determine the signal processing methods for screening. Figure 5a,b show the P_i values for negative swab samples and positive swab samples spiked with 10^3 genome equivalents/mL-SARS-CoV-2 (N = 6), respectively. Overall, the P_2, P_3, and P_4 values of the positive samples were greater than those of negative samples. However, the P_i values were not clearly differentiated in certain cases, which was attributed to sensor production batches and potential errors in washing steps. It was interesting to find that the positive signals showed a larger slope of P_i between prewash (P_1) and the first wash (P_2). Also, the positive signals showed a lower average slope of ($P_2 - P_3$) and ($P_3 - P_4$). According to the results, we defined two parameters to determine the positive screening results as described in the following conditions.

$$\text{If } (P_2 - P_1) > 0.12\text{, a score of } C_1 = 0.5 \text{ is given.} \quad (1)$$

$$\text{If } (P_4 - P_1) > 0.1\text{, a score of } C_2 = 0.5 \text{ is given.} \quad (2)$$

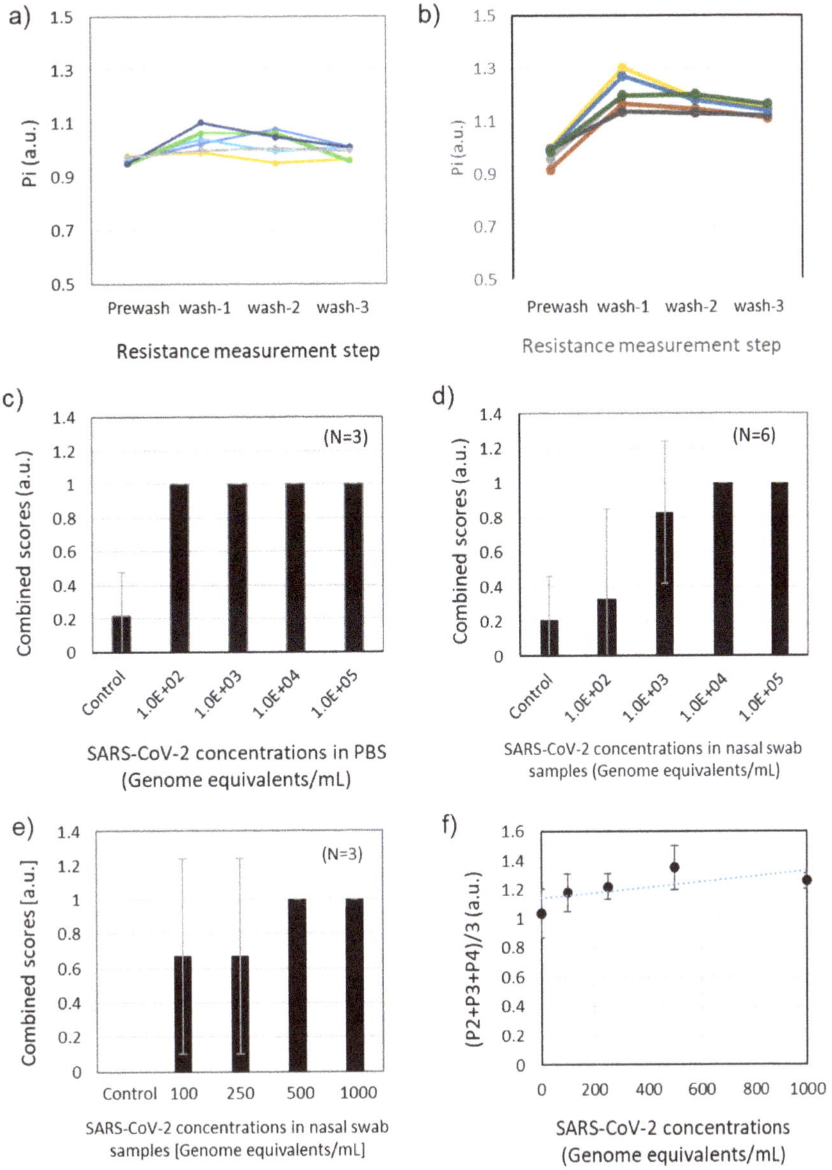

Figure 5. (**a**) Pi changes for negative nasal swab samples (N = 6). (**b**) Pi changes for nasal swab samples spiked with SARS-CoV-2 (1000 genome equivalents/mL). (N = 6) (**c**) Combined scores for various concentrations of SARS-CoV-2 in 1×PBS (N = 3). Negative control (N = 9) (**d**) Combined scores for various concentrations of SARS-CoV-2 in nasal swab samples (N = 6 for positive samples, N = 12 for negative controls). (**e**) Dose response tests for estimating the limit of detection in nasal swab samples spiked with SARS-CoV-2. The concentrations of SARS-CoV-2 are 0, 100, 250, 500, and 1000 genome equivalents/mL (N = 3). (**f**) Average values of P2, P3, and P4 for the SARS-CoV-2 at the concentrations of 0, 100, 250, 500, and 1000 genome equivalents/mL in nasal swab samples (N = 3).

If the combined score of $C_1 + C_2$ was equal to 1, it was positive. If the combined scores were 0 or 0.5, it was negative.

Using the combined scores, the dose response tests of SARS-CoV-2 in PBS were conducted. Figure 5c shows the combined scores for SARS-CoV-2 in PBS at the concentrations of 10^2 and 10^5 genome equivalents/mL. All the signals of the positive samples showed the combined value of 1. When the nasal swab samples spiked with 10^2 and 10^5 genome equivalents/mL were used, two out of six samples showed the combined value of 1 at 10^2 genome equivalents/mL, and five out of six samples showed the combined value of 1 at 10^3 genome equivalents/mL (Figure 5d).

To estimate the LLD in nasal swab samples, further testing was conducted for the SARS-CoV-2 concentrations of 100, 250, 500, and 1000 genome equivalents/mL (Figure 5e). At concentrations of 100 and 250, only one sensor out of three showed the combined score of 1. The combined scores at 500 and 1000 genome equivalents/mL were 1 (N = 3). When the average values of P_2, P_3, and P_4 were used, the linear increase of the resistance ratio was observed (Figure 5f). Based on the linear approximation of the average P_i values, the LOD was 350 genome equivalents/mL. The LOD of 350 genome equivalents/mL was better than typical nucleic amplification-based assays being used for COVID-19 screening. Given that swab samples were replete with human cell fragments, bacteria, and other interferents, these results also demonstrated the specificity of the developed SWCNT sensors.

The average value at 1000 genome equivalents/mL in Figure 5f was a little lower than those of other concentrations, which could be caused by the different fabrication batches. Among the dataset, all the sensors except those used for 1000 genome equivalents/mL were from the same batch. Note that the P_2 value was the parameter that was conventionally used for screening using SWCNT sensors. Due to the batch-to-batch variation, the analog value of the resistance ratio could not be used directly. Instead, the combined scores were better for determining the positive and negative screening results.

3.3. Cross-Reactivity Test

Figure 6 shows the testing of cross-reactivity of the SWCNTs sensors. The nasal swab samples spiked with *S. epidermidis, MTB, H1N1, RSV*, and *S.a.* were used for negative samples and showed no response. The positive samples were nasal swab samples spiked with 10^3 genome equivalents/mL-SARS-CoV-2, S. *epidermidis, MTB, H1N1, RSV*, and *SA*. The combined scores clearly showed the difference between negative and positive samples.

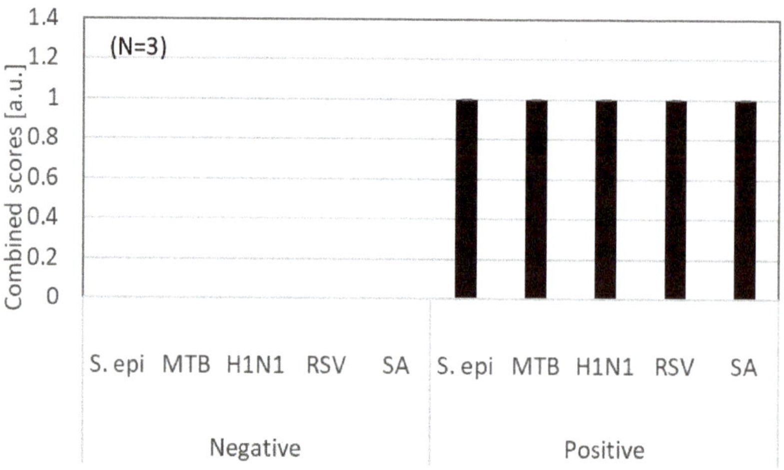

Figure 6. Combined scores for negative and positive nasal swab samples spiked with S. epidermidis, MTB, H1N1, RSV, and SA. The concentration of SARS-CoV-2 was 10^3 genome equivalents/mL. The bacterial concentrations of *S. epidermidis*, MTB, and *S.a* were 10^6 CFU/mL. The viral concentrations of H1N1 and RSV were 10^8 genome equivalents mL (N = 3).

3.4. Clinical Sample Test Results

Clinical testing was performed on previously frozen SARS-CoV2 positive and negative samples collected in TE buffer and tested with RT-PCR. Since only 100 µL of the samples were available in TE buffer, the positive and negative samples were diluted 10-fold using 1×PBS. The PCR test results showed that the positive samples included alpha and delta variants. Among the twelve positive and ten negative samples, an SWCNT sensor showed one false positive result for a negative sample. According to the results, the clinical sensitivity was 100%, and the clinical specificity was 90% (Table 3).

Table 3. Comparison of PCR results and SWCNT sensor results for positive and negative clinical samples (N/A means Ct > 40).

Positive	Reference PCR		* SWCNT	Negative	Reference PCR	* SWCNT
Sample ID	Ct Value	Variants	Sensor	Sample ID	Ct Value (>40)	Sensor
XXXX61b	22.5	alpha	Positive	XXXX8ba7	N/A	Negative
XXXXa4dc	33	alpha	Positive	XXXX4fbd	N/A	Negative
XXXXf041	23.5	alpha	Positive	XXXX6ea9	N/A	Negative
XXXX89d7	30	alpha	Positive	XXXXa467	N/A	Negative
XXXX996	29.4	alpha	Positive	XXXXd9ee	N/A	Negative
XXXXa320	38.5	alpha	Positive	XXXX297e	N/A	Negative
XXXX1b27	31.3	delta	Positive	XXXX4907	N/A	** Positive
XXXXf10e	30.6	delta	Positive	XXXXde69	N/A	Negative
XXXX8c9c	26.5	delta	Positive	XXXX07e3	N/A	Negative
XXXXf06c	31.2	alpha	Positive	XXXX4d9f	N/A	Negative
XXXX5456	30.4	delta	Positive			
XXXX76fb	23.5	alpha	Positive			

* Unblinded trial. ** A PCR negative sample shows the strong positive signal of the SWCNT sensor. The sample collection and testing procedure has been approved by the institutional review board (IRB) at the University of Washington (Husky Testing number: STUDY00011148). The sample IDs are deidentified with XXXX.

4. Conclusions

In summary, an immunoresistive SWCNT sensor was developed to specifically detect SARS-CoV-2 in nasal swab samples. The analytical LOD was 350 genome equivalents/mL with a detection time of 15 min. The analytical LOD was better than point-of-care screening nucleic acid detection assays. In comparison to other antigen detection assays, the detection limit was 2~3 orders of magnitude more sensitive (Figure 7). To achieve such high sensitivity and specificity, the relative resistance change of an SWCNT sensor was measured in comparison to a control sensor. To improve the clinical sensitivity and specificity, a combined score using two parameters based on the resistance ratio was used. According to clinical sample tests, the assay showed 100% sensitivity and 90% specificity. The SWCNT sensors detected both alpha and delta variants. The simple resistive measurement will allow rapid screening by minimally trained personnel. Also, a minimal power requirement (<1 W) will be important for point-of-care (POC) screening in limited-resource settings.

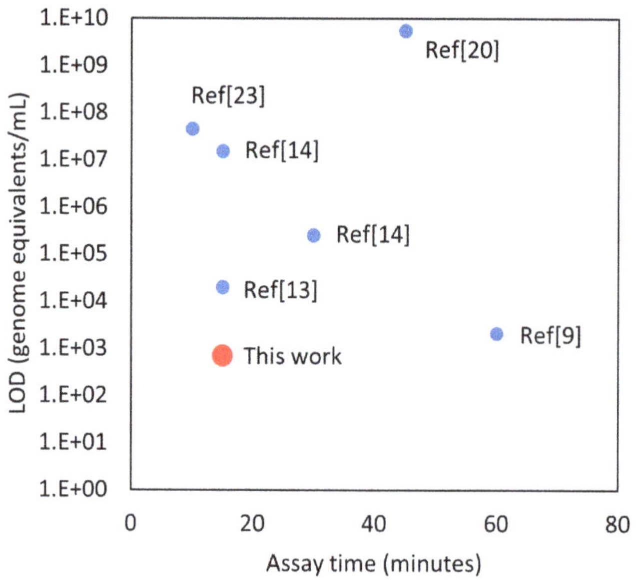

Figure 7. Comparison between this sensor and prior reports in terms of assay time and limit of detection (LOD). Several assumptions have been made to unify the units of LOD. Each virus contains 2 RNA strands. 1 PFU/mL is assumed to be 10,000 RNA copies/mL [37]. One virus is assumed to have 24 Spike Glycoprotein (S) and each of them has a mass of 100 kDa [38]. In reference [7], the reported time is the response time instead of the assay time.

Regarding the analyzer and assay cost, the analyzer was constructed using mass-produced parts to reduce the manufacturing cost. The assay cost was very low due to the plastic film patterned with silkscreened silver electrodes and antibodies. The fabrication yield of the SWCNT sensors was ~70%. The quality control process needs to be improved for a higher fabrication yield. Currently, we are developing a larger scale production of sensors with a quality management system included.

Author Contributions: Conceptualization (J.-H.C.); methodology (T.L., S.D.S., Z.T., V.S., S.-g.A., P.D.H.); software (T.L., Z.T.); data curation (T.L., S.D.S., J.-H.C.); formal analysis (C.E.F., J.-H.K., L.M.S., J.-H.C.); writing (T.L., S.D.S., J.-H.K., J.-H.C.); edit (T.L., C.E.F., J.-H.K., L.M.S., J.Z., J.-H.C.); visualization (T.L., S.-g.A., J.-H.K., J.-H.C.); investigation (T.L., S.D.S., J.-H.C.); resources (C.E.F., S.-g.A., L.M.S., J.Z., J.-H.C.); supervision (C.E.F., L.M.S., J.-H.C.); funding acquisition and project administration (J.-H.C.). All authors have read and agreed to the published version of the manuscript.

Funding: We acknowledge the support by WE-REACH foundation (U01HL152401-S2; WR-20-041-Dx) as a part of an NIH RADx program (project number: 2640).

Institutional Review Board Statement: The sample collection and testing procedure were approved by the institutional review board (IRB) at the University of Washington (Husky Testing number: STUDY00011148).

Informed Consent Statement: Not applicable.

Data Availability Statement: Not available.

Acknowledgments: We appreciate Rodney Ho (Director of WE-REACH), Stephen Flaim (Senior Advisor at NIH), Young-Hoon Kwon (UW Medicine), and Xiaohu Gao (UW BioEngineering) for advice on assay development and optimization.

Conflicts of Interest: The authors declare no conflict of interest.

References

1. Coronavirus Disease (COVID-2019) Situation Reports. Available online: https://www.cmim.org/PDF_covid/Coronavirus_disease2019_COVID-19_UpToDate2.pdf (accessed on 2 January 2022).
2. Pokhrel, P.; Hu, C.P.; Mao, H.B. Detecting the Coronavirus (COVID-19). *ACS Sens.* **2020**, *5*, 2283–2296. [CrossRef] [PubMed]
3. Seshadri, D.R.; Davies, E.V.; Harlow, E.R.; Hsu, J.J.; Knighton, S.C.; Walker, T.A.; Voos, J.E.; Drummond, C.K. Wearable Sensors for COVID-19: A Call to Action to Harness Our Digital Infrastructure for Remote Patient Monitoring and Virtual Assessments. *Front. Digit. Health* **2020**, *2*, 8. [CrossRef]
4. Kumar, S.S.; Dashtipour, K.; Abbasi, Q.H.; Imran, M.A.; Ahmad, W. A Review on Wearable and Contactless Sensing for COVID-19 With Policy Challenges. *Front. Commun. Netw.* **2021**, *2*, 636293. [CrossRef]
5. Gupta, N.; Augustine, S.; Narayan, T.; O'Riordan, A.; Das, A.; Kumar, D.; Luong, J.H.T.; Malhotra, B.D. Point-of-Care PCR Assays for COVID-19 Detection. *Biosensors* **2021**, *11*, 141. [CrossRef] [PubMed]
6. Ulinici, M.; Covantev, S.; Wingfield-Digby, J.; Beloukas, A.; Mathioudakis, A.G.; Corlateanu, A. Screening, Diagnostic and Prognostic Tests for COVID-19: A Comprehensive Review. *Life* **2021**, *11*, 561. [CrossRef]
7. Interim Guidance for Antigen Testing for SARS-CoV-2. Available online: https://www.cdc.gov/coronavirus/2019-ncov/lab/resources/antigen-tests-guidelines.html (accessed on 5 February 2022).
8. Kubina, R.; Dziedzic, A. Molecular and Serological Tests for COVID-19. A Comparative Review of SARS-CoV-2 Coronavirus Laboratory and Point-of-Care Diagnostics. *Diagnostics* **2020**, *10*, 434. [CrossRef] [PubMed]
9. Chow, F.W.N.; Chan, T.T.Y.; Tam, A.R.; Zhao, S.H.; Yao, W.M.; Fung, J.; Cheng, F.K.K.; Lo, G.C.S.; Chu, S.; Aw-Yong, K.L.; et al. A Rapid, Simple, Inexpensive, and Mobile Colorimetric Assay COVID-19-LAMP for Mass On-Site Screening of COVID-19. *Int. J. Mol. Sci.* **2020**, *21*, 5380. [CrossRef] [PubMed]
10. Iravani, S. Nano- and biosensors for the detection of SARS-CoV-2: Challenges and opportunities. *Mater. Adv.* **2020**, *1*, 3092–3103. [CrossRef]
11. Giovannini, G.; Haick, H.; Garoli, D. Detecting COVID-19 from Breath: A Game Changer for a Big Challenge. *ACS Sens.* **2021**, *6*, 1408–1417. [CrossRef]
12. FDA. BinaxNOW COVID-19 Antigen Self Test—Letter of Authorization. Available online: https://www.fda.gov/media/147251/download (accessed on 6 January 2021).
13. Perchetti, G.A.; Huang, M.L.; Mills, M.G.; Jerome, K.R.; Greninger, A.L. Analytical Sensitivity of the Abbott BinaxNOW COVID-19 Ag Card. *J. Clin. Microbiol.* **2021**, *59*, 3. [CrossRef]
14. Corman, V.M.; Haage, V.C.; Bleicker, T.; Schmidt, M.L.; Muhlemann, B.; Zuchowski, M.; Jo, W.K.; Tscheak, P.; Moncke-Buchner, E.; Muller, M.A.; et al. Comparison of seven commercial SARS-CoV-2 rapid point-of-care antigen tests: A single-centre laboratory evaluation study. *Lancet Microbe* **2021**, *2*, E311–E319. [CrossRef]
15. Wolfel, R.; Corman, V.M.; Guggemos, W.; Seilmaier, M.; Zange, S.; Muller, M.A.; Niemeyer, D.; Jones, T.C.; Vollmar, P.; Rothe, C.; et al. Virological assessment of hospitalized patients with COVID-2019. *Nature* **2020**, *581*, 465–469. [CrossRef] [PubMed]
16. Benda, A.; Zerajic, L.; Ankita, A.; Cleary, E.; Park, Y.; Pandey, S. COVID-19 Testing and Diagnostics: A Review of Commercialized Technologies for Cost, Convenience and Quality of Tests. *Sensors* **2021**, *21*, 6581. [CrossRef] [PubMed]
17. FDA. Antibody Testing Is Not Currently Recommended to Assess Immunity after COVID-19 Vaccination: FDA Safety Communication. Available online: https://www.fda.gov/medical-devices/safety-communications/antibody-testing-not-currently-recommended-assess-immunity-after-covid-19-vaccination-fda-safety (accessed on 21 February 2022).
18. Abdelhamid, H.N.; Badr, G. Nanobiotechnology as a platform for the diagnosis of COVID-19: A review. *Nanotechnol. Environ. Eng.* **2021**, *6*, 19. [CrossRef]
19. Seo, G.; Lee, G.; Kim, M.J.; Baek, S.H.; Choi, M.; Ku, K.B.; Lee, C.S.; Jun, S.; Park, D.; Kim, H.G.; et al. Rapid Detection of COVID-19 Causative Virus (SARS-CoV-2) in Human Nasopharyngeal Swab Specimens Using Field-Effect Transistor-Based Biosensor. *ACS Nano* **2020**, *14*, 5135–5142. [CrossRef]
20. Mojsoska, B.; Larsen, S.; Olsen, D.A.; Madsen, J.S.; Brandslund, I.; Alatraktchi, F.A. Rapid SARS-CoV-2 Detection Using Electrochemical Immunosensor. *Sensors* **2021**, *21*, 390. [CrossRef]
21. Yakoh, A.; Pimpitak, U.; Rengpipat, S.; Hirankarn, N.; Chailapakul, O.; Chaiyo, S. Paper-based electrochemical biosensor for diagnosing COVID-19: Detection of SARS-CoV-2 antibodies and antigen. *Biosens. Bioelectron.* **2021**, *176*, 112912. [CrossRef]
22. Hashemi, S.A.; Behbahan, N.G.G.; Bahrani, S.; Mousavi, S.M.; Gholami, A.; Ramakrishna, S.; Firoozsani, M.; Moghadami, M.; Lankarani, K.B.; Omidifar, N. Ultra-sensitive viral glycoprotein detection NanoSystem toward accurate tracing SARS-CoV-2 in biological/non-biological media. *Biosens. Bioelectron.* **2021**, *171*, 112731. [CrossRef]
23. Moitra, P.; Alafeef, M.; Dighe, K.; Frieman, M.B.; Pan, D. Selective Naked-Eye Detection of SARS-CoV-2 Mediated by N Gene Targeted Antisense Oligonucleotide Capped Plasmonic Nanoparticles. *ACS Nano* **2020**, *14*, 7617–7627. [CrossRef]
24. Huang, L.P.; Ding, L.F.; Zhou, J.; Chen, S.L.; Chen, F.; Zhao, C.; Xu, J.Q.; Hu, W.J.; Ji, J.S.; Xu, H.; et al. One-step rapid quantification of SARS-CoV-2 virus particles via low-cost nanoplasmonic sensors in generic microplate reader and point-of-care device. *Biosens. Bioelectron.* **2021**, *171*, 112685. [CrossRef]
25. Asghari, A.; Wang, C.; Yoo, K.M.; Rostamian, A.; Xu, X.C.; Shin, J.D.; Dalir, H.; Chen, R.T. Fast, accurate, point-of-care COVID-19 pandemic diagnosis enabled through advanced lab-on-chip optical biosensors: Opportunities and challenges. *Appl. Phys. Rev.* **2021**, *8*, 031313. [CrossRef] [PubMed]

26. Byon, H.R.; Choi, H.C. Network single-walled carbon nanotube-field effect transistors (SWNT-FETs) with increased Schottky contact area for highly sensitive biosensor applications. *J. Am. Chem. Soc.* **2006**, *128*, 2188–2189. [CrossRef] [PubMed]
27. Li, C.; Curreli, M.; Lin, H.; Lei, B.; Ishikawa, F.N.; Datar, R.; Cote, R.J.; Thompson, M.E.; Zhou, C.W. Complementary detection of prostate-specific antigen using ln2O3 nanowires and carbon nanotubes. *J. Am. Chem. Soc.* **2005**, *127*, 12484–12485. [CrossRef] [PubMed]
28. Heller, I.; Janssens, A.M.; Mannik, J.; Minot, E.D.; Lemay, S.G.; Dekker, C. Identifying the mechanism of biosensing with carbon nanotube transistors. *Nano Lett.* **2008**, *8*, 591–595. [CrossRef]
29. Allen, B.L.; Kichambare, P.D.; Star, A. Carbon nanotube field-effect-transistor-based biosensors. *Adv. Mater.* **2007**, *19*, 1439–1451. [CrossRef]
30. Lee, D.J.; Chander, Y.; Goyal, S.M.; Cui, T.H. Carbon nanotube electric immunoassay for the detection of swine influenza virus H1N1. *Biosens. Bioelectron.* **2011**, *26*, 3482–3487. [CrossRef]
31. Wasik, D.; Mulchandani, A.; Yates, M.V. A heparin-functionalized carbon nanotube-based affinity biosensor for dengue virus. *Biosens. Bioelectron.* **2017**, *91*, 811–816. [CrossRef]
32. Singh, R.; Sharma, A.; Hong, S.; Jang, J. Electrical immunosensor based on dielectrophoretically-deposited carbon nanotubes for detection of influenza virus H1N1. *Analyst* **2014**, *139*, 5415–5421. [CrossRef]
33. Kahng, S.; Soelberg, S.; Fongdjo, F.; Kim, J.; Furlong, C.E.; Chung, J.-H. Carbon nanotube-based thin-film resistive sensor for point-of-care screening of tuberculosis. *Biomed. Microdevices* **2020**, *22*, 50. [CrossRef]
34. Hermanson, G.T. *Bioconjugate Techniques*; Elsevier Inc.: Amsterdam, The Netherlands, 2013.
35. Stevens, R.C.; Soelberg, S.D.; Eberhart, B.T.L.; Spencer, S.; Wekell, J.C.; Chinowsky, T.M.; Trainer, V.L.; Furlong, C.E. Detection of the toxin domoic acid from clam extracts using a portable surface plasmon resonance biosensor. *Harmful Algae* **2007**, *6*, 166–174. [CrossRef]
36. Srivatsan, S.; Heidl, S.; Pfau, B.; Martin, B.K.; Han, P.D.; Zhong, W.Z.; van Raay, K.; McDermot, E.; Opsahl, J.; Gamboa, L.; et al. SwabExpress: An End-to-End Protocol for Extraction-Free COVID-19 Testing. *Clin. Chem.* **2022**, *68*, 143–152. [CrossRef] [PubMed]
37. Sender, R.; Bar-On, Y.M.; Gleizer, S.; Bernshtein, B.; Flamholz, A.; Phillips, R.; Milo, R. The total number and mass of SARS-CoV-2 virions. *Proc. Natl. Acad. Sci. USA* **2021**, *118*, e2024815118. [CrossRef] [PubMed]
38. Ke, Z.L.; Oton, J.Q.; Qu, K.; Cortese, M.; Zila, V.; McKeane, L.; Nakane, T.; Zivanov, J.; Neufeldt, C.J.; Cerikan, B.; et al. Structures and distributions of SARS-CoV-2 spike proteins on intact virions. *Nature* **2020**, *588*, 498–502. [CrossRef] [PubMed]

biosensors

Article

A Computational Modeling and Simulation Workflow to Investigate the Impact of Patient-Specific and Device Factors on Hemodynamic Measurements from Non-Invasive Photoplethysmography

Jesse Fine [1], Michael J. McShane [1,2,3], Gerard L. Coté [1,2,*] and Christopher G. Scully [4]

1 Department of Biomedical Engineering, Texas A&M University, College Station, TX 77843, USA
2 Center for Remote Health Technologies and Systems, Texas A&M Engineering Experiment Station, Texas A&M University, College Station, TX 77843, USA
3 Department of Materials Science and Engineering, Texas A&M University, College Station, TX 77843, USA
4 Office of Science and Engineering Laboratories, Division of Biomedical Physics, Center for Devices and Radiological Health, Food and Drug Administration, Silver Spring, MD 20993, USA
* Correspondence: gcote@tamu.edu

Citation: Fine, J.; McShane, M.J.; Coté, G.L.; Scully, C.G. A Computational Modeling and Simulation Workflow to Investigate the Impact of Patient-Specific and Device Factors on Hemodynamic Measurements from Non-Invasive Photoplethysmography. *Biosensors* **2022**, *12*, 598. https://doi.org/10.3390/bios12080598

Received: 6 June 2022
Accepted: 27 July 2022
Published: 4 August 2022

Abstract: Cardiovascular disease is the leading cause of death globally. To provide continuous monitoring of blood pressure (BP), a parameter which has shown to improve health outcomes when monitored closely, many groups are trying to measure blood pressure via noninvasive photoplethysmography (PPG). However, the PPG waveform is subject to variation as a function of patient-specific and device factors and thus a platform to enable the evaluation of these factors on the PPG waveform and subsequent hemodynamic parameter prediction would enable device development. Here, we present a computational workflow that combines Monte Carlo modeling (MC), gaussian combination, and additive noise to create synthetic dataset of volar fingertip PPG waveforms representative of a diverse cohort. First, MC is used to determine PPG amplitude across age, skin tone, and device wavelength. Then, gaussian combination generates accurate PPG waveforms, and signal processing enables data filtration and feature extraction. We improve the limitations of current synthetic PPG frameworks by enabling inclusion of physiological and anatomical effects from body site, skin tone, and age. We then show how the datasets can be used to examine effects of device characteristics such as wavelength, analog to digital converter specifications, filtering method, and feature extraction. Lastly, we demonstrate the use of this framework to show the insensitivity of a support vector machine predictive algorithm compared to a neural network and bagged trees algorithm.

Keywords: photoplethysmography; remote monitoring; computational modeling and simulation; medical device design

1. Introduction

Cardiovascular disease (CVD) is the leading cause of death globally, with an estimated 17.9 million people dying from CVD in 2019 [1]. Of these deaths nearly 85% were due to heart attack or stroke [1]. Nearly half of all adults in the United States (116 million or 47%) have hypertension, commonly referred to as high blood pressure [2]. Studies show that every 10 mmHg drop in systolic BP reduces the probability of heart attack and stroke by ~50% for all age groups [3]. Lowering systolic BP from 140 to 120 mmHg has also shown to reduce the risk of death by ~27% [4]. Thus, monitoring blood pressure to identify and subsequently address hypertension is a common and effective way to reduce risk of developing CVD [5]. Monitoring these parameters noninvasively and continuously could provide additional insight into a patient's blood pressure over time to enable earlier detection and improved management of hypertension [6–8]. Noninvasive and continuous methods to monitor blood pressure are thus of great interest to the healthcare community to provide care to individuals with CVD or those at-risk of developing CVD.

Photoplethysmography (PPG) is a non-invasive optical technique that has been extensively studied for its potential to non-invasively monitor blood pressure [9,10]. By illuminating the skin and recording the light that reaches nearby photodetectors, the PPG waveform resulting from diffusely reflected photons that interact with blood and tissue are collected. The PPG waveform has a large "quasi-DC" component from static absorption and scattering from tissue and blood, as well as a much smaller "AC" component that is of great interest because it correlates to the pulsatile local blood volume dynamics of microvasculature and/or macrovasculature—depending on the device wavelength and target anatomy [11].

The PPG waveform is most often collected with a sampling frequency between ~120–1000 Hz, which enables Pulse Wave Analysis (PWA) of the AC component [12,13]. Through PWA, the PPG waveform is processed through feature extraction to derive the values of specific characteristics of the waveform. Some PPG waveform features commonly studied are listed in Table 1, and an example waveform with labeled systolic peak, dicrotic notch, and pulse onset is shown in Figure 1. These features are studied as inputs to models that estimate cardiovascular parameters such as blood pressure [14]. However, the PPG waveform is subject to added variability and uncertainty from numerous sources. These factors originate from patient physiology as well as environmental factors and device designs [11]. For similar PPG-like optical absorption measurements such as SpO2, differences in measurement performance has been observed between patient skin tones [15,16]. Additionally, the changes in skin thickness and vessel compliance that accompany age also affect the PPG waveform and signal quality [11]. Other factors such as device wavelength, device analog-to-digital converter specifications, and filtering methodology can alter the recorded PPG waveform and manipulate device signal quality [17,18], potentially impacting if algorithms developed from one device are applicable to another. Thus, as efforts continue to utilize PPG for hemodynamic monitoring applications, quantification of effects of age-related changes, patient skin-tone, and device designs on PPG features can improve robustness and generalizability. Additionally, resources that enable systematic assessment of algorithmic performance on data that are inclusive of these factors could provide more robust design of such devices.

Table 1. Common PPG Features.

Feature Name	Definition
Pulse Rise Time	Difference in time from pulse onset to systolic peak
Peak Amplitude	Difference in signal amplitude between systolic peak and onset (AC component)
"X"% Systolic Width	Difference in time between "Y" and the systolic peak, where "Y" is the time at which "X"% of the peak amplitude is achieved before the systolic peak [19]
"X"% Diastolic Width	Difference in time between "Y" and the systolic peak, where "Y" is the time at which "X"% of the peak amplitude is achieved after the systolic peak [19]
Inflection Point Area	The ratio a2/a1, where a2 is the area under the PPG waveform from the dicrotic notch to the next onset and a1 is the area under the PPG waveform from the onset to the dicrotic notch [18]
Pulse Rate	The number of systolic peaks observed over 60 s

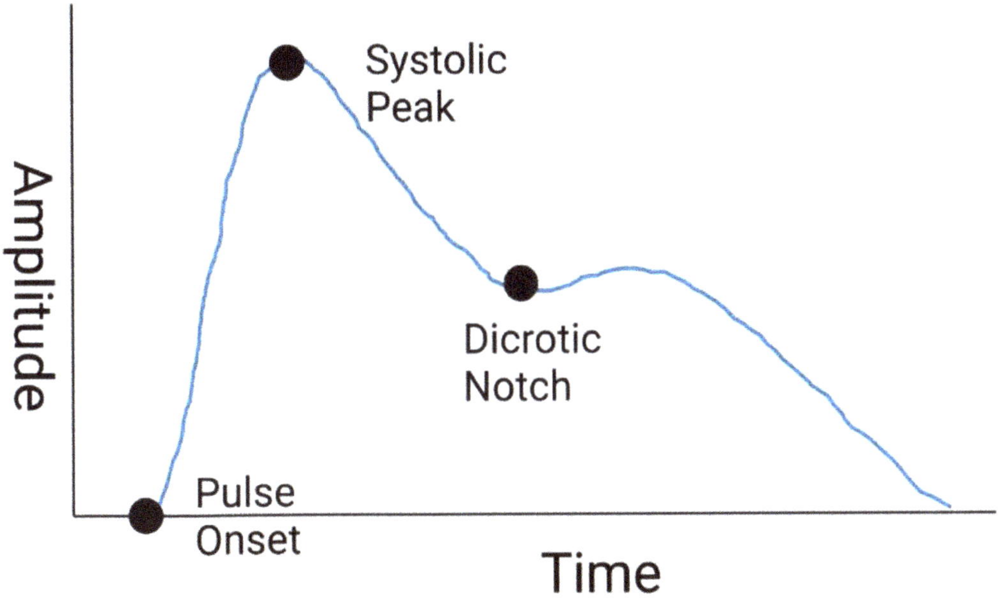

Figure 1. Sample PPG Waveform. Created with BioRender.com (accessed on 26 May 2022).

While available clinical monitoring databases such as the MIMIC-III Waveform Database enable testing of algorithms on data from tens of thousands of patients, insufficient data on patient characteristics such as skin tone can limit the utility to understanding specific factors that may affect the performance of a new measurements [20,21]. Additionally, important information on the devices used during clinical monitoring and characteristics of those devices such as signal filter type and schematics of the light emitting diode (LED) and photodiode (PD) may be unknown. Thus, the data available to support algorithm development and how they can be applied to different device designs are limited. Computational modeling is a powerful tool to fill this gap as any permutation of factors can be incorporated and explored.

Monte Carlo modeling (MC) of the optical path and statistical modeling of waveform morphology (e.g., through Gaussian combinations) are tools that have been used to evaluate the effects of physiology or device parameters on raw PPG signal strength [22–24]. Chatterjee et al. have used MC for this purpose [25]. MC results from Oxygen saturation simulations at 660 nm and 880 nm across skin tone and source/detector separation were compared to experimentally collected data, the model was validated and the origin of the PPG signal was explored [24–26]. Boonya-ananta et al. focused on individuals with dark skin tone and obesity, using MC to generate a single PPG period and then quantified the impact those features have on PPG AC/DC ratio [22].

Despite such advances, it is noteworthy that the use of MC has not yet been extended to evaluate the downstream effects these factors have on algorithm performance or clinical action. One reason why this is the case is because computational time prevents large windows of data from being created. Further, MC for photon propagation is inherently limited in its inability to represent other necessary factors such as motion artifacts that do not manifest in simulation geometry or optical properties. Gaussian combination is a previously reported methodology to generate PPG waveforms over a larger window of time [23]. Tang et al. improved on this work by publishing "PPGSynth" in 2020: a toolbox that uses Gaussian combination to generate arrhythmic PPG signals with a specified sampling frequency, length, heart rate, and noise with an easy-to-use user interface [27]. Gaussian combination, however, is limited by its inability to represent the effect that physiological/anatomical factors have on the PPG waveform. Thus, both of these techniques face limitations to simulate PPG waveforms across populations considering different device designs.

In this work, we combine MC and Gaussian combination to create a platform to assess the impact of device wavelength, device analog to digital converter (ADC) resolution, patient age, and patient skin-tone against PPG feature extraction. By leveraging the ability of MC to represent patient-specific factors and the ability of gaussian combination to generate entire waveforms without utilizing extensive computational resources, we propose that the combination of these two methodologies will enable creation of physiologically and anatomically accurate waveforms to evaluate patient and device specific effects on the PPG waveform. The main purpose of the simulation tool is to generate databases of synthetic PPG signals with customizable parameters that represent a diverse cohort. This will enable end users who are currently developing blood pressure predictive algorithms to use this tool as a cost-effective and accessible methodology to test the robustness of algorithms to these factors. Additionally, as an example test case of this framework, synthesized data are passed through feature extraction tools to study how the patient and device factors impact the waveform characteristics. We then present a case example with different machine learning models (Neural Network, Bagged Trees algorithm, Support Vector Machine) trained to estimate blood pressure from PPG waveforms to show how such an approach can be used to evaluate hemodynamic measurement performance changes as a function of the aforementioned parameters.

2. Materials and Methods

2.1. Schema Overview

This workflow, conceptually illustrated in Figure 2, involves creating and processing synthetic PPG waveforms with two primary components: the PPG signal generator and the device algorithm simulator. Small icons indicate where a process (such as filtering) or parameter (such as age or skin tone) is relevant. The PPG signal generator creates a 30 s window of data with a sampling frequency of 120 Hz that is representative of a PPG derived from an individual of a specified skin tone and age and taken with a device of a specified wavelength. The PPG signal generator has two sub-components: a Monte Carlo (MC) model and a PPG waveform generator. The MC model estimates the AC and DC components of a PPG signal derived from a combination of the above three factors by simulating photon propagation through tissue, where the dimensions of the tissue and its optical properties change as a function of the age, skin tone, and wavelength being simulated. These AC and DC values are used as inputs into the PPG waveform generator, which uses Gaussian combination and a generalized reduced gradient (GRG) solver to create a waveform that is very similar to an input PPG wave shape from a template pulse. By using Gaussian combination, the end user is able to explore any interpolated PPG waveform morphology. PPG noise can be added to create PPG waveforms under various conditions. Within the device algorithm simulator, these data are filtered, segmented into 30 s windows, and re-scaled to be passed through feature extraction where fiducial points are calculated and used as inputs for blood pressure prediction algorithms. In the current study, device filters are applied to the generated PPG waveforms.

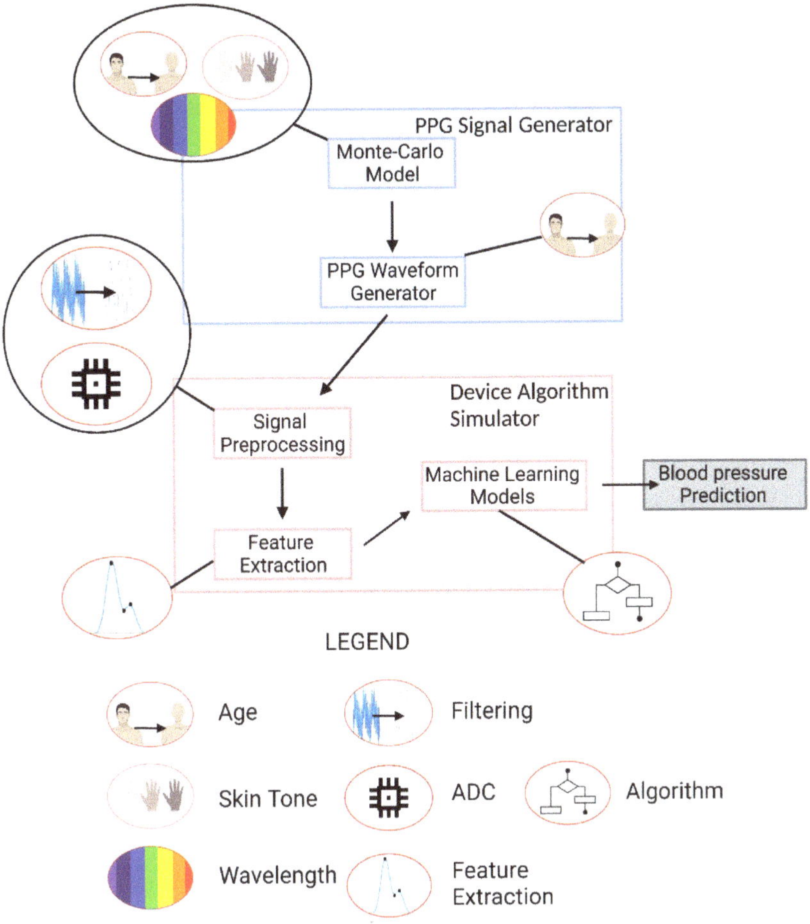

Figure 2. Computational Workflow. Created with Biorender.com (accessed on 26 May 2022).

2.2. PPG Signal Generator

2.2.1. Monte Carlo Model

A six-layer MC model of the volar fingertip consisting of the epidermis, papillary dermis, upper blood net dermis, reticular dermis, deep blood net dermis, and subcutaneous fat was constructed using MCmatlab (Figure 3, isometric view) [24,28,29]. MCmatlab was chosen due to its ability to simply manipulate geometrical and optical properties of the models developed, as well as ease of use by someone not intimately familiar with MATLAB or Monte Carlo. The isometric view in Figure 3 provides a graphical illustration of the multi-layered model and a legend that names each layer based on the color used. The geometrical and optical properties of the model were dependent on the simulated device wavelength, patient age, and patient skin tone; and are listed in Table 2 [30–35]. A cardiac pulse is simulated in the Monte Carlo model by completing two simulations for a given combination of parameters: a first simulation where the optical properties are representative of tissue at rest ("rest"), and a second simulation where the optical properties of the dermal layer are changed to represent an increased blood volume ("pulse"). The result of the first simulation is the DC value, and the result of the second simulation is the AC + DC.

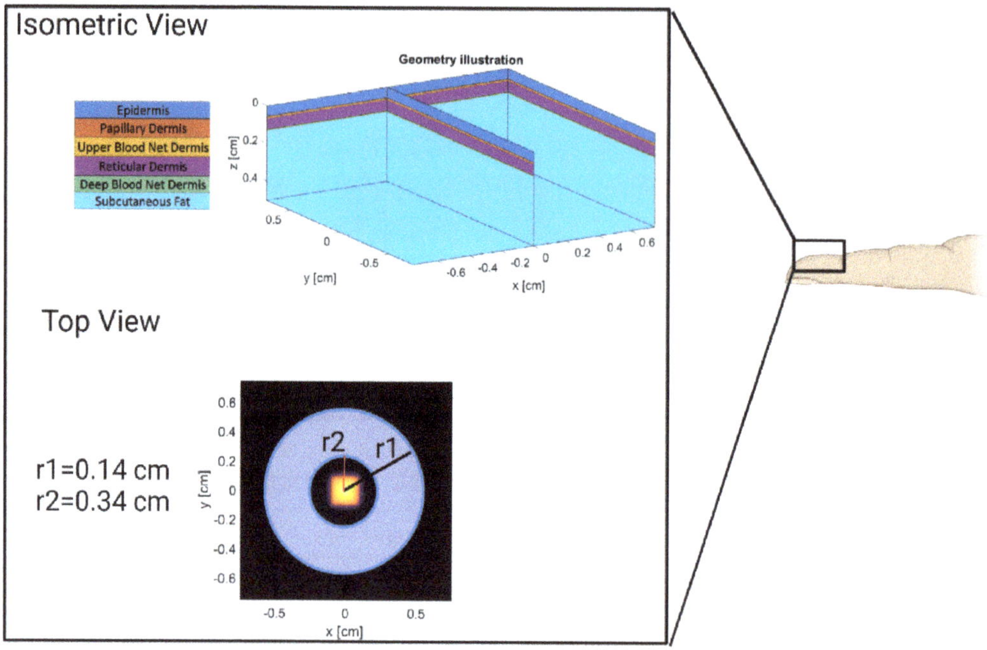

Figure 3. Model Geometry and Source/Detector Geometry. Created with Biorender.com (accessed on 26 May 2022).

Table 2. Model Optical and Geometric Properties.

	Age (Years)					Wavelength (nm)					
	23	34.4	44.8	55		515		660		880	
	Thickness (mm)/Starting Depth (mm)					μ_a (cm^{-1})	μ_s (cm^{-1})	μ_a (cm^{-1})	μ_s (cm^{-1})	μ_a (cm^{-1})	μ_s (cm^{-1})
Epidermis	0.55/0.00	0.55/0.00	0.55/0.00	0.55/0.00	**(0.03/0.10/ 0.20/0.30 VFM)**	1.96/6.28/ 12.43/18.58	388.35	0.86/2.75/ 5.44/8.13	303.03	0.33/1.06/ 2.09/3.13	227.27
Papillary Dermis	0.075/0.55	0.071/0.55	0.067/0.55	0.064/0.55	**Rest**	1.2166	389.99	0.5249	208.65	0.2344	118.94
					Pulsed	1.2202		0.5250		0.2346	
Upper Blood Net Dermis	0.04/0.63	0.038/0.62	0.036/0.62	0.033/0.61	**Rest**	1.5328	389.99	0.5398	208.65	0.2546	118.94
					Pulsed	1.5593		0.5410		0.2558	
Reticular Dermis	0.75/0.67	0.71/0.66	0.67/0.65	0.64/0.65	**Rest**	1.2167	389.99	0.5256	208.65	0.2456	118.94
					Pulsed	1.2202		0.5257		0.2458	
Deep Blood Net Dermis	0.05/1.42	0.05/1.37	0.04/1.33	0.04/1.28	**Rest**	1.2896	389.99	0.5288	208.65	0.2462	118.94
					Pulsed	1.2985		0.5292		0.2466	
Subcutaneous Tissue	2.00/1.47	2.00/1.42	2.00/1.37	2.00/1.33	n/a	6.0798	336.18	0.2827	249.74	0.3195	191.53

Skin layer thickness are derived from previously published literature [31–33]. First, the epidermal thickness was found in literature to be 0.055 cm and the total dermal thickness for a control cohort (termed "healthy") within a systemic sclerosis study of 61-year-old subjects (4 male, 33 female) was found to be 0.075 cm [32,33]. Then, using data collected by Shuster et al., a line of best fit correlating age to dermal thickness allows estimation of appropriate dermal thickness for subjects of any age. In this work, the line of best fit yielded an annual average decrease of 0.00044 mm [31]. Of the entire dermal thickness, the papillary dermis is 8.2%, the upper blood net dermis is 4.37%, the reticular dermis is

81.97%, and the deep blood net is 5.46% [28]. From this, the thickness of each sublayer at the simulated ages are calculated and can be seen in Table 2.

The Monte Carlo model layers are derived from previous literature: Meglinski et al. created a four-layer dermis for MC modeling, and modifying the blood volume fraction to represent the systolic peak of a PPG waveform has been done previously by Fine et al. and Chatterjee et al. [26,28,36]. Additionally, the optical properties of these layers are derived from Jacques et al. [30]. The model presented herein differs from previous literature by being the first to incorporate patient age by varying dermal layer thickness and vessel compliance.

Many tissue optical properties are included natively in MCmatlab (as derived from Jacques et al.) [29,30]. The epidermal absorption coefficient is changed to account for volume fraction melanosomes (VFM) on the volar fingertip that for this work we used the range from 0.03 to 0.30, shown to be within physiological range for other body sites [37]. The range 0.03 to 0.30 was chosen for this work instead of the typical 0.03 to 0.43 because fingertips have less melanin than most body sites; however, it is a limitation that there is not a direct reference for experimental values at this site. Additionally, the default MCmatlab subcutaneous fat absorption coefficient is multiplied by 0.10 to be respective of values found in literature [38].

In the case of the pulse Monte Carlo model, the absorption coefficient of the dermal sublayers is increased to represent an additional absorptive contribution by oxygenated blood. Modifying the magnitude of increase also allows simulating changes in vessel compliance that accompany age, as the volar fingertip is vascularized by a subungual arcade instead of a discrete artery. The increase in blood volume is calculated based on values from literature. The change in carotid artery diameter during the cardiac cycle across ages was converted to a change in area [34]. Next, the change in area of the carotid artery as a function of age was assumed to be constant for the largest artery supplying the subungual arcade of the fingertip- the proper digital artery, which increases in diameter 6% and has a cross sectional area change of 12% for a healthy ~20 year old subject [39]. Finally, it was estimated that the increase in blood volume at the systolic peak is approximately 1.124× for a 23-year-old, 1.099× for a 34.4-year-old, 1.083× for a 44.8-year-old, and 1.073× for a 55-year-old.

For this study, the Monte Carlo model used a square LED-type emitter (top-hat distribution in the near field and Lambertian distribution in the far field) with a side length of 1.0 mm and a half angle of 2.4 radians. The photodiode is donut-shaped surrounding the emitter with an inner radius of 0.0071 mm and an outer radius of 0.0091 mm. However, photodiode and LED size, half angles, and distributions can be changed as needed for the end user. These use-case values were chosen to be similar to the existing Apple Watch LED/PD configuration.

The simulations were completed on a PowerSpec G900 (Micro Electronics Inc, Hilliard, OH, USA) and were parallelized to the GPU: an NVIDIA GeForce RTX 3070 8 GB (NVIDIA Corporation, Santa Clara, CA, USA). To determine the number of photons required for each simulation, every simulation was completed in triplicate (a given combination of parameters required 3 rest simulations and 3 pulse simulations) and repeated with an increasing number of photons until the coefficient of variation of the AC across the triplicate results was less than 10%. The AC is defined as the result of the pulse simulation minus the result of the rest simulation, whereas the DC is the result of the rest simulation. This value was found to be dependent on the parameters of a given simulation, ranging from 5×10^8 photons for the case of device wavelength of 515 nm and volume fraction melanosomes 0.03 to 1×10^{11} photons in the case of device wavelength of 880 nm and volume fraction melanosomes 0.30. In total, 96 simulations were completed at the sufficient number of photons, requiring approximately 3.5 weeks.

The outputs of these simulations are synthetic AC and DC amplitudes. To enable comparison of AC values across wavelength, age, and skin tone as well as assess the simulated results with respect to other works; the AC values were normalized to the maximum value such that the largest AC value has a normalized value of 1. Lastly, a blue/white colormap was applied to enable qualitative comparisons such that the maximum value is blue and the minimum value is white. The same procedure was applied to the DC amplitudes.

2.2.2. PPG Waveform Generator

The PPG waveform generator creates a continuous and synthetic PPG waveform intended to represent a combination of patient- and device- specific factors. For this work, the shape of a single waveform period was derived from Allen and Murray, which details the average volar fingertip PPG waveform from individuals that are 23 years-old (YO), 34.4 YO, 44.8 YO, and 55 YO [40]. These four waveforms were chosen as they represent morphologically different waveforms observed in PPG data analysis: namely, loss of diastolic peak and dicrotic notch. Other waveforms were not included to maintain a reasonable length work and limit time needed to run all simulations. To generate full waveforms representative of patients with various ages for the study, the PPG Waveform Generator utilizes an input waveform collected from the volar fingertip with an infrared LED found in literature [41]. A generalized reduced gradient (GRG) solver native to Microsoft excel was used to determine the amplitude (a1, a2, a3), bias (b1, b2, b3) and width (c1, c2, c3) of three Gaussians that additively combine and minimize relative error when compared to the input waveforms from the literature, and enables creation of PPG waveforms by the end user not included within this work.

After a single 0.8 s period of the PPG waveform is created, a heart rate (75 beats per minute), and sampling frequency (120 Hz) are specified and the waveform is repeated for a specified signal length. Finally, any second waveform or noise, including noise from real PPG data, can be added to the waveform to imitate noise. Here, the noise waveform is constructed via adding sinusoids of customizable frequencies and relative amplitudes to mimic common noise frequencies for PPG signals. Specifically, in this work, three noise sinusoids at 20 Hz, 40 Hz, and 60 Hz and amplitudes 38%, 59%, and 59% of the AC amplitude were used, as measured in previous literature [42].

To analyze the accuracy of the waveform generator, one period of the resultant waveform for each of the four ages is compared to the waveform derived from literature [41]. Median relative error was the chosen statistical measure to make this comparison, as it provides the ability to compare difference between the input and output waveforms while also being robust to larger relative differences at the tail ends of the waveforms that would have their relative difference overrepresented with other measures, such as mean relative error.

2.3. *Device Algorithm Simulator*

2.3.1. Signal Preprocessing

The main components of signal preprocessing simulated here includes high level components: filtering, ADC simulation, and rescaling. The data is filtered by one of the following: a 0.1–7 Hz 4th order Butterworth Bandpass, a 0.1–7 Hz 4th order Inverse Chebyshev bandpass with a 10-element moving average filter, and a 7 Hz 4th order Inverse Chebyshev lowpass with a 10-element moving average filter. ADC simulation is completed by allowing the user to specify an ADC resolution in bits, a reference current in amps, and LED power in Watts. The ADC value is found by using Equation (1):

$$\text{ADC Values} = \text{MC\_Out} \times (2\text{\^{}ADC Resolution})/\text{Reference Current} \tag{1}$$

where MC_Out is the output AC of the MC simulation modified by:

$$\text{MC\_Out} = 10 \times \text{AC} \times \text{LED power} \times \text{photodiode area} \tag{2}$$

The morphology of the PPG waveforms with the smallest and largest AC amplitudes are evaluated across ADC values. First, an assumed reference current of 32 uA and an assumed LED power of 50 mW are used. PPG waveform data is simulated with an ADC from 1 bit to 25 bits for the patient-specific and device factors that yield the highest and lowest AC amplitudes. Next, waveforms collected with select simulated ADC resolutions are qualitatively compared to determine the impact that insufficient ADC resolution can have on PPG morphology. The percent difference between a PPG waveform at a given ADC resolution and the PPG waveform at an ADC resolution of 25 bits is compared as a suggested methodology for end users to identify sufficient ADC resolutions. Lastly, all data taken from a single combination of parameters (i.e., 23 years old, 515 nm, 0.03 VFM, Chebyshev Bandpass) is rescaled to range from 0.5 to 2.7 via MATLAB's rescale function. This was performed to match the approximate range of values seen in the training data for feature extraction and machine learning.

2.3.2. Feature Extraction

PPG feature extraction was performed in Python using in-house code and the heartPy library to extract the systolic peak and onset [43]. The feature extraction identifies 30 s of data wherein heartPy successfully extracts >90% of the expected number of systolic peaks and rejects fewer than 10% of the expected number of systolic peaks. Then, 38 features found in Table A1 are calculated with 3 fiducial points: the systolic onset determined from heartPy, the systolic peak determined from heartPy, and the dicrotic notch determined by identifying the "c" peak in the second derivative of the PPG waveform [44]. The second derivative is smoothed and scaled to enable easier detection for PPGs with less-visible dicrotic notches. Once all of the 38 features were extracted, we aimed to determine the effect of patient-specific and device factors on the value of these features. This was done by comparing the mean and standard deviation of each feature across each factor. Then, a colormap that shows the range of values for each feature across each factor was created to enable visual inspection of the data.

2.3.3. Machine Learning Algorithms

As an example use-case of this framework, three separate models were trained to estimate blood pressure from PPG-derived features with MATLAB 2020b (The Mathworks, Natick, MA, USA). A Support Vector Machine (SVM) and Bagged Trees algorithm were developed with MATLAB's Regression Learning Application and a Neural Network was developed with MATLAB's Neural Network Fitting Application.

All models were trained with data from the publicly available and deidentified MIMIC III Matched Data Set [20]. From this database, 40,000 patient data samples from 2437 patients that included arterial blood pressure (ABP) measured from an invasive arterial line and PPG waveforms were identified via stratified random sampling and 17,517 data samples, 30 s in length, were passed to feature extraction. The systolic peak and diastolic peak within the ABP data over 30 s was used to determine the systolic and diastolic blood pressure, respectively. Extracted features were then pre-processed as follows: data with systolic/diastolic ranges greater than 20 mmHg/12 mmHg within the 30 s were discarded and statistical outliers (defined as samples with data beyond 3 standard deviations) were removed. PPG feature values were then rescaled from zero to one. These methods are derived from ISO-81060-2 standard [45].

The SVM was trained on 70% of the MIMIC-III data with 10-fold validation, and then tested on the remaining 30% of the data. All data were standardized together to have a mean of zero and standard deviation of one. A fine Gaussian kernel function with a kernel scale of 1.5 was used. The artificial neural network was trained on 70% of the data, tested on 15% of the data, and validated on the remaining 15% of the data. Levenberg-Marquardt backpropagation was used with 100 hidden layers and mean squared error as an error function. The bagged trees algorithm was trained on 70% of the MIMIC-III data with 10-fold cross-validation and tested on the remaining 30% of the data. After training the algorithms, features originating from the synthetic data were used to predict systolic and diastolic blood pressure and the standard deviations of these predictions were analyzed as a way to assess the sensitivity of these algorithms to patient and device specific factors. Lastly, the predicted blood pressure is analyzed via mean error and standard deviation.

This decision was informed by "ISO-81060-2, Non-invasive Sphygmamonometers—Part 2: Clinical investigation of intermittent automated measurement type" [45].

3. Results and Discussion

3.1. PPG Signal Generator Verification

3.1.1. Monte Carlo Model

Figure 4 shows changes in PPG normalized AC and DC amplitudes with respect to wavelength, VFM, and age relative to the maximum amplitude (515 nm, 0.03 VFM, 23 years old for AC and 880 nm, 0.03 VFM, 23 years old for DC). Note that while AC and DC amplitudes are shown separately, the AC/DC ratio is another parameter discussed in literature to gauge PPG waveform signal quality. However, it was not used here since the smaller AC/DC values in dark skin tones require more photons to precisely and accurately resolve than what was used in this work. Since a target coefficient of variation of less than 10% was set as a target for simulation precision, the derived value AC/DC would have a coefficient of variation greater than 10% because it is a derived value consisting of the AC divided by the DC. This limitation is caused by the computational complexity of these simulations wherein it would take weeks to properly simulate this scenario. Differences between this work and others with respect to simulated conditions (age, wavelengths, etc.) and the lack of details in other work prevent exact comparisons from being made. However, it is valuable to demonstrate agreement of trends between the simulations presented here and data collected elsewhere.

Experimental and in silico research has been published exploring the relationship between PPG wavelength and amplitude. Moco et al. observed a decrease of PPG amplitude from 515 nm to 660 nm by 55% and then a subsequent 150% increase in signal from 660 nm to 880 nm [46]. We observed a similar trend, namely a 59% decrease in PPG amplitude from 515 nm to 600 nm and a 107% increase in signal from 660 nm to 880 nm. Factors such as skin thickness and device characteristics explain the absolute differences in results from 660 nm to 880 nm.

The second variable explored in Figure 4 is the impact of VFM on the PPG signal. Ajmal et al. used MC modeling to explore the impact of skin tone on the wrist, an anatomy with more melanin than the fingertip. Specifically, they explored the impact of Fitzpatrick Skin Tone I (set by Ajmal et al. to be 0.03 VFM) and Fitzpatrick Skin Tone VI (set by Ajmal et al. to be 0.42 VFM), on the AC/DC ratio of various commercial PPG-based heart rate monitors [47]. While error propagation in this study limits conclusions regarding the AC/DC ratio on dark skin tones, our results agree with those presented in the literature as AC/DC ratio does not change in 0.03 and 0.10 VFM [47]. Ajmal et al. presented that AC/DC ratio decrease as a function of skin tone ranged from less than 1% to approximately 15% depending on the wearable source/detector configuration. This study is different from the current effort, as Ajmal et al. performed their work at the wrist with different source to detector configurations.

The last variable shown in Figure 4 is age. The effect of age on PPG signal amplitude is largely unexplored, however previous work showed that at least two physiological changes create an effect: (1) decrease in skin thickness, and (2) decrease in vessel compliance. The former increases PPG signal amplitude and the later decreases PPG signal amplitude by reducing the change in blood volume caused by the cardiac cycle [11]. Both of these factors are included in determining the effect of age on PPG amplitude in Figure 4. In previous literature, the significant decrease in vessel compliance observed with age supports the trend observed in the results of a decrease in PPG amplitude [34]. To increase the accuracy of the model with respect to varying age, the epidermal layer should also decrease in thickness as age changes. This factor was not included in this work, as decreasing epidermal thickness would require increasing simulation resolution and to substantially increase the time required to collect results. It is hypothesized that decreased epidermal thickness would increase PPG signal, however it is unknown whether this effect would negate the decrease in signal caused by changes in vessel compliance. However, PPG amplitude is not the only change that age causes in PPG feature extraction, rather the main change is morphological [41].

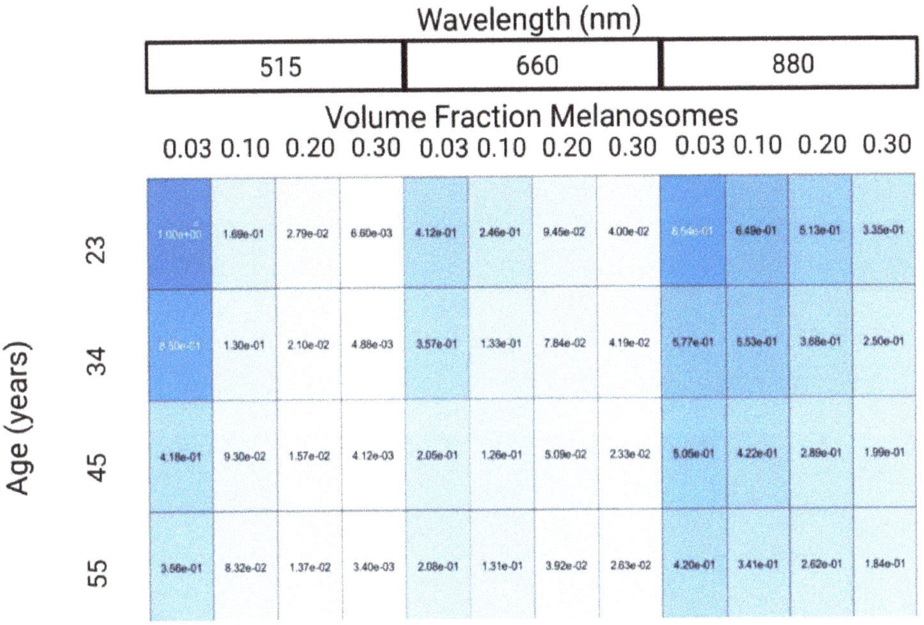

(**a**)

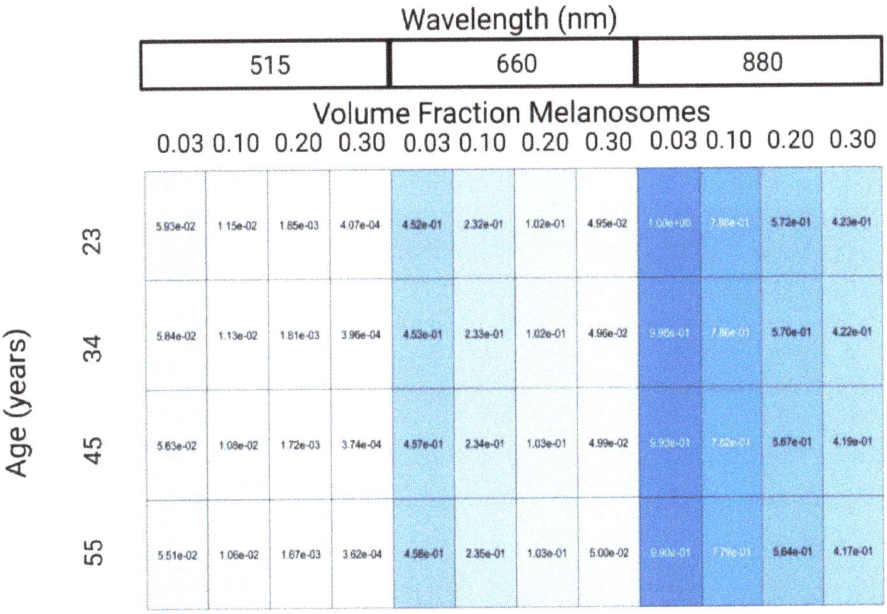

(**b**)

Figure 4. Normalized PPG AC amplitude (**a**) and PPG DC amplitude (**b**) from Monte-Carlo Simulation Results. Made with Biorender.com (accessed on 26 May 2022).

3.1.2. PPG Waveform Generator

The ability of the workflow to replicate PPG waveforms was assessed. Table 3 shows the Gaussian parameters used to generate waveforms across four ages. To analyze the ability of the gaussian combination method to replicate literature-sourced waveforms, median relative error was chosen as it is robust to large percent differences when the waveforms approach zero. In all cases, between 23 and 55 years old, median relative error was below 5% indicating strong ability to generate data derived from waveforms supplied by the end user or specified in this work. Qualitatively, as depicted in Figure 5, these waveforms also demonstrated well-studied morphological changes in PPG waveforms as a function of subject age: the dicrotic notch and diastolic peak become less noticeable as age increases [18]. These individual waveforms are repeated over a window of time to generate continuous data for signal processing, an example of this is shown in Figure 6.

Table 3. PPG Waveform Gaussian Parameters and Median Relative Error for GRG nonlinear solver.

Age (Years)	Gaussian 1 Parameters (a1, b1, c1)	Gaussian 2 Parameters (a2, b2, c2)	Gaussian 3 Parameters (a3, b3, c3)	Median Relative Error (%)
23	0.57,0.19,0.09	0.47,0.11,0.05	0.77,0.39,0.30	3.58
34.4	0.80,0.28,0.25	0.77,0.59,0.44	0.74,0.13,0.11	2.12
44.8	0.59,0.21,0.12	0.38,0.11,0.06	0.75,0.40,0.29	4.14
55.0	0.77,0.28,0.25	0.67,0.14,0.13	0.79,0.58,0.44	1.79

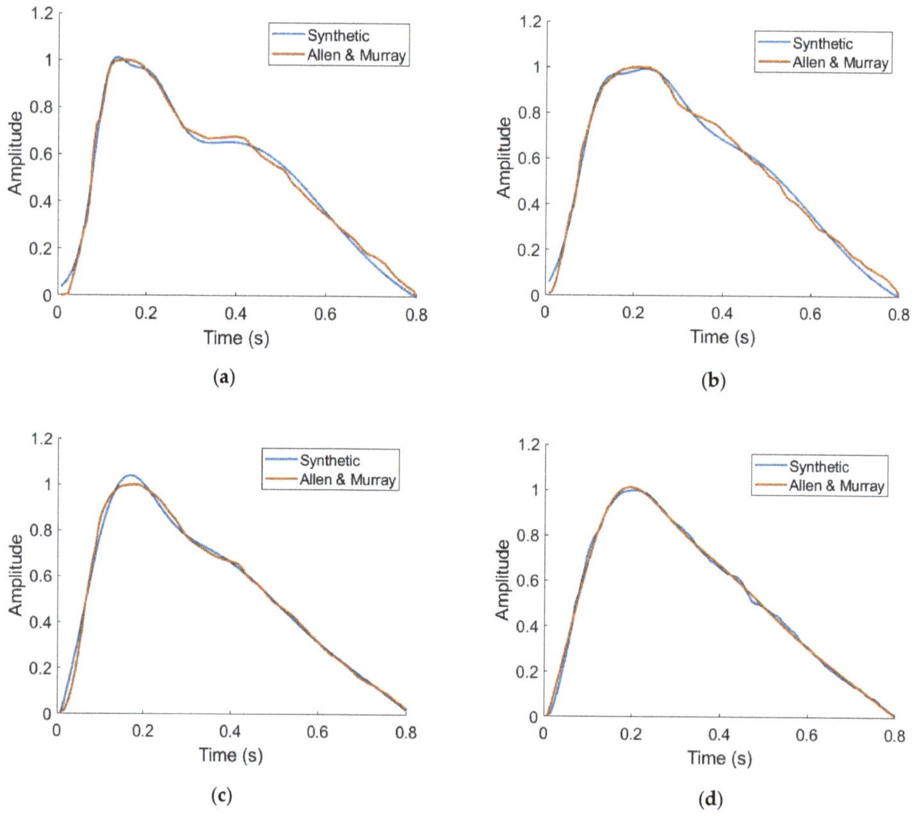

Figure 5. Synthetic vs. literature-derived PPG waveforms for 23 years old (**a**), 34 years old (**b**), 45 years old (**c**), and 55 years old (**d**) [41].

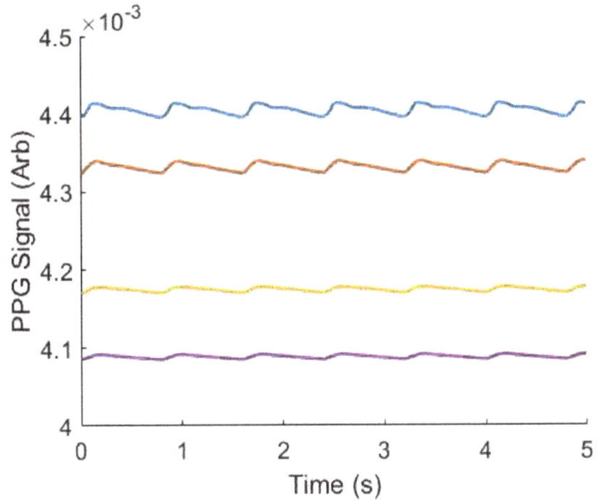

(**a**)

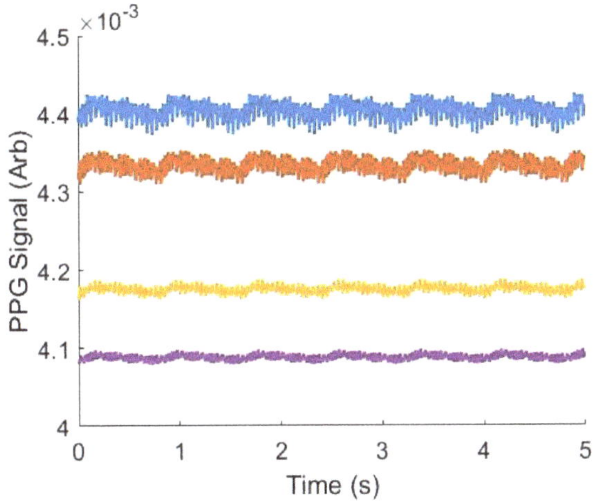

(**b**)

Figure 6. Example synthetic data across wavelengths and ages (VFM = 0.03, Wavelength = 515 nm), without (**a**) and with (**b**) noise. Blue is 23 years old, orange is 34 years old, yellow is 45 years old and purple is 55 years old.

3.2. Impact on PPG Morphology and Features

A simple ADC simulation component was included in the Device Algorithm Simulator to be able to study the minimum resolution needed to accurately resolve the PPG waveform features. Figure 7a,b shows a PPG waveform originating from a synthetic patient with an excitation wavelength of 515 nm, 0.30 VFM (b) or 0.03 VFM (a) and 23 years old (a) or 55 years old (b). This synthetic data was filtered through a bandpass Butterworth and then put through the ADC simulator. The lowest ADC resolution, shown in blue, has false features in both subfigures after the systolic peak that were artificially added by the filter in an attempt to process a digitized signal. Additionally, the systolic onset is greater and the systolic peak is less than their high-resolution counterparts. This waveform would be unable to undergo feature extraction, or would yield incorrect feature values if processed. However, as the resolution increases, the waveform regains its morphology. Figure 7c demonstrates the framework's ability to analyze the impact of ADC resolution on waveform morphology. This data illustrates the relative percent difference between the PPG waveform at a given ADC resolution, compared to the same waveform at the high resolution of 25 bits which serves as a near-perfect waveform for this analysis. According to Figure 4, the synthetic data yielding the black curve is approximately 300× greater in amplitude than the magenta curve. This amplitude difference manifests itself in ADC resolution necessary to sufficiently resolve the signal. In order to obtain a signal <1% different than the high-resolution signal, a 10-bit resolution is necessary for the 23 year old, whereas the synthetic data yielding the magenta curve (55 year old) requires a 19-bit resolution. This functionality can also be used to evaluate appropriate LED intensity, as it is expected that increasing the LED intensity to yield a matching PPG amplitude across features would potentially yield equivalently resolved features, even though this action would similarly amplify noise and the DC component of the PPG waveform.

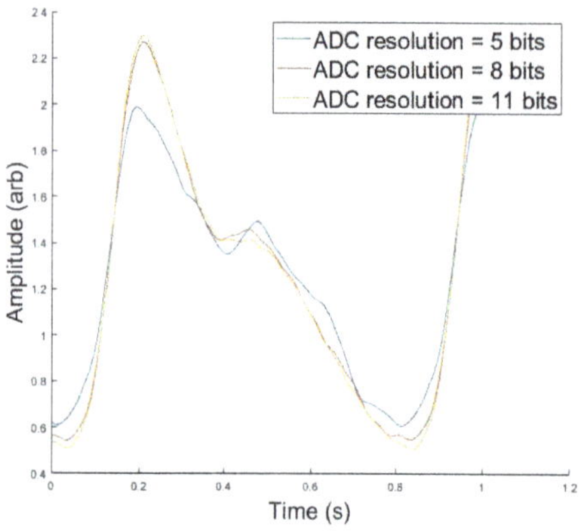

(**a**)

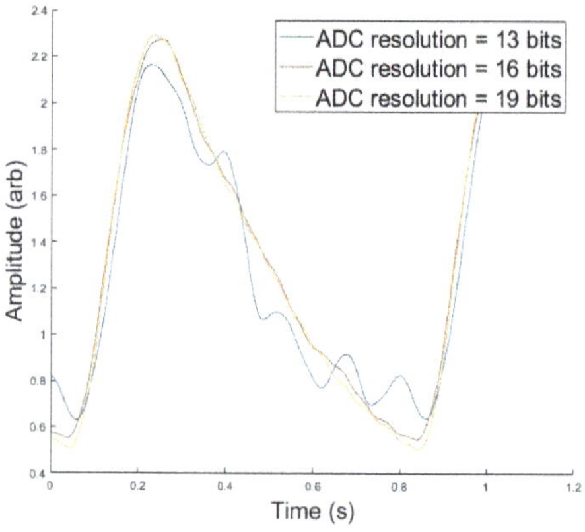

(**b**)

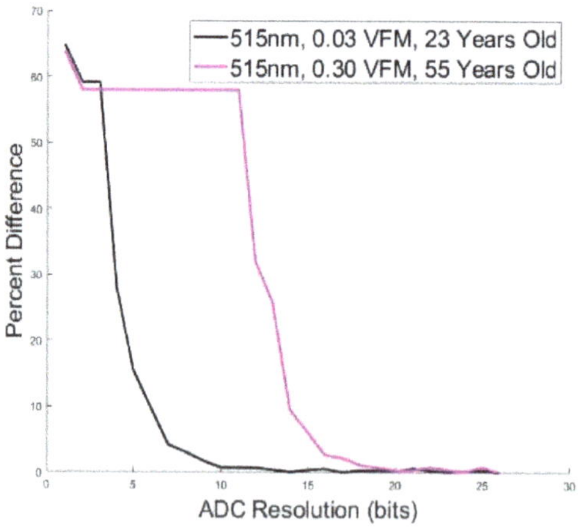

(**c**)

Figure 7. (**a**) PPG Morphology at Different ADC Resolutions (blue = 5 bits, red = 8 bits, orange = 11 bits) for 515 nm, 0.03 VFM, and 23 Years old. (**b**) PPG Morphology at Different ADC Resolutions (blue = 13 bits, red = 16 bits, orange = 19 bits) for 515 nm, 0.30 VFM, and 55 years old. (**c**) Median Percent Difference Between PPG Morphologies for Large and Small ADC Resolution for two simulated data.

Figure 8, an abbreviated version of Figure A1, illustrates that by comparing values of a given feature within a patient-specific or device facto, we can study which factors modulate which features. Skin tone, or rather VFM from 0.03 to 0.30, and wavelength did not significantly impact any feature measured. This intuitively makes sense, as their representation within this framework is through changing optical properties of tissue and thus their impact is in the amplitude of the PPG waveform (shown in Figure 4). Dicrotic notch height, an amplitude-based feature in Figure 8, does not change as one of the aforementioned components of signal processing was data rescaling. There is very limited evidence suggesting that skin tone or wavelength may impact the PPG waveform, but such an effect would largely be caused by changes in optical properties of tissue leading to manipulating whether the PPG signal is predominately provided by superficial arterioles or deeper arteries [48]. However, in this work, where the simulated anatomy is primarily vascularized by superficial arterioles in the form of subungual arcades and their branches, this is not a likely outcome [49]. Filter methodology and age are shown to have significant impacts on extracted feature values. Specifically, "DivWidthTime" features decrease as age increases, and most "WidthTime" features increase as a function of age. As the target percentage for the WidthTime features decrease, the impact of age also decreases. For example, x75WidthTime increases from 0.16 to 0.23 for 23-year old's to 55-year old's, but x10WidthTime changes from 0.67 to 0.68 as age increases. This effect is inverted for "DivWidthTime" features as a higher target percentage changes less as a function of age. X75DivWidthTime changes from 2.53 to 2.12 as age increases and X10DivWidthTime changes from 4.68 to 3.26 as age increases. Signal filtering is shown to impact extracted feature values. The inverse Chebyshev bandpass has the least accurate performance, consistently leading to underestimated features values compared to the control data when the feature is related to timing. However, these waveforms assume that ADC resolution is sufficiently high. Identifying the appropriate ADC resolution is a key component of device design.

	Filter				Age				VFM				Wavelength (nm)		
	1	2	3	4	23	34	45	55	0.03	0.10	0.20	0.30	515	660	880
MeanPulseRisingTime	0.20 (0.02)	0.20 (0.03)	0.19 (0.02)	0.19 (0.04)	0.17 (0.03)	0.19 (0.02)	0.21 (0.02)	0.20 (0.02)	0.19 (0.03)	0.20 (0.03)	0.19 (0.03)	0.19 (0.03)	0.19 (0.03)	0.19 (0.03)	0.19 (0.03)
x75SystolicWidthTime	0.06 (0.01)	0.05 (0.01)	0.06 (0.01)	0.08 (0.03)	0.05 (0.01)	0.06 (0.01)	0.08 (0.03)	0.07 (0.01)	0.06 (0.02)	0.06 (0.02)	0.06 (0.02)	0.06 (0.02)	0.06 (0.02)	0.06 (0.02)	0.06 (0.02)
x75DiastolicWidthTime	0.13 (0.03)	0.11 (0.02)	0.15 (0.03)	0.15 (0.01)	0.11 (0.02)	0.12 (0.02)	0.16 (0.02)	0.15 (0.02)	0.14 (0.03)	0.13 (0.03)	0.14 (0.03)	0.14 (0.03)	0.14 (0.03)	0.14 (0.03)	0.14 (0.03)
x75WidthTime	0.19 (0.03)	0.17 (0.03)	0.21 (0.04)	0.22 (0.04)	0.16 (0.02)	0.18 (0.02)	0.24 (0.02)	0.23 (0.02)	0.20 (0.04)	0.20 (0.04)	0.20 (0.04)	0.20 (0.04)	0.20 (0.04)	0.20 (0.04)	0.20 (0.04)
x75DivWidthTime	2.26 (0.59)	2.30 (0.48)	2.33 (0.54)	2.32 (1.05)	2.53 (0.88)	2.20 (0.42)	2.34 (0.82)	2.12 (0.51)	2.35 (0.71)	2.23 (0.70)	2.31 (0.70)	2.31 (0.70)	2.27 (0.70)	2.29 (0.71)	2.33 (0.70)
WidthDifference	0.21 (0.04)	0.16 (0.03)	0.23 (0.04)	0.23 (0.08)	0.26 (0.07)	0.20 (0.03)	0.21 (0.04)	0.18 (0.03)	0.22 (0.06)	0.21 (0.06)	0.21 (0.06)	0.21 (0.06)	0.21 (0.06)	0.21 (0.06)	0.22 (0.06)
MeanMaxSlope	14.10 (2.76)	18.10 (1.51)	17.49 (1.00)	18.44 (4.42)	19.93 (1.46)	16.28 (1.96)	16.61 (2.51)	14.58 (2.13)	16.92 (3.23)	17.02 (3.14)	16.87 (3.34)	16.81 (3.42)	17.72 (2.44)	16.59 (3.51)	16.38 (3.62)
InflectionPointArea	0.68 (0.41)	0.46 (0.24)	0.74 (0.45)	0.87 (0.22)	1.07 (0.22)	0.91 (0.25)	0.32 (0.15)	0.44 (0.22)	0.71 (0.39)	0.70 (0.38)	0.70 (0.38)	0.70 (0.38)	0.69 (0.38)	0.70 (0.38)	0.71 (0.39)
DiastolicTime	0.60 (0.02)	0.60 (0.03)	0.61 (0.02)	0.62 (0.04)	0.63 (0.03)	0.61 (0.02)	0.59 (0.02)	0.60 (0.02)	0.61 (0.03)	0.61 (0.03)	0.61 (0.03)	0.61 (0.03)	0.61 (0.03)	0.61 (0.03)	0.61 (0.03)
HeartRate	82.99 (21.25)	74.65 (0.95)	88.42 (28.76)	75.04 (1.00)	80.53 (19.77)	79.23 (17.79)	80.52 (19.55)	83.26 (23.57)	80.02 (18.98)	82.70 (22.92)	81.10 (20.67)	79.82 (18.52)	81.01 (20.48)	80.58 (19.85)	81.15 (20.78)
p2p1Mean	0.61 (0.05)	0.51 (0.03)	0.65 (0.04)	0.68 (0.02)	0.61 (0.06)	0.66 (0.06)	0.60 (0.07)	0.61 (0.07)	0.62 (0.07)	0.62 (0.07)	0.62 (0.07)	0.62 (0.07)	0.62 (0.07)	0.62 (0.07)	0.62 (0.07)
DicroticNotchHeight	0.85 (0.17)	0.90 (0.06)	1.13 (0.07)	1.28 (0.06)	1.03 (0.13)	1.06 (0.16)	0.99 (0.20)	1.01 (0.22)	1.02 (0.18)	1.03 (0.17)	1.02 (0.19)	1.02 (0.19)	1.07 (0.13)	1.01 (0.20)	0.99 (0.20)
MeanTimeBetweenPeakAndNextNotch	26.47 (5.95)	28.27 (4.22)	26.37 (5.83)	24.51 (2.54)	23.89 (3.21)	22.03 (2.30)	31.83 (5.00)	28.09 (3.00)	26.44 (5.19)	26.17 (5.09)	26.37 (5.05)	26.29 (5.07)	26.40 (5.11)	26.28 (5.05)	26.28 (5.14)
CardiacPeriod	0.80 (0.00)	0.80 (0.00)	0.80 (0.00)	0.81 (0.01)	0.80 (0.01)	0.80 (0.00)	0.80 (0.01)	0.80 (0.01)	0.80 (0.01)	0.80 (0.01)	0.80 (0.01)	0.80 (0.01)	0.80 (0.01)	0.80 (0.01)	0.80 (0.01)
OnsetPeriod	0.80 (0.00)	0.80 (0.00)	0.80 (0.00)	0.80 (0.00)	0.80 (0.00)	0.80 (0.00)	0.80 (0.00)	0.80 (0.00)	0.80 (0.00)	0.80 (0.00)	0.80 (0.00)	0.80 (0.00)	0.80 (0.00)	0.80 (0.00)	0.80 (0.00)
PPGIntegral	66.88 (11.96)	75.16 (4.56)	88.09 (3.21)	92.09 (8.11)	80.28 (10.33)	74.76 (10.31)	85.87 (14.08)	81.14 (13.82)	80.53 (12.44)	80.73 (12.13)	80.31 (13.16)	79.98 (13.39)	84.43 (2.70)	78.69 (13.88)	77.93 (14.70)

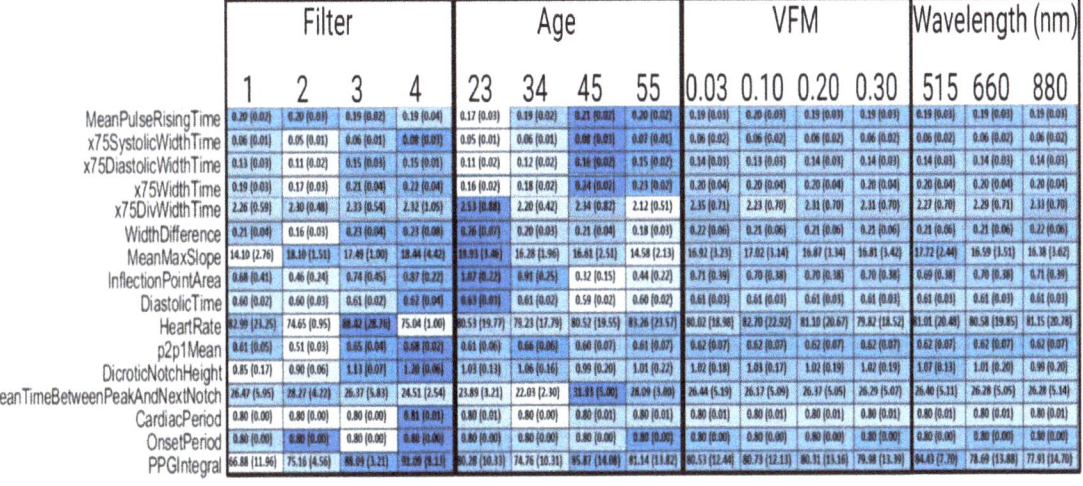

Figure 8. Selected Synthetic PPG Feature Values Across Parameters. Filter 1 is a 4th order bandpass Butterworth (0.1–0.7 Hz), Filter 2 is a 4th order bandpass Inverse Chebyshev (0.1–0.7 Hz), Filter 3 is a 4th order Low pass Inverse Chebyshev, and Filter 4 is control data that has no noise and no filters applied. Colormap was determined by normalizing each row. Standard deviations are in parentheses.

3.3. *Blood Pressure Estimation from Synthetic PPG Features*

A number of machine learning approaches have been studied for non-invasive blood pressure (BP) prediction from PPG [19,50,51]. This includes variations in features as well as variation in methodology/algorithms. As a test case of utilizing this framework to evaluate the robustness of trained algorithms against patient and device specific factors, a Support Vector Machine (SVM) algorithm, a Bagged Trees (BT) algorithm, and a Neural Network (NN) were developed. The algorithms were selected after analyzing commonly used techniques to predict blood pressure from PPG data in the literature. Similar to previous work, each model was trained using 70% of data extracted from the MIMIC-III dataset and tested on the remaining 30% of extracted data (15% for the NN, as 15% was withheld for validation) [52]. Table 4 displays the mean average error and standard deviation of error for the trained models on the MIMIC dataset in the first two rows, and the standard deviation of predicted values for each algorithm on the synthetic dataset in the bottom two rows. The bottom two rows show the standard deviation of prediction because the true blood pressure values in the synthetic data are unknown. Mean average error on the test data was found to be within ISO-81060-2 standards of <5 mmHg, and the standard deviation of the error was found to be greater than the ISO-81060-2 threshold of 8 mmHg for these example algorithms [45]. However, the purpose of this test case is to examine the variation of predicted blood pressures across synthetic data for each trained model, not to develop models for blood pressure prediction; thus we do not anticipate the standard deviation of error to impact conclusions derived within this work. While the true blood pressure of the synthetic data is unknown, the standard deviation of predictions from each algorithm can be used to assess sensitivity or insensitivity to the factors discussed in this work. It was found that the SVM had a low standard deviation of measurement of 0.10 mmHg and 0.12 mmHg for diastolic and systolic BP, respectively across synthetic data. In contrast, the NN had much greater standard deviations of prediction 14.53 mmHg and 9.44 mmHg for systolic and diastolic BP, respectively. Thus, this workflow was able to show that the systolic and diastolic outputs of the SVM models developed in this work were less sensitive to the diverse cohort of synthetic PPG signals, compared to the NN or Bagged Trees models.

Table 4. Algorithm Mean Error and Standard Deviation.

	Support Vector Machine		Bagged Trees		Neural Network	
	Mean Error (mmHg)	**Standard Deviation (mmHg)**	**Mean Error (mmHg)**	**Standard Deviation (mmHg)**	**Mean Error (mmHg)**	**Standard Deviation (mmHg)**
Systolic	0.55	11.56	−0.02	12.4	−0.36	15.53
Diastolic	−0.72	8.24	−0.11	8.63	−0.16	10.75
Systolic-Synthetic	N/A	0.12	N/A	3.46	N/A	14.53
Diastolic-Synthetic	N/A	0.10	N/A	4.34	N/A	9.44

4. Conclusions

Due to the number of anatomical, physiological, and device recording factors that can impact the morphology of a PPG waveform, it is important to have tools to enable the systematic assessment of hemodynamic measurement algorithms to these factors. We considered a framework and developed an initial software implementation towards this purpose. We demonstrated how this can be used to generate synthetic data specific to device characteristics and inclusive of patient-specific factors, one can systematically evaluate feature and algorithm robustness across a range of patient and device-specific characteristics. This type of framework can enable rapid development of algorithms and devices that aim to predict blood pressure, or potentially other hemodynamic measurements, from pulse wave analysis of the PPG waveform by combining in silico developmental tools to overcome individual limitations. Namely, this research includes both physiological and anatomical considerations in designing PPG-based medical devices and external sources of noise. Other frameworks that are Monte Carlo based explored changes in PPG amplitude caused by physiological factors, and frameworks that were Gaussian combination -based explored noise-based changes in the PPG waveform. The framework described here enables studying the impact of both categories on the PPG waveform. It also allows the understanding of how the effects may propagate through data recording and processing algorithms to the end clinical parameters by performing feature extraction on the simulated waveforms. This study presented the use of this framework for a single anatomy due to the computational power of the computers used for simulations. Increasing the computational power, and consequently the number of photons used in the Monte Carlo simulations would enable evaluation of derived parameters such as AC/DC, particularly for darker skin tones. The simulated PPG waveforms presented herein assume physiotypical subjects and are created/validated with data from literature, which limits control over the health of patients from which the data originated. It is anticipated that nonhealthy patients may present changes to the model that may include but are not limited to changes in skin thickness, optical properties of the skin layers, and vessel compliance. Thus, future work might include conducting studies to gather the parameters such as skin thickness used in this work that are controlled to important variables such as cardiovascular health. Additionally, some works used as reference have uneven gender distributions that might impact the results incorporated to build the simulations presented herein. Generalized signal processing was performed in this work that does not represent the full processing of any known device. Additionally, the research presented herein uses a single source/detector configuration as a case study and is not representative of any specific product configuration. Lastly, increased validation and uncertainty quantification would further enable functionalities such as including template PPG waveforms for patients of any age.

Author Contributions: Conceptualization, J.F. and C.G.S.; methodology, J.F.; software, J.F.; validation, J.F.; formal analysis, J.F.; investigation, J.F.; resources, J.F and C.G.S., G.L.C. and M.J.M.; data curation, J.F.; writing—original draft preparation, J.F.; writing—review and editing, C.G.S., G.L.C. and M.J.M.; visualization, J.F.; supervision, C.G.S., G.L.C. and M.J.M.; project administration, J.F.; funding acquisition, J.F., G.L.C. and M.J.M. All authors have read and agreed to the published version of the manuscript.

Funding: This research was funded by the National Science Foundation as a National Science Foundation INTERN supplement to the Engineering Research Center for Precise Advanced Technologies and Health Systems for Underserved Populations (PATHS-UP), #1648451.

Institutional Review Board Statement: This research used deidentified and publicly available data determined to meet the definition of non-human subject research.

Informed Consent Statement: Not applicable.

Data Availability Statement: Software and Data used in this work will be provided by the authors upon reasonable request.

Acknowledgments: The authors acknowledge and thank Zane Arp.

Conflicts of Interest: The authors declare no conflict of interest.

Disclaimer: The mention of commercial products, their sources, or their use in connection with material reported herein is not to be construed as either an actual or implied endorsement of such products by the Department of Health and Human Services.

Appendix A

Table A1. PPG Features. The left column is the name of the PPG feature, and the right column is a brief description of the associated feature.

Feature Name	Definition
Mean Peak Amplitude	distance from systolic onset to systolic peak over 30 s window
Mean Pulse Rising Time	time from systolic onset to systolic peak over 30 s window
x75 Systolic Width Time	Time from systolic peak to the point before the systolic peak with amplitude of 75% of peak amplitude

Table A1. *Cont.*

Feature Name	Definition
X75 Diastolic Width Time	Time from systolic peak to the point after the systolic peak with amplitude of 75% of peak amplitude
X66 Systolic Width Time	Time from systolic peak to the point before the systolic peak with amplitude of 66% of peak amplitude
X66 Diastolic Width Time	Time from systolic peak to the point after the systolic peak with amplitude of 66% of peak amplitude
X50 Systolic Width Time	Time from systolic peak to the point before the systolic peak with amplitude of 50% of peak amplitude
X50 Diastolic Width Time	Time from systolic peak to the point after the systolic peak with amplitude of 50% of peak amplitude
X33 Systolic Width Time	Time from systolic peak to the point before the systolic peak with amplitude of 33% of peak amplitude
X33 Diastolic Width Time	Time from systolic peak to the point after the systolic peak with amplitude of 33% of peak amplitude
X25 Systolic Width Time	Time from systolic peak to the point before the systolic peak with amplitude of 25% of peak amplitude
X25 Diastolic Width Time	Time from systolic peak to the point after the systolic peak with amplitude of 25% of peak amplitude
X10 Systolic Width Time	Time from systolic peak to the point before the systolic peak with amplitude of 10% of peak amplitude
X10 Diastolic Width Time	Time from systolic peak to the point after the systolic peak with amplitude of 10% of peak amplitude
X75 Width Time	Time from the point on systolic rising edge to the point after the systolic rising edge where 75% of peak amplitude occurs
X66 Width Time	Time from the point on systolic rising edge to the point after the systolic rising edge where 66% of peak amplitude occurs
X50 Width Time	Time from the point on systolic rising edge to the point after the systolic rising edge where 50% of peak amplitude occurs
X33 Width Time	Time from the point on systolic rising edge to the point after the systolic rising edge where 33% of peak amplitude occurs
X25 Width Time	Time from the point on systolic rising edge to the point after the systolic rising edge where 25% of peak amplitude occurs
X10 Width Time	Time from the point on systolic rising edge to the point after the systolic rising edge where 10% of peak amplitude occurs
X75 Div Width Time	X75 Systolic Width Time/X75 Diastolic Width Time
X66 Div Width Time	X66 Systolic Width Time/X66 Diastolic Width Time
X50 Div Width Time	X50 Systolic Width Time/X50 Diastolic Width Time
X33 Div Width Time	X33 Systolic Width Time/X33 Diastolic Width Time
X25 Div Width Time	X25 Systolic Width Time/X25 Diastolic Width Time
X10 Div Width Time	X10 Systolic Width Time/X10 Diastolic Width Time
Width Difference	The absolute difference of X50 Systolic Width Time and X50 Diastolic Width Time

Table A1. *Cont.*

Feature Name	Definition
Mean Max Slope	The maximum slope observed across 3 points in the systolic rising edge
Inflection Point Area	The integral of the PPG waveform from the dicrotic notch to the next systolic onset divided by the integral of the PPG waveform from the onset to the dicrotic notch
Diastolic Time	Time from the systolic peak to the next systolic onset
Heart Rate	Systolic peaks identified over 30 s × 2
P2p1 Mean	The ratio of dicrotic notch amplitude to systolic peak amplitude
Dicrotic Notch Height	Dicrotic notch amplitude
Mean Time Between Peak and Next Notch	Time between the systolic peak and dicrotic notch
Cardiac Period	Average time between systolic peaks
Onset Period	Average time between systolic onsets
PPG Integral	Area under the PPG waveform

Appendix B

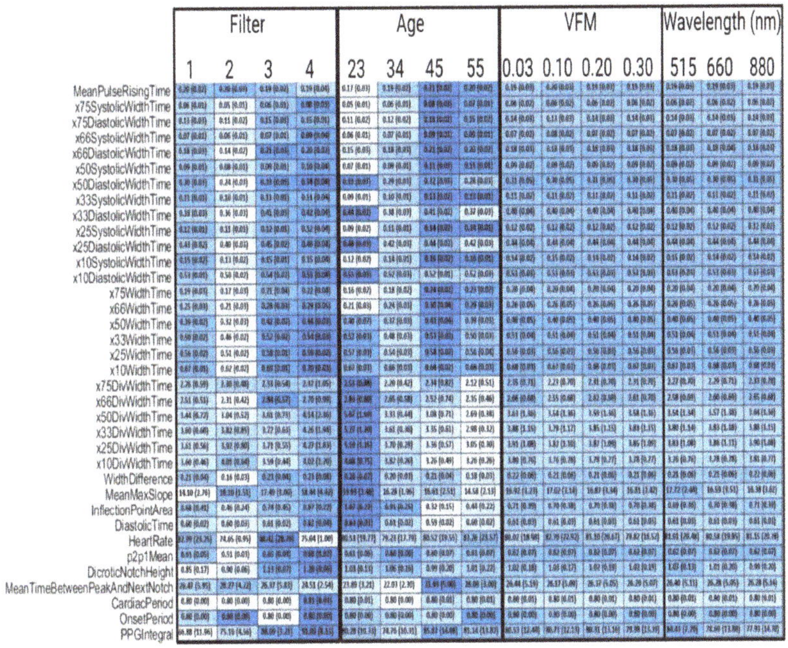

Figure A1. Synthetic PPG Feature Values Across Parameters, Filter 1 is a 4th order bandpass Butterworth (0.1–0.7 Hz), Filter 2 is a 4th order bandpass Inverse Chebyshev (0.1–0.7 Hz), Filter 3 is a 4th order Low pass Inverse Chebyshev, and Filter 4 is control data that has no noise and no filters applied. Colormap was determined by normalizing each row. Standard deviations are in parentheses.

References

1. Cardiovascular Diseases (CVDs). Available online: https://www.who.int/news-room/fact-sheets/detail/cardiovascular-diseases-(cvds)#:~{}:text=Cardiovascular%20diseases%20(CVDs)%20are%20the,%2D%20and%20middle%2Dincome%20countries (accessed on 26 May 2022).
2. Hypertension Cascade: Hypertension Prevalence, Treatment and Control Estimates among U.S. Adults Aged 18 Years and Older Applying the Criteria from the American College of Cardiology and American Heart Association's 2017 Hypertension Guideline—NHANES 2015–2018. Available online: https://millionhearts.hhs.gov/data-reports/hypertension-prevalence.html (accessed on 26 May 2022).
3. Lewington, S.; Clarke, R.; Qizilbash, N.; Peto, R.; Collins, R. Age-specific relevance of usual blood pressure to vascular mortality: A meta-analysis of individual data for one million adults in 61 prospective studies. *Lancet* **2002**, *360*, 1903–1913. [CrossRef] [PubMed]
4. Group, S.R. A randomized trial of intensive versus standard blood-pressure control. *N. Engl. J. Med.* **2015**, *373*, 2103–2116. [CrossRef] [PubMed]
5. Wu, C.-Y.; Hu, H.-Y.; Chou, Y.-J.; Huang, N.; Chou, Y.-C.; Li, C.-P. High blood pressure and all-cause and cardiovascular disease mortalities in community-dwelling older adults. *Medicine* **2015**, *94*, e2160. [CrossRef]
6. Woo, S.H.; Choi, Y.Y.; Kim, D.J.; Bien, F.; Kim, J.J. Tissue-informative mechanism for wearable non-invasive continuous blood pressure monitoring. *Sci. Rep.* **2014**, *4*, 1–6. [CrossRef] [PubMed]
7. Mukherjee, R.; Ghosh, S.; Gupta, B.; Chakravarty, T. A literature review on current and proposed technologies of noninvasive blood pressure measurement. *Telemed. e-Health* **2018**, *24*, 185–193. [CrossRef]
8. Kim, B.J.; Park, J.-M.; Park, T.H.; Kim, J.; Lee, J.; Lee, K.-J.; Lee, J.; Chae, J.E.; Thabane, L.; Lee, J. Remote blood pressure monitoring and behavioral intensification for stroke: A randomized controlled feasibility trial. *PLoS ONE* **2020**, *15*, e0229483. [CrossRef]
9. Castaneda, D.; Esparza, A.; Ghamari, M.; Soltanpur, C.; Nazeran, H. A review on wearable photoplethysmography sensors and their potential future applications in health care. *Int. J. Biosens. Bioelectron.* **2018**, *4*, 195.
10. Elgendi, M.; Fletcher, R.; Liang, Y.; Howard, N.; Lovell, N.H.; Abbott, D.; Lim, K.; Ward, R. The use of photoplethysmography for assessing hypertension. *NPJ Digit. Med.* **2019**, *2*, 1–11. [CrossRef] [PubMed]
11. Fine, J.; Branan, K.L.; Rodriguez, A.J.; Boonya-Ananta, T.; Ramella-Roman, J.C.; McShane, M.J.; Coté, G.L. Sources of inaccuracy in photoplethysmography for continuous cardiovascular monitoring. *Biosensors* **2021**, *11*, 126. [CrossRef]
12. Gircys, R.; Liutkevicius, A.; Kazanavicius, E.; Lesauskaite, V.; Damuleviciene, G.; Janaviciute, A. Photoplethysmography-based continuous systolic blood pressure estimation method for low processing power wearable devices. *Appl. Sci.* **2019**, *9*, 2236. [CrossRef]
13. Fujita, D.; Suzuki, A. Evaluation of the possible use of PPG waveform features measured at low sampling rate. *IEEE Access* **2019**, *7*, 58361–58367. [CrossRef]
14. Maqsood, S.; Xu, S.; Springer, M.; Mohawesh, R. A Benchmark Study of Machine Learning for Analysis of Signal Feature Extraction Techniques for Blood Pressure Estimation Using Photoplethysmography (PPG). *IEEE Access* **2021**, *9*, 138817–138833. [CrossRef]
15. Bickler, P.E.; Feiner, J.R.; Severinghaus, J.W. Effects of skin pigmentation on pulse oximeter accuracy at low saturation. *J. Am. Soc. Anesthesiol.* **2005**, *102*, 715–719. [CrossRef] [PubMed]
16. Feiner, J.R.; Severinghaus, J.W.; Bickler, P.E. Dark skin decreases the accuracy of pulse oximeters at low oxygen saturation: The effects of oximeter probe type and gender. *Anesth. Analg.* **2007**, *105*, S18–S23. [CrossRef]
17. Maeda, Y.; Sekine, M.; Tamura, T. Relationship between measurement site and motion artifacts in wearable reflected photoplethysmography. *J. Med. Syst.* **2011**, *35*, 969–976. [CrossRef]
18. Elgendi, M. On the analysis of fingertip photoplethysmogram signals. *Curr. Cardiol. Rev.* **2012**, *8*, 14–25. [CrossRef]
19. Kılıçkaya, S.; Güner, A.; Dal, B. Comparison of different machine learning techniques for the cuffless estimation of blood pressure using PPG signals. In Proceedings of the 2020 International Congress on Human-Computer Interaction, Optimization and Robotic Applications (HORA), Ankara, Turkey, 9–11 June 2022; pp. 1–6.
20. Johnson, A.E.; Pollard, T.J.; Shen, L.; Li-Wei, H.L.; Feng, M.; Ghassemi, M.; Moody, B.; Szolovits, P.; Celi, L.A.; Mark, R.G. MIMIC-III, a freely accessible critical care database. *Sci. Data* **2016**, *3*, 1–9. [CrossRef] [PubMed]
21. Moody, B.; Moody, G.; Villarroel, M.; Clifford, G.D.; Silva, I. MIMIC-III Waveform Database Matched Subset (Version 1.0). PhysioNet. 2020. Available online: https://doi.org/10.13026/c2294b (accessed on 26 May 2022).
22. Boonya-Ananta, T.; Rodriguez, A.J.; Ajmal, A.; Du Le, V.N.; Hansen, A.K.; Hutcheson, J.D.; Ramella-Roman, J.C. Synthetic Photoplethysmography (PPG) of the radial artery through parallelized Monte Carlo and its correlation to Body Mass Index (BMI). *bioRxiv* **2020**, *11*, 1–11. [CrossRef] [PubMed]
23. Martin-Martinez, D.; Casaseca-de-la-Higuera, P.; Martin-Fernandez, M.; Alberola-López, C. Stochastic modeling of the PPG signal: A synthesis-by-analysis approach with applications. *IEEE Trans. Biomed. Eng.* **2013**, *60*, 2432–2441. [CrossRef] [PubMed]
24. Chatterjee, S.; Kyriacou, P.A. Monte Carlo analysis of optical interactions in reflectance and transmittance finger photoplethysmography. *Sensors* **2019**, *19*, 789. [CrossRef]
25. Chatterjee, S.; Abay, T.Y.; Phillips, J.P.; Kyriacou, P.A. Investigating optical path and differential pathlength factor in reflectance photoplethysmography for the assessment of perfusion. *J. Biomed. Opt.* **2018**, *23*, 075005. [CrossRef]

26. Chatterjee, S.; Budidha, K.; Kyriacou, P.A. Investigating the origin of photoplethysmography using a multiwavelength Monte Carlo model. *Physiol. Meas.* **2020**, *41*, 084001. [CrossRef] [PubMed]
27. Tang, Q.; Chen, Z.; Allen, J.; Alian, A.; Menon, C.; Ward, R.; Elgendi, M. PPGSynth: An innovative toolbox for synthesizing regular and irregular photoplethysmography waveforms. *Front. Med.* **2020**, *7*, 735. [CrossRef] [PubMed]
28. Meglinski, I.V.; Matcher, S. Computer simulation of the skin reflectance spectra. *Comput. Methods Programs Biomed.* **2003**, *70*, 179–186. [CrossRef]
29. Marti, D.; Aasbjerg, R.; Andersen, P.E.; Hansen, A.K. MCmatlab: An open-source user-friendly MATLAB-integrated 3D Monte Carlo light transport solver with heat diffusion and tissue damage. In Proceedings of the Optical Interactions with Tissue and Cells XXX, San Francisco, CA, USA, 2–3 February 2019; p. 108760T.
30. Jacques, S.L. Optical properties of biological tissues: A review. *Phys. Med. Biol.* **2013**, *58*, R37. [CrossRef] [PubMed]
31. Shuster, S.; BLACK, M.M.; McVitie, E. The influence of age and sex on skin thickness, skin collagen and density. *Br. J. Dermatol.* **1975**, *93*, 639–643. [CrossRef]
32. Lin, Y.; Li, D.; Liu, W.; Zhong, Z.; Li, Z.; He, Y.; Wu, S. A measurement of epidermal thickness of fingertip skin from OCT images using convolutional neural network. *J. Innov. Opt. Health Sci.* **2021**, *14*, 2140005. [CrossRef]
33. Sulli, A.; Ruaro, B.; Alessandri, E.; Pizzorni, C.; Cimmino, M.A.; Zampogna, G.; Gallo, M.; Cutolo, M. Correlations between nailfold microangiopathy severity, finger dermal thickness and fingertip blood perfusion in systemic sclerosis patients. *Ann. Rheum. Dis.* **2014**, *73*, 247–251. [CrossRef]
34. Reneman, R.S.; Van Merode, T.; Hick, P.; Muytjens, A.M.; Hoeks, A.P. Age-related changes in carotid artery wall properties in men. *Ultrasound Med. Biol.* **1986**, *12*, 465–471. [CrossRef]
35. Meglinski, I.V.; Matcher, S.J. Quantitative assessment of skin layers absorption and skin reflectance spectra simulation in the visible and near-infrared spectral regions. *Physiol. Meas.* **2002**, *23*, 741. [CrossRef]
36. Fine, J.; Boonya-ananta, T.; Rodriguez, A.; Ramella-Roman, J.C.; McShane, M.; Cote, G.L. Parallelized multi-layered Monte Carlo model for evaluation of a proximal phalanx photoplethysmograph. In Proceedings of the Optical Diagnostics and Sensing XX: Toward Point-of-Care Diagnostics, San Francisco, CA, USA, 3 February 2020; p. 1124702.
37. Jacques, S.L. Optical Absorption of Melanin. In *Oregon Medical Laser Center Monthly News and Articles on Biomedical Optics and Medical Lasers*. 1998. Available online: http://omlc.ogi.edu/news/jan98/skinoptics.html (accessed on 26 May 2022).
38. Anderson, R.; Parrish, J. Optical properties of human skin. In *The Science of Photomedicine*; Springer: Berlin/Heidelberg, Germany, 1982; pp. 147–194.
39. Blanco, P.J.; Watanabe, S.M.; Passos, M.A.R.; Lemos, P.A.; Feijóo, R.A. An anatomically detailed arterial network model for one-dimensional computational hemodynamics. *IEEE Trans. Biomed. Eng.* **2014**, *62*, 736–753. [CrossRef]
40. Allen, J.; O'Sullivan, J.; Stansby, G.; Murray, A. Age-related changes in pulse risetime measured by multi-site photoplethysmography. *Physiol. Meas.* **2020**, *41*, 074001. [CrossRef] [PubMed]
41. Allen, J.; Murray, A. Age-related changes in the characteristics of the photoplethysmographic pulse shape at various body sites. *Physiol. Meas.* **2003**, *24*, 297. [CrossRef] [PubMed]
42. Li, S.; Liu, L.; Wu, J.; Tang, B.; Li, D. Comparison and noise suppression of the transmitted and reflected photoplethysmography signals. *BioMed Res. Int.* **2018**, *2018*, 4523593. [CrossRef]
43. van Gent, P.; Farah, H.; van Nes, N.; van Arem, B. Analysing noisy driver physiology real-time using off-the-shelf sensors: Heart rate analysis software from the taking the fast lane project. *J. Open Res. Softw.* **2019**, *7*, 32. [CrossRef]
44. Ab Hamid, H.; Nayan, N.A.; Suboh, M.Z.; Aminuddin, A. Second Derivatives of Photoplethysmogram for Hyperuricemia Classification using Artificial Neural Network. In Proceedings of the 2020 IEEE-EMBS Conference on Biomedical Engineering and Sciences (IECBES), Langkawi, Malaysia, 1 December 2020–3 March 2021; pp. 494–498.
45. *ISO 81060-2:2018*; Noninvasive Sphygmomanometers—Part 2: Clinical Investigation of Intermittent Automated Measurement Type. ISO: Geneva, Switzerland, 2018.
46. Moço, A.V.; Stuijk, S.; de Haan, G. New insights into the origin of remote PPG signals in visible light and infrared. *Sci. Rep.* **2018**, *8*, 1–15. [CrossRef] [PubMed]
47. Ajmal, A.; Boonya-Ananta, T.; Rodriguez, A.J.; Du Le, V.N.; Ramella-Roman, J.C. Investigation of optical heart rate sensors in wearables and the influence of skin tone and obesity on photoplethysmography (PPG) signal. In *Proceedings of the Biophotonics in Exercise Science, Sports Medicine, Health Monitoring Technologies, and Wearables II*; SPIE: Bellingham, DC, USA, 2021; p. 1163808.
48. Asare, L.; Kviesis-Kipge, E.; Rubins, U.; Rubenis, O.; Spigulis, J. Multi-spectral photoplethysmography technique for parallel monitoring of pulse shapes at different tissue depths. In Proceedings of the European Conference on Biomedical Optics, Munich, Germany, 26–29 April 2022; p. 80872E.
49. Abood, M.H.; Daood, A.S. A comparative study of the supraperiosteal and the subperiosteal dissection in the VY advancement (atasoy) flap for the management of fingertip injury. *Basrah J. Surg.* **2007**, *13*, 1–11.
50. Schrumpf, F.; Frenzel, P.; Aust, C.; Osterhoff, G.; Fuchs, M. Assessment of Non-Invasive Blood Pressure Prediction from PPG and rPPG Signals Using Deep Learning. *Sensors* **2021**, *21*, 6022. [CrossRef]
51. Monte-Moreno, E. Non-invasive estimate of blood glucose and blood pressure from a photoplethysmograph by means of machine learning techniques. *Artif. Intell. Med.* **2011**, *53*, 127–138. [CrossRef]
52. El-Hajj, C.; Kyriacou, P.A. Cuffless blood pressure estimation from PPG signals and its derivatives using deep learning models. *Biomed. Signal Process. Control.* **2021**, *70*, 102984. [CrossRef]

biosensors

MDPI

Communication

Wearable Biosensor with Molecularly Imprinted Conductive Polymer Structure to Detect Lentivirus in Aerosol

Jaskirat Singh Batra [1], Ting-Yen Chi [1], Mo-Fan Huang [2,3,†], Dandan Zhu [2,†], Zheyuan Chen [4], Dung-Fang Lee [2,3] and Jun Kameoka [4,5,*]

1 Department of Materials Science and Engineering, Texas A&M University, College Station, TX 77840, USA; jbatra@tamu.edu (J.S.B.); kevin0149@tamu.edu (T.-Y.C.)

2 Department of Integrative Biology and Pharmacology, McGovern Medical School, The University of Texas Health Science Center at Houston, Houston, TX 77030, USA; mo-fan.huang@uth.tmc.edu (M.-F.H.); dandan.zhu@uth.tmc.edu (D.Z.); dung-fang.lee@uth.tmc.edu (D.-F.L.)

3 The University of Texas MD Anderson Cancer Center UTHealth Graduate School of Biomedical Sciences, Houston TX 77030, USA

4 Department of Electrical and Computer Engineering, Texas A&M University, College Station, TX 77843, USA; zychen@tamu.edu

5 Graduate School of Information, Production and System Research, Waseda University, Fukuoka 808-0135, Japan

* Correspondence: jkameoka@waseda.jp

† These authors contributed equally to this work.

Abstract: The coronavirus disease (COVID-19) pandemic has increased pressure to develop low-cost, compact, user-friendly, and ubiquitous virus sensors for monitoring infection outbreaks in communities and preventing economic damage resulting from city lockdowns. As proof of concept, we developed a wearable paper-based virus sensor based on a molecular imprinting technique, using a conductive polyaniline (PANI) polymer to detect the lentivirus as a test sample. This sensor detected the lentivirus with a 4181 TU/mL detection limit in liquid and 0.33% to 2.90% detection efficiency in aerosols at distances ranging from 30 cm to 60 cm. For fabrication, a mixture of a PANI monomer solution and virus were polymerized together to form a conductive PANI sensing element on a polyethylene terephthalate (PET) paper substrate. The sensing element exhibited formation of virus recognition sites after the removal of the virus via ultrasound sonication. A dry measurement technique was established that showed aerosol virus detection by the molecularly imprinted sensors within 1.5 h of virus spraying. This was based on the mechanism via which dispensing virus droplets on the PANI sensing element induced hybridization of the virus and molecularly imprinted virus recognition templates in PANI, influencing the conductivity of the PANI film upon drying. Interestingly, the paper-based virus sensor was easily integrated with a wearable face mask for the detection of viruses in aerosols. Since the paper sensor with molecular imprinting of virus recognition sites showed excellent stability in dry conditions for long periods of time, unlike biological reagents, this wearable biosensor will offer an alternative approach to monitoring virus infections in communities.

Keywords: wearable paper sensor; molecular imprinting; conductive polymer; lentivirus; virus sensor

Citation: Batra, J.S.; Chi, T.-Y.; Huang, M.-F.; Zhu, D.; Chen, Z.; Lee, D.-F.; Kameoka, J. Wearable Biosensor with Molecularly Imprinted Conductive Polymer Structure to Detect Lentivirus in Aerosol. *Biosensors* **2023**, *13*, 861. https://doi.org/10.3390/bios13090861

Received: 3 July 2023
Revised: 26 August 2023
Accepted: 27 August 2023
Published: 31 August 2023

1. Introduction

The global health threat from COVID-19 has raised attention regarding the need for low-cost, rapid, sensitive, compact, and selective detection platforms for viruses. In particular, keeping viral diseases from spreading into the community relies heavily on the detection of such viruses at the initial stages of an outbreak. Individual personal virus testing and aerosol virus detection can trace the spread of infection, minimizing virus outbreaks and preventing city lockdowns. Currently, virus detection relies on conventional approaches such as serological [1] and viral nucleic acid tests [2]. Serological tests include antibody and antigen detection in immune chromatography formats. Antibody detection involves detecting antibodies produced by the immune system once it is exposed to a virus. This approach often shows false-negative results for actively infected persons. Antigen testing uses the same platform as antibody testing and can rapidly detect virus markers that are virus surface proteins. This serological platform is mostly built on a paper substrate with a sample pad, gold-conjugated pad, capture/test line, and control line [3]. Once the sample solution is dispensed onto the sample pad, target molecules (either antigens or antibodies) are conjugated with target antibodies bound with gold nanoparticles. Molecular complexes are also conjugated with antigen/antibody-specific antibodies at the testing line, visually indicating the existence of antibodies/antigens. These approaches are generally less sensitive than nucleic acid tests and can show false-negative results at the early stages of diagnosis. Currently, quantitative reverse transcription polymerase chain reaction (qRT-PCR), a viral nucleic test, is the gold standard for detecting viruses. It operates by amplifying virus DNA or RNA after extracting a virus gene, and then measuring the fluorescence intensities from the amplified virus gene to detect the virus. Many commercial qRT-PCR kits are available, even for COVID-19 [4]. The drawback of this approach is that it is time-consuming, demands high costs for reagents and bulky detection equipment, and requires trained lab personnel [5].

In an effort to reduce sensing cost, improve convenience, and provide a more compact design, various new virus sensing approaches have been put forth. Electrochemical detection through low-cost paper substrates is one of the most popular for detecting viruses [6,7]. Reference, counter, and working electrodes are screen-printed on paper or polymer substrates, and reagents such as antibodies or aptamers immobilized on the working electrode. Hybridization of target molecules on working electrodes via a reagent induces an impedance change between the reference and working electrodes. The detection of viruses such as H1N1 [8–10], H5N1 [11], SARS-CoV-2 [12], and H7N9 [11,13,14] has been demonstrated using this approach. However, electrochemical detection still requires costly reagents such as antibodies, peptides, and aptamers, as well as makes it challenging to detect aerosol viruses.

To replace the costly biological reagents, molecularly imprinted electrodes for electrochemical detection have also been suggested. Instead of the metal or carbon working electrode, a conductive polymer electrode with target molecule templates was used to detect the Zika virus [15,16]. In this process, the Zika virus was molded onto the surface of a graphene oxide (GO) polymer composite solution and templates formed by eliminating the virus from the composite for detection purposes. Hybridization of the virus on the working electrode influenced the electrochemical impedance. The molecular imprinting approach has also been shown to detect other viruses such as water-borne viruses [17], influenza A [18,19], HIV [6], Japanese encephalitis [20], dengue virus [21], and hepatitis C [22]. The drawback of the molecularly imprinted polymer (MIP) electrochemical approach is that it still requires bulky potentiostat detection equipment, and detection requires a liquid environment. Thus, it is still challenging to detect viruses under dry conditions and in aerosol formats.

The present research demonstrated a low-cost MIP lentivirus sensor that requires no biological reagent and enables virus detection in liquid and aerosol phases without bulky equipment. We previously developed glucose and perfluorooctanesulfonic acid (PFOS) conductive molecularly imprinted paper sensors [23–25] and expanded this approach to the detection of viruses. Lentivirus was used as a proof-of-concept test sample because it can be used in biosafety level 2 labs and is considered a safe alternative to live coronavirus. To form the molecular imprinting template for lentivirus, the virus was blended with a conductive monomer solution polymerized on a polyethylene terephthalate (PET) paper substrate. The lentivirus was then removed from the molecularly imprinted template by ultrasonication. Edges of the conductive MIP sensing paper were connected using two copper metal tapes as electrodes to measure the conductance of the MIP sensing structures. Since the electrical resistance of the conductive polymer polyaniline (PANI) relied on the polaron hopping through π–π stacking, the absorption of virus in the MIP sensing structure modulated the conductance of the paper sensor.

We established a dry measurement technique for virus detection that includes the process of the virus and molecularly imprinted cavity hybridization and sensor element drying. The electrical resistance of the sensor, fabricated from the conductive polymer, enabled the passive measurement of the resistivity ratio over time through the use of a portable multimeter. With this approach, we were able to demonstrate detection of the lentivirus on the sensing element (i) within 1 h by simply dispensing liquid, and (ii) within 1.5 h after spraying a virus solution. This simple and low-cost approach can potentially detect viruses from liquid and aerosol samples in a short period of time. To the best of our knowledge, this is the first attempt to demonstrate the detection of viruses directly in aerosols. The stability of the molecularly imprinted structure in the air [24] will possibly reduce outbreaks and prevent large-scale lockdowns in the future.

2. Materials and Methods

2.1. Materials

Aniline and ammonium persulfate (APS) acting as the monomer and the oxidant, along with phosphate-buffer saline (PBS) for adjusting the virus concentration, were purchased from Sigma-Aldrich (St. Louis, MO, USA). Acidic stock solutions including hydrochloric acid (HCl, 36–38%) and acetic acid were acquired from Macron (Center Valley, PA, USA). Methanol was ordered from VWR Chemicals (Radnor, PA, USA). Polyethylene terephthalate paper and silver conductive paste (Cat# 125-15) were provided by Xerox (Norwalk, CT, USA) and Creative Materials (Ayer, MA, USA), respectively.

The generation of lentiviruses was described previously [26], and the detailed protocol is included in the Supplemental Materials of this paper. Briefly, HEK-293T cells were maintained in DMEM supplemented with 10% (vol/vol) Opti-Gold fetal bovine serum (FBS, GenDEPOT, Katy, TX, USA), L-glutamine, and penicillin/streptomycin. pLKO.pig, pCMV-VSVG (envelope, Addgene plasmid #8454), and pCMV-dR8.2 (packaging; Addgene plasmid #8455) plasmids were co-transfected into HEK-293T cells by the PEI transfection reagent. After 18 h transfection, the fresh medium was replaced. At day 3 post transfection, the supernatant containing lentiviral particles was collected. The entire synthesis was performed under a biosafety level 2 environment. The virus concentration of the stock vial was estimated to be 2.2×10^5 TU/mL, where TU denotes the transducing units of viral particles. Retro-CMV-GFP retroviruses (RVP003, Applied Biological Materials, Vancouver, BC, Canada), polystyrene latex beads (0.1 μm mean particle size, Sigma-Aldrich, St. Louis, MO, USA), and human whole blood (stocked in EDTA K2, BioChemed Services, Winchester, VA, USA) were used as selectivity references. Phosphate-buffered saline (PBS) for adjusting the virus concentration was diluted from concentrated PBS (10×) purchased from Sigma-Aldrich (St. Louis, MO, USA).

2.2. Synthesis of Virus-Imprinted Polyaniline Structure

The synthesis of the virus-imprinted PANI followed the protocol detailed in the previous study [24]. Briefly, 200 μL of aniline and 500 μL of the virus stock solution (2.2×10^5 TU/mL) as the molecular imprinting template were blended into 1 M HCl with a final volume of 5 mL as the monomer solution. The final virus concentration in the polymer solution was 1.1×10^4 TU/mL. Paper strips (1 cm × 0.5 cm) were dipped into the monomer solution for 5 min to saturate the solution on the paper. The oxidant solution prepared by mixing 409 mg of APS with 5 mL of 1 M HCl was then added drop by drop to initiate polymerization for 10 min. After the bulk polymerization, the PANI strips were taken out from the solution and rinsed with deionized water until the eluent showed no excess PANI particles. The virus templates were removed by sonicating the strips in acetic acid/methanol solution (vol/vol = 1:6) for 4 h, followed by rinsing the strips until the pH value of the eluent reached to 7. The resulted lentivirus molecularly imprinted (MIP) PANI paper strips were air-dried at ambient temperature overnight. The monomer solution without lentiviruses was synthesized as non-molecularly imprinted (NIP) control devices. NIP preparation without virus followed the same treatment as MIP.

2.3. Fabrication of Virus MIP Paper Sensor

To fabricate the duplex sensor device, one NIP and another MIP strip were integrated with a plastic stencil substrate (2 cm × 2.5 cm) using double-sided tape, with copper tape (1 cm × 0.635 cm) as the contact electrode. The strip and electrode were separated by a 1 mm gap which was then filled with silver conductive paste. The silver paste was cured at 25 °C for at least 12 h to ensure optimal conductivity, and the resulting device was used to measure the resistivity responses of NIP and MIP to lentiviruses on a single device. The surfaces of NIP and MIP PANI were investigated by scanning electron microscopy, and the result is shown in Supplement 5.

2.4. Lentivirus Detection and Resistance Measurement

To test the detection efficacy of virus MIP sensor, virus samples with different concentrations were prepared. Specifically, for the selectivity test, the virus concentration of lentivirus and Retro-CMV-GFP retrovirus was set at 1.65 × 10^5 TU/mL. Then, an aliquot of 30 μL virus solution was dispensed in the middle of the PANI sensing element (0.5 cm × 0.5 cm) and saturated for 30 min, followed by gentle aspiration and air-drying at 25 °C for 30 min. For virus detection in aerosol, virus contained in DMEM solution was sprayed onto the PANI sensing element, as described in detail in Supplement 6, and the resistance measurements were conducted.

To obtain the virus concentration calibration curve, the resistance of the PANI electrode was measured using a multimeter (8846A, Fluke, Everett, WA, USA) in direct current mode after a drying time of 30 min. This was the time needed to air-dry the sensor surface after 30 μL of virus solution was dispensed and aspirated until no visible moisture was found. Resistance was converted to resistivity as shown in Equation (1).

$$\rho = \frac{R\,A}{L} \tag{1}$$

In this equation, A and L are the cross-sectional area and the longitudinal length of the PANI sensing element, respectively. In addition, the resistivity after virus exposure was divided by the resistivity before virus exposure to determine the resistivity ratio which is the output signal of the sensor calculated using Equation (2) [24].

$$Resistivity\ Ratio\ (RR) = \frac{\rho_{\ after\ virus}}{\rho_{\ before\ virus}} \tag{2}$$

To investigate the effect of non-specific bonding, the resistivity ratio of NIP were subtracted from that of MIP as shown in Equation (3).

$$\text{Specific binding} = \text{RR}_{\text{MIP}} - \text{RR}_{\text{NIP}} \tag{3}$$

The limit of detection (LoD) was estimated using Equation (4), where the slope (m) was obtained from the linear regression fit of specific binding. σ is the standard error of blank samples that were exposed to PBS [27].

$$LoD = \frac{3\sigma}{m} \tag{4}$$

To study the stability of the PANI electrode, PANI was first synthesized on paper specimens (1 cm × 1 cm) using the same synthetic protocol above. The resistance was then measured weekly at room temperature (25 °C) for 13 weeks after the fabrication (total of 14 weeks), and the normalized resistivity was calculated.

3. Results and Discussion

3.1. Calibration Curve: Lentivirus Concentration from Liquid on Virus MIP Sensors

The resistivity ratios of the MIP and non-molecularly imprinted polymer (NIP) electrodes (as shown in Figure 1a) after being exposed to the lentivirus in liquid form and dried for 30 min are plotted as a function of virus concentration in Figure 1b. After sensor drying, the 24 h observation of resistance showed stable values, as displayed in Supplement 7. The I–V curve for this sensor is shown in Supplement 8.

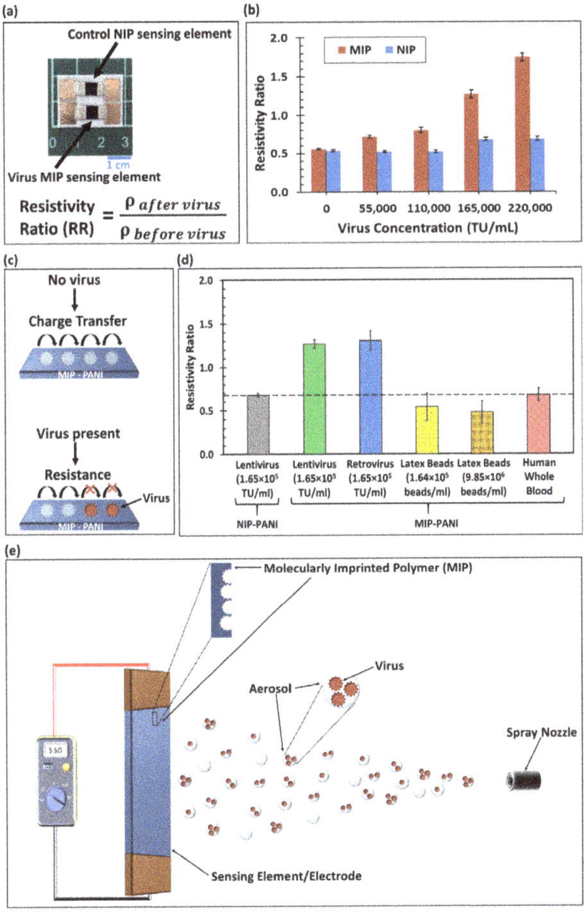

Figure 1. (**a**) Photographic image of virus sensor with MIP and NIP electrodes. Scale is 1 cm. (**b**) Resistivity ratio of the MIP and NIP electrodes as a function of the lentivirus concentration (n = 3, RSD avg. = 3.0%). For calibration, the lentivirus was detected after a 30 min liquid saturation, aspiration, and 30 min natural drying process. (**c**) Schematic of virus detection mechanism showing polaron hopping and charge transfer in MIP-conductive PANI. The electrical resistance increased from the virus present in the molecularly imprinted cavity. (**d**) Selectivity test of MIP electrode and comparison to NIP control (represented by dashed line). The resistivity ratios of the lentivirus, retrovirus, latex beads, and human whole blood were calculated from resistance measurements ($n \geq 5$, RSD avg. = 13.7%). (**e**) Diagram of MIP sensing electrode with molecularly imprinted cavities inside the conductive polymer and virus aerosol sprayed onto the sensing element. TU = transducing units; RSD = relative standard deviation.

The MIP and NIP resistivity ratios were identical at zero virus concentration. As the virus concentration increased, the MIP electrode showed an increase in the resistivity ratio (Figure 1b), which was much larger than the NIP value. PANI conductivity relies on polaron hopping through π–π stacking, as shown in Figure 1c, which is generated by acidic doping in its emeraldine form. When the negatively charged viruses in a neutral pH condition [28] were captured on the MIP electrodes, the virus particles electrostatically neutralized the polaron hopping in the electrode (see Figure 1c). Therefore, this virus-capturing process obscured the charge transfer route, increasing the resistivity of the MIP electrode.

In the experiment, the NIP resistivity ratio remained constant for lentivirus concentrations up to 1.1×10^5 TU/mL (TU = transducing units of viral particles). At high lentivirus concentrations (1.65×10^5 TU/mL and 2.2×10^5 TU/mL), there was a slight increment in the NIP resistivity ratio. However, this extremely small signal increment (attributable to non-specific binding) was removed from the overall sensor signal (see Supplement 1, Figure S1 in Supplementary Materials). The limit of detection for lentivirus sensing by the MIP sensor was estimated to be 4181 TU/mL (or 125 TU virus particles). The sensor made from polyaniline was stable at temperatures between 11.0 °C and 41.5 °C and relative humidities ranging from 15% to 85% for 11 weeks (see Supplement 2, Figures S2–S4).

Even though the MIP sensor demonstrated a promising virus detection efficacy as compared to the NIP control, a small increase in the non-specific binding of the lentivirus was found on the NIP electrode at high virus concentrations. This could be due to the lentivirus–polyaniline material interactions and some of the virus adhering to the surface, despite the absence of molecularly imprinted templates in the NIP electrode (since the PANI surface was not smooth). To eliminate such bias from the total sensor response, the subtracted (i.e., MIP–NIP) data were essential, accounting for the specific recognition of the lentivirus by the MIP sensor. The significant difference in resistivity ratio between the MIP and NIP responses supports the strategy of molecular imprinting technology.

The lentivirus served as an effective template for fabricating the molecular imprinting virus sensor. The sensor's virus-capturing efficiency and detection limit could be further improved by increasing the concentration of the virus used for fabrication, which would amplify the number of MIP cavities. Further surface investigation is needed to visualize the functional groups and intermolecular interactions between the virus particles and MIP polyaniline matrix. Studies of the viability and possible structural transition of the lentivirus during synthesis are also necessary to reveal the detailed mechanisms of molecular imprinting associated with microorganisms.

3.2. Sensor Selectivity

We investigated the selectivity of the MIP sensor by comparing the resistivity ratios of the lentivirus, retrovirus, latex beads, and human blood. The results are shown in Figure 1d. The MIP sensor demonstrated a promising selectivity for detection of the lentivirus, as compared to other nanoparticles and whole blood.

The MIP sensor detected the Retro-CMV-GFP retrovirus (1.65×10^5 TU/mL virus concentration), in addition to the lentivirus, since the resistivity ratios on the MIP sensors were similar. Because the lentivirus and retrovirus belong to the same virus family and their viral envelope structures are almost identical, the retrovirus was also captured by the MIP structure synthesized with the lentivirus template. This shows the ability of the sensor to capture the same family of viruses. Future investigations will compare the selectivity of different families of viruses.

Moreover, the detection of 100 nm polystyrene latex beads roughly the same size as the lentivirus were investigated at the same concentration of 1.64×10^5 beads/mL as an analogue of virus particles. The resistivity ratio for the MIP electrodes with regard to latex bead detection showed no significant difference from the NIP control results. Even with a much higher concentration of beads (9.85×10^6 beads/mL, 60 times the virus concentration), no difference from the control in terms of resistivity ratio was observed. This confirmed that the MIP electrode did not respond to the beads, even though they were the same size as the virus. Additionally, no significant MIP resistivity change was found with the human whole blood sample containing potential contaminants such as plasma and blood cells. The resistivity ratio for the blood sample on the MIP electrode was close to that of the NIP control. Even though the geometric shapes of polystyrene nanoparticles and blood proteins are roughly spherical, similar to the lentivirus shape, they may lack the surface interactions found in the lentivirus. The absence of surface interactions with the molecularly imprinted cavities may have prevented nanoparticles and blood proteins from being captured on the molecularly imprinted sensor.

Due to the presence of MIP cavities for virus capturing, this sensing device exhibited more substantial responses to the lentiviruses than did the NIP device. Although the strongly acidic condition of the monomer solution remains a concern with regard to preventing the lentiviruses from maintaining viability, the geometric structure may still be maintained during the molecular imprinting process, since it is of a short duration. More characterizations are needed to acquire further evidence and visualize the formation related to the molecularly imprinted structures.

3.3. Lentivirus Detection from Aerosol on Virus MIP Sensors

The resistivity ratio of the MIP sensor for the lentivirus in aerosol form was measured from multiple spray distances (between 30 cm and 60 cm) to investigate the feasibility of the sensor (detailed procedure shown in Supplement 6). The conceptual diagram and experimental setup are shown in Figures 1e and 2a, respectively. The results of the resistivity ratio as a function of time with different distances are shown in Figure 2b.

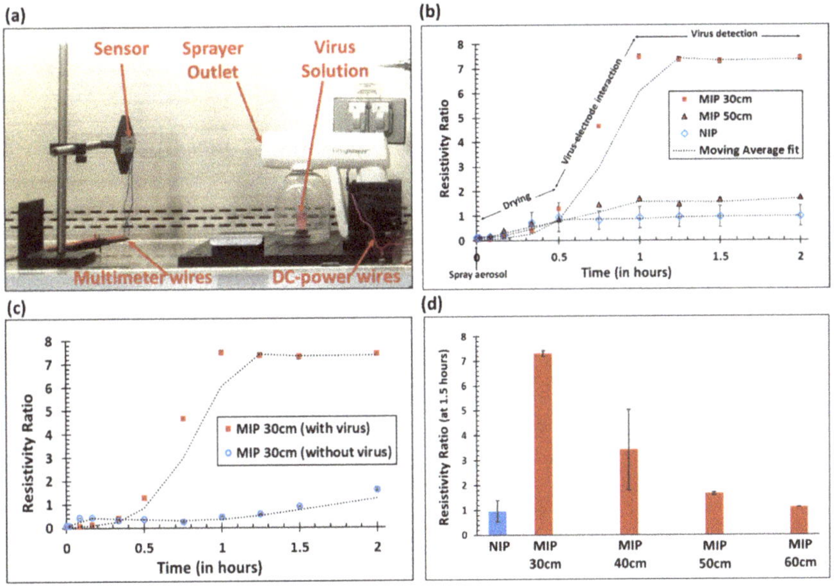

Figure 2. Resistivity ratio as a function of time and distance ($n \geq 5$, RSD avg. = 13.3%). Lentivirus aerosol was sprayed for 10 to 12 s (initial volume of lentivirus solution = 2.65 ± 0.15 mL; approximate virus concentration = 2.2×10^5 TU/mL). (**a**) Photographic image of the aerosol sprayer and virus detection using sensing electrodes. (**b**) Resistivity ratios for the MIP and NIP sensing elements as a function of time. (**c**) Resistivity ratio for the MIP sensing element with and without the virus. DMEM was used as a control without the virus. (**d**) The resistivity ratio (time = 1.5 h) for the MIP sensing element as a function of sprayer distance. The resistivity ratio for the NIP control was averaged across various distances.

The resistivity ratio increased over time and reached the saturation value at which the resistivity ratio detects viruses. In this graph, from 0 to 0.5 h, the resistivity ratio increased slightly, which can mainly be attributed to the drying of the sensing surface that was wetted by the aerosol particles. A sharp increase in the sensor response from 0.5 to 1 h was observed. This was primarily because of hybridization of the virus with the MIP templates; there was very little contribution from the drying of the sensor. According to the humidity experiment (see Figure S4), the sensor resistivity remained constant for a relative humidity between 15% and 85%. In Figure 2b, the resistivity ratio increased over time, as the conductive polymer's electrical path was obstructed by the virus. After 1 h, the resistivity ratio reached saturation because all of the virus particles present on the surface were electrically detected by the molecularly imprinted conductive polymer and the surface was visibly dried. The NIP control electrode showed very little response to the lentivirus aerosol (as compared to the MIP sensing electrode) at 30 cm and 50 cm, which is consistent with lentivirus detection in liquid. Further, the resistivity ratio of the MIP sensor at 30 cm was significantly higher than at 50 cm. This was due to the higher volume of aerosol virus deposited on the sensing element since the distance between the sensor and sprayer outlet was shorter. The NIP resistivity ratio value over various distances was averaged, resulting in a higher standard deviation of NIP (see Figure 2b). When the MIP sensing element sprayed with the lentivirus was compared to the MIP sprayed with DMEM without the virus, the resistivity ratio was significantly higher in the presence of virus particles after saturation (see Figure 2c). This further exemplifies the functionality of the MIP sensor in the presence of the virus.

Since the resistivity ratio remained constant after 1 h, a fixed time of 1.5 h was used to compare the resistivity ratio as a function of distance (see Figure 2d). The MIP resistivity ratios at a distance between 30 cm and 60 cm decreased as the sensor moved further away from the sprayer. This was due to the reduction in virus aerosol volume reaching the sensing element as the distance was increased. At a short distance from the sprayer (less than 30 cm), a very high volume of virus aerosol was sprayed, resulting in excessive wetting of the sensing electrode, not a realistic situation. Therefore, a minimum distance of 30 cm was selected. Far away from the sprayer (up to 60 cm), a very small amount of virus aerosol reached the MIP sensing electrode, resulting in a resistivity ratio that approached the NIP control value. On the basis of this result, we concluded that the lentivirus could be detected in an aerosol format using the virus MIP sensor at distances between 30 cm and 60 cm from the virus source.

In Figure 2d, the MIP resistivity ratio at 40 cm had a large standard deviation, which could be due to variations in the total volume of aerosol particles reaching the electrodes at this distance. Even though the maximum distance of the aerosol spray was 60 cm, the aerosol distribution in the air from 30 cm to 60 cm was not uniform, due to fluidic instability [29]. At a critical distance of 40 cm away from the sprayer, the fluctuation in aerosol volume reaching the electrodes may have affected the resistivity ratio measurements, leading to a large standard deviation. To verify, the aerosol spray characteristics were visualized using a colored dye sprayed on white paper (see Supplement 3, Figure S5). Additionally, compared to lentivirus detection in liquid at 1 h (30 min of liquid saturation, gentle aspiration, and an additional 30 min of drying time), lentivirus detection in aerosol form required a slightly longer duration of 1.5 h, due to the additional time needed to dry the sensing elements. Detection of virus aerosol using the passive resistance method discussed in this paper simplifies the virus detection process significantly as compared to the costly electrochemical method; however, the trade-off is a longer detection time due to complete drying required for virus effects to become evident in the MIP sensing layer. This detection time using resistance measurement could be significantly reduced using a faster convective evaporation approach. The evaporation rate for the MIP sensor and its impact on the resistivity ratio will need to be further studied in detail in the future.

To confirm lentivirus detection in aerosol form, the resistivity ratio of the lentivirus sprayed at 50 cm was compared with the calibration curve trendline fit (see Figure S1) and the amount of lentivirus calculated. Using the MIP and NIP resistivity ratios, the number of lentivirus particles detected in aerosol at 50 cm was found to be 5275 TU. Since the total number of particles at the spray source was 5.8×10^5 TU, this meant that only 0.90% of the lentivirus was detected by the sensor at a 50 cm distance. As a function of the spraying area characteristics (see Figure S5), the theoretical amount of lentivirus reaching the sensing element was calculated to be 74,566 TU, assuming all aerosols from the sprayer reached the 50 cm sensing position. Even though 12.79% of the total virus reached the sensing element area, only 0.90% of the total virus was electrically detected. This calculation resulted in a 7.07% hybridization efficiency from the 50 cm spray distance. This could have been due to the specific detection of only those viruses on the sensor trapped inside the molecularly imprinted cavities. From the 30 cm to 60 cm sprayer distance, the virus detection efficiency was found to be between 0.33% and 2.90% (see Figure S6). At 60 cm, the amount of lentivirus calculated from calibration curves was 1953 TU, which approached the limit of detection (4181 TU/mL) for this sensor.

3.4. Face Mask Application and Sensor Accuracy, Sensitivity, and Specificity

A wearable virus sensor application was demonstrated by attaching the NIP and MIP sensing electrodes to a face mask to detect the lentivirus in aerosol form (see Figure 3a). The maximum dimensions of the face mask were 16 cm × 11 cm.

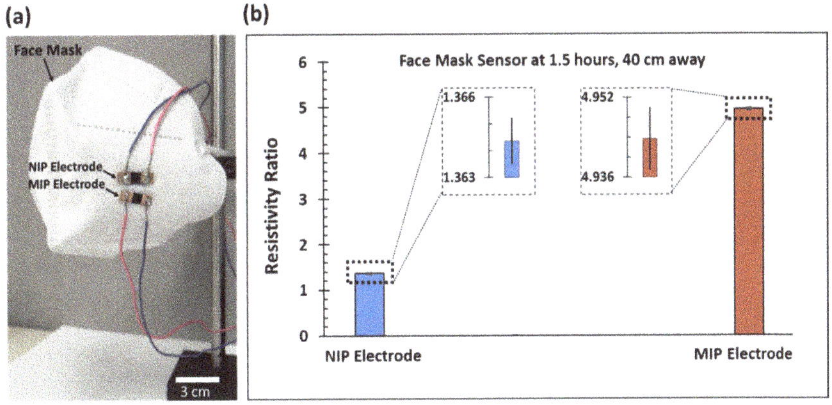

(c)

		Actual value	
		Positive	Negative
Sensor value	Positive	True positive = 6	False positive = 6
	Negative	False negative = 2	True negative = 6

Accuracy = 60.0 % ; Sensitivity = 75.0 % ; Specificity = 50.0 %

Figure 3. Lentivirus detection using face mask virus sensor. (**a**) Image of the face mask sensor with NIP and MIP electrodes attached using epoxy. The scale bar is 3 cm. A video is available for download from the Supplemental Materials. (**b**) The resistivity ratio (time = 1.5 h) of the NIP and MIP electrodes when the face mask was placed 40 cm away from the aerosol sprayer (n = 5, RSD avg. = 0.1%). The inset shows the error bars. (**c**) Diagnostic test parameters for the virus MIP sensor (n = 20).

At a detection time of 1.5 h and with the face mask sensor placed 40 cm away from the aerosol sprayer, the resistivity ratios of the NIP and MIP electrodes were found to be 1.364 ± 0.001 and 4.944 ± 0.006, respectively (as shown in Figure 3b), with a virus concentration of 2.2×10^5 TU/mL. The resistivity ratio of this sensor was within the standard deviation at a 40 cm distance (see Figure 2d). This 40 cm distance for the face mask experiment was selected because it is a similarly close distance to two people standing next to each other. The fluctuation in aerosol volume reaching the face mask sensor electrodes at 40 cm, which is the critical spray distance, could have caused the $MIP_{face\ mask}$ value to be at the extreme end of the $MIP_{40\ cm}$ aerosol detection curve.

Using the specific binding curve (see Figure S1 and Equation (S8)), the amount of lentivirus on the face mask sensor was calculated to be 12,600 TU. This meant that 2.16% of lentivirus was detected by the face mask sensor at 40 cm, as compared to the total amount of virus. With 13.74% of the total virus aerosol reaching a sensor element placed at a 40 cm distance, a virus hybridization efficiency of ~15.73% for the face mask sensor was calculated. The virus detection efficiency at 40 cm was approximately twice the value for a sensor placed at a 50 cm distance (i.e., 2.16% vs. 0.90%). Overall, the virus detection efficiency decreased as the sensor was placed further away from the sprayer, which is illustrated in Figure S6.

A preliminary determination of diagnostic test parameters for the virus MIP sensor was achieved by comparing the MIP sensor output with the known experimental conditions (presence or absence of the virus, control, etc.). Figure 3c is a summary of the sensor parameters resulting in 60.0% accuracy, 75.0% sensitivity, and 50.0% specificity, illustrating the potential of the low-cost virus MIP sensor to provide clinically useful results with relatively high accuracy and sensitivity. Additional investigations with a larger sample size are needed to confirm the diagnosis of a virus using this aerosol sensor.

While the importance of aerosol virus detection is enhanced by the urgent need to slow down and prevent the respiratory transmission of infectious viruses such as COVID-19 [30], there is still a lack of tools available to efficiently capture viruses from aerosols [31]. Our virus MIP sensor integrates the virus capturing and detection processes in a single platform. To improve the virus detection efficiency from aerosol particles on the sensor surface, a highly porous membrane or molecular absorbent layer made from a metal–organic framework [32] could be used on top of the molecularly imprinted polymer sensor. Viruses in electrostatically charged aerosols could further be attracted to the sensing surface by applying a small voltage near the sensor region, which would further enhance the virus capture efficiency of the sensor.

4. Conclusions and Future Directions

We designed a low-cost paper-based virus sensor with a detection limit of 4181 TU/mL using the molecularly imprinted polymer technique. We also demonstrated virus detection in aerosols using our paper-based MIP sensor, as well as a wearable sensor application in the form of a face mask, which will be critical in future public health and safety. In the aerosol experiments, we detected the lentivirus at distances ranging from 30 cm to 60 cm away from the virus sprayer. The sensor showed a virus detection efficiency of 0.33% to 2.90% from the lentivirus present in the aerosol. The dry measurement of the virus was obtained within 1.5 h after spraying the virus aerosol solution onto the sensor electrode. Furthermore, our paper-based MIP sensor was easily integrated with a wearable face mask for the future detection of viruses in aerosols.

A few limitations regarding this MIP sensor still exist. It took 1.5 h to detect the lentivirus in aerosol form. In the future, the drying time of aerosols on sensing electrodes could be reduced by using a convection evaporation process, in addition to drying using diffusion [33,34] resulting in a 3–5-fold reduction in drying time. More importantly, by using a highly conductive PEDOT:PSS [poly(3,4-ethylenedioxythiophene)-poly(styrenesulfonate)] polymer material instead of polyaniline, we may be able to obtain an even better detection limit and faster response rate. This could also circumvent acidic pH problems with the virus molecular imprinting process. In our experience, high-conductivity grade commercial PEDOT:PSS showed ≥200 S/cm electrical conductivity compared to <1 S/cm obtained from polyaniline. PEDOT:PSS may result in a 200-fold improvement in sensitivity or response time of the virus MIP sensor. With these improvements, virus aerosol detection could be achieved in under 10 min, where the limiting factor is the drying time.

Further improvements could be made by integrating this sensor with artificial intelligence (AI) and machine learning. With a humidity sensor and the addition of an AI algorithm, the virus detection time could be significantly reduced. Lastly, the MIP and NIP sensing electrodes were connected to a multimeter via electrical wires, limiting their real-world use. This could be overcome by wirelessly connecting the wearable MIP and NIP sensing electrodes to a smartphone app or cloud server, employing the Internet of things (IoT) in healthcare.

Supplementary Materials: The following are available online at https://www.mdpi.com/article/10.3390/bios13090861/s1: Figure S1. The specific and non-specific binding of lentivirus on the sensor; Figure S2. The stability test of the PANI electrode on the PET paper substrate; Figure S3. Photo of the experimental setup for temperature and humidity experiments; Figure S4. Humidity and temperature effects on the normalized resistivity of the polyaniline sensing electrode; Figure S5. Aerosol spray characteristics; Figure S6. Sensor performance in the virus aerosol environment; Figure S7. SEM images of sensor surface after virus exposure; Figure S8. Photographic image of aerosol virus detection experimental setup; Figure S9. Resistance data over time for lentivirus detection from the liquid; Figure S10. Current–voltage relationship for the MIP electrode; Video S1. Spraying virus on polyaniline electrode; Video S2. Face mask sensor. Reference [35] is cited in Supplementary Materials.

Author Contributions: Conceptualization, D.-F.L. and J.K.; methodology, J.S.B., T.-Y.C. and J.K.; investigation, J.S.B., T.-Y.C. and Z.C.; resources, M.-F.H., D.Z., D.-F.L. and J.K.; data curation, J.S.B. and T.-Y.C.; writing—original draft preparation, J.S.B., T.-Y.C., D.Z., Z.C. and J.K.; writing—review and editing, J.S.B., T.-Y.C., D.Z., Z.C., D.-F.L. and J.K.; visualization, J.S.B., T.-Y.C., Z.C. and J.K.; supervision, D.-F.L. and J.K.; project administration, D.-F.L. and J.K.; funding acquisition, D.-F.L. and J.K. All authors have read and agreed to the published version of the manuscript.

Funding: This research was funded by the Bill and Melinda Gates Foundation (Grant #1199456 (J.K) and the Department of Integrative Biology and Pharmacology of the University of Texas Health Science Center at Houston (Grant Start-Up-Fund #37516-11998 (D.-F.L.).

Institutional Review Board Statement: Not applicable.

Informed Consent Statement: Not applicable.

Data Availability Statement: The data presented in this study are available on request from the corresponding author.

Conflicts of Interest: The authors declare no conflict of interest.

References

1. Greer, S.; Alexander, G.J. Viral serology and detection. *Baillière's Clin. Gastroenterol.* **1995**, *9*, 689–721. [CrossRef]
2. Gullett, J.C.; Nolte, F.S. Quantitative nucleic acid amplification methods for viral infections. *Clin. Chem.* **2015**, *61*, 72–78. [CrossRef] [PubMed]
3. Huang, L.; Xiao, W.; Xu, T.; Chen, H.; Jin, Z.; Zhang, Z.; Song, Q.; Tang, Y. Miniaturized paper-based smartphone biosensor for differential diagnosis of wild-type pseudorabies virus infection versus vaccination immunization. *Sens. Actuators B Chem.* **2021**, *327*, 128893.
4. Mahendra, C.; Kaisar, M.M.M.; Vasandani, S.R.; Surja, S.S.; Tjoa, E.; Chriestya, F.; Junusmin, K.I.; Widowati, T.A.; Irwanto, A.; Ali, S. Wide Application of Minimally Processed Saliva on Multiple RT-qPCR Kits for SARS-CoV-2 Detection in Indonesia. *Front. Cell. Infect. Microbiol.* **2021**, *11*, 691538. [CrossRef] [PubMed]
5. Heid, C.A.; Stevens, J.; Livak, K.J.; Williams, P.M. Real time quantitative PCR. *Genome Res.* **1996**, *6*, 986–994. [CrossRef] [PubMed]
6. Ma, Y.; Shen, X.-L.; Zeng, Q.; Wang, H.-S.; Wang, L.-S. A multi-walled carbon nanotubes based molecularly imprinted polymers electrochemical sensor for the sensitive determination of HIV-p24. *Talanta* **2017**, *164*, 121–127. [CrossRef]
7. Mojsoska, B.; Larsen, S.; Olsen, D.A.; Madsen, J.S.; Brandslund, I.; Alatraktchi, F.A. Rapid SARS-CoV-2 detection using electrochemical immunosensor. *Sensors* **2021**, *21*, 390. [CrossRef]

8. Li, J.; Lin, R.; Yang, Y.; Zhao, R.; Song, S.; Zhou, Y.; Shi, J.; Wang, L.; Song, H.; Hao, R. Multichannel Immunosensor Platform for the Rapid Detection of SARS-CoV-2 and Influenza A (H1N1) Virus. *ACS Appl. Mater. Interfaces* **2021**, *13*, 22262–22270. [CrossRef]
9. Bhardwaj, J.; Sharma, A.; Jang, J. Vertical flow-based paper immunosensor for rapid electrochemical and colorimetric detection of influenza virus using a different pore size sample pad. *Biosens. Bioelectron.* **2019**, *126*, 36–43. [CrossRef]
10. Ferguson, B.S.; Buchsbaum, S.F.; Wu, T.-T.; Hsieh, K.; Xiao, Y.; Sun, R.; Soh, H.T. Genetic analysis of H1N1 influenza virus from throat swab samples in a microfluidic system for point-of-care diagnostics. *J. Am. Chem. Soc.* **2011**, *133*, 9129–9135. [CrossRef]
11. Han, J.-H.; Lee, D.; Chew, C.H.C.; Kim, T.; Pak, J.J. A multi-virus detectable microfluidic electrochemical immunosensor for simultaneous detection of H1N1, H5N1, and H7N9 virus using ZnO nanorods for sensitivity enhancement. *Sens. Actuators B Chem.* **2016**, *228*, 36–42. [CrossRef]
12. Eissa, S.; Alhadrami, H.A.; Al-Mozaini, M.; Hassan, A.M.; Zourob, M. Voltammetric-based immunosensor for the detection of SARS-CoV-2 nucleocapsid antigen. *Microchim. Acta* **2021**, *188*, 199.
13. Zhou, C.H.; Wu, Z.; Chen, J.J.; Xiong, C.; Chen, Z.; Pang, D.W.; Zhang, Z.L. Biometallization-Based Electrochemical Magnetoimmunosensing Strategy for Avian Influenza A (H7N9) Virus Particle Detection. *Chem. –Asian J.* **2015**, *10*, 1387–1393.
14. Dong, S.; Zhao, R.; Zhu, J.; Lu, X.; Li, Y.; Qiu, S.; Jia, L.; Jiao, X.; Song, S.; Fan, C.; et al. Electrochemical DNA biosensor based on a tetrahedral nanostructure probe for the detection of avian influenza A (H7N9) virus. *ACS Appl. Mater. Interfaces* **2015**, *7*, 8834–8842. [CrossRef]
15. Tancharoen, C.; Sukjee, W.; Thepparit, C.; Jaimipuk, T.; Auewarakul, P.; Thitithanyanont, A.; Sangma, C. Electrochemical biosensor based on surface imprinting for zika virus detection in serum. *ACS Sens.* **2018**, *4*, 69–75.
16. Afsahi, S.; Lerner, M.B.; Goldstein, J.M.; Lee, J.; Tang, X.; Bagarozzi, D.A., Jr.; Pan, D.; Locascio, L.; Walker, A.; Barron, F.; et al. Novel graphene-based biosensor for early detection of Zika virus infection. *Biosens. Bioelectron.* **2018**, *100*, 85–88. [CrossRef]
17. Altintas, Z.; Gittens, M.; Guerreiro, A.; Thompson, K.-A.; Walker, J.; Piletsky, S.; Tothill, I.E. Detection of waterborne viruses using high affinity molecularly imprinted polymers. *Anal. Chem.* **2015**, *87*, 6801–6807. [CrossRef]
18. Wangchareansak, T.; Thitithanyanont, A.; Chuakheaw, D.; Gleeson, M.P.; Lieberzeit, P.A.; Sangma, C. Influenza A virus molecularly imprinted polymers and their application in virus sub-type classification. *J. Mater. Chem. B* **2013**, *1*, 2190–2197.
19. Sukjee, W.; Thitithanyanont, A.; Wiboon-Ut, S.; Lieberzeit, P.A.; Gleeson, M.P.; Navakul, K.; Sangma, C. An influenza A virus agglutination test using antibody-like polymers. *J. Biomater. Sci. Polym. Ed.* **2017**, *28*, 1786–1795. [CrossRef]
20. Liang, C.; Wang, H.; He, K.; Chen, C.; Chen, X.; Gong, H.; Cai, C. A virus-MIPs fluorescent sensor based on FRET for highly sensitive detection of JEV. *Talanta* **2016**, *160*, 360–366. [CrossRef]
21. Navakul, K.; Warakulwit, C.; Yenchitsomanus, P.-t.; Panya, A.; Lieberzeit, P.A.; Sangma, C. A novel method for dengue virus detection and antibody screening using a graphene-polymer based electrochemical biosensor. *Nanomed. Nanotechnol. Biol. Med.* **2017**, *13*, 549–557. [CrossRef] [PubMed]
22. Ghanbari, K.; Roushani, M. A nanohybrid probe based on double recognition of an aptamer MIP grafted onto a MWCNTs-Chit nanocomposite for sensing hepatitis C virus core antigen. *Sens. Actuators B Chem.* **2018**, *258*, 1066–1071. [CrossRef]
23. Chen, Z.; Wright, C.; Dincel, O.; Chi, T.-Y.; Kameoka, J. A Low-Cost Paper Glucose Sensor with Molecularly Imprinted Polyaniline Electrode. *Sensors* **2020**, *20*, 1098. [CrossRef] [PubMed]
24. Chi, T.-Y.; Chen, Z.; Kameoka, J. Perfluorooctanesulfonic Acid Detection Using Molecularly Imprinted Polyaniline on a Paper Substrate. *Sensors* **2020**, *20*, 7301. [CrossRef]
25. Chen, Z.; Chi, T.-Y.; Dincel, O.; Tong, L.; Kameoka, J. A Low-cost and Enzyme-free Glucose Paper Sensor. In Proceedings of the 2020 42nd Annual International Conference of the IEEE Engineering in Medicine & Biology Society (EMBC), Montreal, QC, Canada, 20–24 July 2020; pp. 4097–4100.
26. Lee, D.-F.; Su, J.; Ang, Y.-S.; Carvajal-Vergara, X.; Mulero-Navarro, S.; Pereira, C.F.; Gingold, J.; Wang, H.-L.; Zhao, R.; Sevilla, A.; et al. Regulation of embryonic and induced pluripotency by aurora kinase-p53 signaling. *Cell Stem Cell* **2012**, *11*, 179–194. [CrossRef]
27. Panggabean, A.S.; Silaban, H.S.; Pasaribu, S.P.; Alimuddin. Method validation of Cd (II) determination in lubrication oil by direct dilution method using atomic absorption spectrophotometer. *J. Phys. Conf. Ser.* **2019**, *1277*, 012004. [CrossRef]
28. Arkhipenko, M.V.; Nikitin, N.A.; Baranov, O.A.; Evtushenko, E.A.; Atabekov, J.G.; Karpova, O.V. Surface charge mapping on virions and virus-like particles of helical plant viruses. *Acta Naturae* **2019**, *11*, 73–78. [CrossRef]
29. Tsuda, A.; Henry, F.S.; Butler, J.P. Particle Transport and Deposition: Basic Physics of Particle Kinetics. *Compr. Physiol.* **2013**, *3*, 1437–1471.
30. Wang, C.C.; Prather, K.A.; Sznitman, J.; Jimenez, J.L.; Lakdawala, S.S.; Tufekci, Z.; Marr, L.C. Airborne transmission of respiratory viruses. *Science* **2021**, *373*, eabd9149. [CrossRef]
31. Breshears, L.E.; Nguyen, B.T.; Robles, S.M.; Wu, L.; Yoon, J.-Y. Biosensor detection of airborne respiratory viruses such as SARS-CoV-2. *SLAS Technol.* **2022**, *27*, 4–17. [CrossRef]
32. Wang, Y.; Hu, Y.; He, Q.; Yan, J.; Xiong, H.; Wen, N.; Cai, S.; Peng, D.; Liu, Y.; Liu, Z. Metal-organic frameworks for virus detection. *Biosens. Bioelectron.* **2020**, *169*, 112604. [CrossRef] [PubMed]
33. Kelly-Zion, P.L.; Batra, J.; Pursell, C.J. Correlation for the convective and diffusive evaporation of a sessile drop. *Int. J. Heat Mass Transf.* **2013**, *64*, 278–285. [CrossRef]

34. Kelly-Zion, P.L.; Pursell, C.J.; Vaidya, S.; Batra, J. Evaporation of sessile drops under combined diffusion and natural convection. *Colloids Surf. A Physicochem. Eng. Asp.* **2011**, *381*, 31–36. [CrossRef]
35. Olad, A.; Khatamian, M.; Naseri, B. Removal of toxic hexavalent chromium by polyaniline modified clinoptilolite nanoparticles. *J. Iran. Chem. Soc.* **2011**, *8*, S141–S151. [CrossRef]

MDPI
St. Alban-Anlage 66
4052 Basel
Switzerland
www.mdpi.com

Biosensors Editorial Office
E-mail: biosensors@mdpi.com
www.mdpi.com/journal/biosensors

www.ingramcontent.com/pod-product-compliance
Lightning Source LLC
LaVergne TN
LVHW070647100526
838202LV00013B/900
* 9 7 8 3 0 3 6 5 9 1 5 8 2 *